MRCPsych:
Passing the CASC Exam

n Trust;

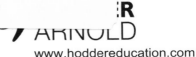

ARNOLD

www.hoddereducation.com

First published in Great Britain in 2009 by
Hodder Arnold, an imprint of Hodder Education,
an Hachette UK Company, 338 Euston Road, London NW1 3BH

http://www.hoddereducation.com

Hachette UK's policy is to use papers that are natural, renewable and recyclable products and made from wood grown in sustainable forests. The logging and manufacturing processes are expected to conform to the environmental regulations of the country of origin.

Whilst the advice and information in this book are believed to be true and accurate at the date of going to press, neither the author[s] nor the publisher can accept any legal responsibility or liability for any errors or omissions that may be made. In particular, (but without limiting the generality of the preceding disclaimer) every effort has been made to check drug dosages; however it is still possible that errors have been missed. Furthermore, dosage schedules are constantly being revised and new side-effects recognized. For these reasons the reader is strongly urged to consult the drug companies' printed instructions before administering any of the drugs recommended in this book.

British Library Cataloguing in Publication Data
A catalogue record for this book is available from the British Library

Library of Congress Cataloging-in-Publication Data
A catalog record for this book is available from the Library of Congress

ISBN-13   978-0-340-98194-8

2 3 4 5 6 7 8 9 10

Commissioning Editor: Philip Shaw
Project Editor: Amy Mulick
Production Controller: Karen Tate
Cover Design: Laura DeGrasse
Cover image © Pasieka/Science Photo Library

Typeset in 8 on 10 Stone Serif by Dorchester Typesetting Group Ltd
Printed and bound in Great Britain by CPI Antony Rowe

What do you think about this book? Or any other Hodder Arnold title?
Please visit our website: www.hoddereducation.com

Dedication

To the Sauers north and the Agarwals south of the river.

Contents

Contributors

Sangita Agarwal MBBS BSc MSc MRCP
Consultant Rheumatologist
Department of Rheumatology
Guy's Hospital
London, UK

Jayati Das-Munshi MBBS BSc(Hons) MRCPsych
Honorary Specialist Registrar and
MRC Special Training Fellow in Health Service Research
Section of Epidemiology
Department of Health Service & Population Research
Institute of Psychiatry
King's College
London, UK

Russell Foster BSc BA CandMag MSc PhD MBBS MRCPsych
Honorary Consultant Psychiatrist
Institute of Liver Studies
King's College Hospital
London, UK

Virupakshi Jalihal MBBS DCP DPM MRCPsych
Specialist Registrar
South London and Maudsley NHS Foundation Trust
London, UK

Marc Lyall MBBS BSc MRCPsych LLM
Consultant Forensic Psychiatrist
Centre for Forensic Mental Health
John Howard Centre
London, UK

David Okai MBBS BMedSci MRCPsych
Clinical Research Worker and Honorary Specialist Registrar
Section of Cognitive Neuropsychiatry
Institute of Psychiatry
King's College
London, UK

Dennis Ougrin MBBS MRCPsych
Kraupl Taylor Research Fellow
Department of Child and Adolescent Psychiatry
Institute of Psychiatry
London, UK

Armin Raznahan MBBS(Hons) MRCPCH MRCPsych
MRC Clinical Research Training Fellow
Department of Child and Adolescent Psychiatry
Institute of Psychiatry
London, UK

Justin Sauer MBBS BSc MRCPsych
Consultant Psychiatrist
South London and Maudsley NHS Foundation Trust; and
Honorary Lecturer
Institute of Psychiatry
London, UK

Dinesh Sinha MBBS MRCPsych MSc
Consultant Psychiatrist in Psychotherapy
Cambridge and Peterborough NHS Foundation Trust
Cambridge, UK

Derek Tracy MB BCh BAO MSc MRCPsych
Specialist Registrar in Neuropsychiatry
King's College Hospital
London, UK

Foreword

The establishment of professional guilds between 1100 and 1500 led to setting standards for training and assessment. National standards measure the quality of training and examinations. In 2005, when the Postgraduate Medical Education Training Board (PMETB) was set up, as one of its early tasks the Board produced standards of assessment. All medical Royal Colleges had to comply with these standards. All examinations had to meet these criteria. Consequently, the Royal College of Psychiatrists, in line with other medical Royal Colleges, modified its assessment systems, introducing Work Place Based Assessments. The MRCPsych examination was also modified radically. Among the changes was the introduction of CASC (Clinical Assessment of Skills and Competencies) component at the old level of MRCPsych Part II examination. This also replaced OSCEs and the uncertainty of seeing a long case under examination conditions. CASC assesses competencies *and* skills in a structured way so that as far as possible like is compared with like. Dr Sauer has produced a lucid book which the trainees taking the exam will find helpful in their preparation. The structure - using case vignettes, setting the scene, possible questions and additional information with references – is clearly expressed. Trainees will find this book useful in their preparation.

Dinesh Bhugra
Professor of Mental Health & Cultural Diversity
Institute of Psychiatry, King's College London

Preface

Royal College membership exams have significant financial, emotional and career implications, which is why leaving them to chance is unwise. Trainees who have taken into consideration exam deadlines, planned their preparation carefully and maximized their clinical rehearsal stand the greatest chances of success.

The CASC or 'Clinical Assessment of Skills and Competencies' is a series of complex OSCE scenarios and this book guides you through over 100 stations, coaching you along the way. I hope that this book will become a dear friend to you during your exam preparation and that, used correctly, it should significantly increase your chances of success.

Justin Sauer

Acknowledgements

I am grateful to the contributors for their time and effort. I would like to thank Philip Shaw, Amy Mulick and the rest of the team at Hodder Arnold for their commitment to this project from the start.

Thank you also to the OSCE Course trainers and all the trainees for their invaluable contributions over the years.

Exam guidance

Use the stations in this book for practice with colleagues and for individual rehearsal. Refer to the Royal College website for any CASC updates. Currently you need to pass 12 out of 16 stations. All stations have equal weighting towards the total number required to pass. Half of the stations (8 in total) are single stations lasting seven minutes, with one minute to read the scenario. The other half are linked stations lasting ten minutes each, with two minutes to read (4 linked scenarios, 8 stations in total). Linked stations are designed so the task in the first station is followed by a related task in the second. Single stations are run in the same way as the old part 1 OSCE. Some of the scenarios may be similar to the OSCE, but a higher performance standard will be required. Don't be surprised to find two examiners in the station, one marking and one playing a medical role (who will not contribute to the marking).

The CASC standards are high and as a more senior trainee you will be expected to show competence in management issues. However, you will still need to demonstrate ability in history taking, assessment and formulation of cases. Diagnosis, aetiology and prognosis will similarly be assessed. Without doubt, the most important skill is clear and effective communication and it is here that candidates usually fall down, rather than lack of knowledge. Clarity when communicating in lay terms or when dealing with a colleague is crucial. Showing genuine empathy where appropriate is similarly important. If communication is a weakness, you must rehearse intensely to change your style – which is difficult a few weeks before the exam. It can take time and hard work. If English is not your first language ask colleagues how they might 'phrase' questions or demonstrate empathy. If you are able to act, like the actors in the scenarios, you will also be at an advantage. Treat the scenarios as real, and you will perform better.

The marks given for each station are as follows:
- PASS
- BORDERLINE PASS
- BORDERLINE FAIL
- FAIL

The chances are that a poor performance in one station does not mean complete failure. You are unlikely to be in a good position to judge your own performance, so do not dwell on this. Concentrate on the job at hand and carry on!

A list of some top tips

In your preparation consider how you would manage disorders using the following matrix or something similar. It is important to have a structure in your mind for the common scenarios:

Management	Short term	Medium term	Long term
Biological			
Psychological			
Social			

In aetiological scenarios consider the predisposing, precipitating and perpetuating factors.

Examiners are looking for:
- Competence in your assessment and management
- Structure
- Logic
- Safety
- Emotional intelligence

Examiners do not like:
- Repetition
- Waffle
- Poor communication skills
- Poor listening skills
- Disorganization
- Arrogance
- Arguments

Consider your own

Appearance and behaviour
- Confident, professional, but not arrogant
- Don't panic – rehearse opening phrases for different scenarios to build initial confidence
- If you are anxious, the examiners become anxious too
- Dress smart, formal – like a future colleague!
- Body language – stop any habits – ask colleagues to comment – your nonverbal communication should be of someone who is calm, interested and supportive.

Speech
- Should be clear, confident and unrushed – many of us have a tendency to speak faster when anxious
- Verbal habits – again ask colleagues or record your interview – addressing your 'ums' or similar can make a huge difference in how you come across
- Where possible start with an open question
- Avoid swing questions
- Avoid leading questions

- Speak in lay terms to patients – avoid psychobabble
- The use of silence, where appropriate, can be very valuable.

Interview technique

- Read the scenario carefully
- Answer the tasks that have been set you and not what you want to talk about (a common error)
- Clarification is important if you are unsure
- Introduce yourself to the patient
- Ask if it would be alright to 'talk to them/ask some questions etc.'
- Reassure/empathize where appropriate
- Use of normalization where appropriate
- Learn stock phrases in case you run dry e.g. 'Do you have any questions for me at this point?' 'So to summarize...'
- Don't end the station until you are told to end – if you get the timing wrong it can feel very awkward
- If running short of time, explain this to the patient/relative
- Better to say you don't know, than to get it very wrong
- Always be polite and courteous throughout – even if you've had a hard time – and thank the actor at the end
- Don't take the actors' behaviour personally
- Smiling can put everyone at ease
- Know the ICD-10 diagnostic criteria for the main conditions as these will instruct your assessments
- Do not ignore nonverbal cues – e.g. EPSE, agitation
- Listen to what the patient or relative is saying. It is a common mistake to ignore valuable information and to talk 'at' people rather than enter into a dialogue.
- Always consider risk
- Practise with a stopwatch and Dictaphone.

Chapter 1
General adult psychiatry Dr David Okai

O LINKED STATION 1

1a.

A 21-year-old woman (Miss Lara Tracey) has been referred to your service with bouts of depression lasting a few weeks at a time. She takes mirtazapine and has reported no change in her depressive symptoms. You have inherited this patient from your predecessor's outpatient clinic.

Take a history of her mood and find out more about her symptoms.
Explain to the patient what you think the problem is.

1b.

You decide from your history that the patient has bipolar II and is a rapid cycler with several cases of depression each year and previously unobserved episodes of hypomania. She is currently hypomanic. The patient says she would be willing to take lithium now that you have explained the illness more.

Prepare to discuss the case with your consultant, including your management plan.

O LINKED STATION 2

2a.

You are asked to see a patient for a second opinion. She has a longstanding history of low mood and several admissions with suicidal thoughts and plans. She is currently prescribed amitriptyline.

Take a history of her mood symptoms and explore her previous psychiatric history.

2b.

The lady you have just seen is depressed with an atypical depression. She has symptoms of variability of mood, tension, overeating, oversleeping and fatigue.

She has also expressed thoughts of self-harm. She lost her job as she was not performing (due to depression). She has a partner who is not supportive and drinks heavily. He has been both verbally and physically abusive in the past.

Explain to your consultant how you will manage her condition.

○ LINKED STATION 3

3a.

An 18-year-old university student is referred for assessment by his general practitioner (GP). The patient is perplexed, frightened and expresses ideas of persecution. He is willing to be admitted to hospital. He has no previous psychiatric history.

Your consultant catches you before you see the patient and wants to discuss the differential diagnosis and how you intend to proceed over the next 48 hours.

3b.

The patient's mother turns up and asks what is going on. She saw a programme on bipolar disorder the other day and wonders if this is what her son has. She wants to know what the management plan is and if he will be able to go back to university. If not, should she take him home? She has also heard of early-onset services, and wonders if this is an option or what other options may be available.

○ LINKED STATION 4

4a.

You are asked to assess Mr Jones, a 63-year-old doctor who took early retirement. Concerns have been raised by his family that he is collecting refuse in his house. You attend with a social worker (following a previous visit from the GP) to find the house in abject squalor with large collections of paper and magazines lying around.

Assess this gentleman. Towards the end of the scenario the examiner will ask your preferred diagnosis.

4b.

You discover that this gentleman collects items that he finds in his day-to-day life and subsequent thoughts of removing said items appear to generate a level of distress (i.e. where to put them, whether they are needed). He avoids such problems by setting them aside. He says he is happy to work with you as he has been reading lots about talking therapies and is particularly interested in the works of Freud. He does not believe hoarding to be the same as obsessive compulsive disorder (OCD).

Explain to the social worker how you should manage this gentleman.

SINGLE STATIONS

5.

You are asked to see a 19-year-old African man who, one month ago, witnessed the death of someone sitting next to him on a train. He has since complained of fears of going mad and poor sleep.

Assess him and manage the situation.

6.

A 34-year-old African female presents with a degree of confusion, variable agitation, distress and perplexity. It is difficult to get a clear history of her symptoms from the notes as they seemed to vary from day to day. She currently believes that she has water and electricity moving through her veins. She was admitted under the team 6 months previously. At the time, she had a full psychotic work-up. Organic causes were excluded. Her husband discharged her home after a failed trial of three different antipsychotics. She is currently on quetiapine. It seems from her history that she then lost contact with her community mental health team (CMHT). The GP has sent a letter requesting an urgent assessment. Her husband reports that she has not been well since her discharge and he can now no longer cope.

Your consultant is on the phone. He has heard the history and wishes to know what you would do next with this lady. He is thinking about starting clozapine.

7.

You are asked to see 60-year-old female twins who believe they are being visited by aliens from Jupiter. The GP mentions in his referral that they believe the aliens are controlling them in some way. The twins have only recently starting living together.

How would you proceed in the short and long term? Explain your management to the examiner.

STATION 1

1a: Bipolar disorder

> **KEY POINTS**
> History of presenting complaint
> ICD-10 categories of depression, bipolar and mood disorder
> Exploration of differentials
> Exploration of risks
> Avoiding the use of jargon
> Empathy and sensitivity

INTRODUCE YOURSELF

The candidate may wish to start the station by explaining who they are and why the GP has referred them.

SET THE SCENE

This station is of a patient with bouts of depression alternating with bouts of hypomania i.e. rapid cycling. The antidepressant is not helping matters and may be contributing to her instability. She previously also discontinued lithium (prescribed by your predecessor for treatment-resistant depression). The GP and then your colleague have tried several antidepressants, none of which really seems to have improved her mood symptoms.

On history today, the patient appears euthymic but on closer questioning will slowly reveal that she is overactive, restless and irritable. She also has problems sleeping.

Questions to start should be open ended but then gradually focus on depressive (and other affective) symptoms with some degree of structure.

'I understand you've been referred to me by your GP because of mood problems? Is that correct? Can you tell me a little more about this?'

COMPLETING THE TASKS

The candidate will gain marks first for demonstrating the core features of depression (low mood, anergia, anhedonia) along with additional symptoms that indicate the level of severity (ICD-10 DCR). The candidate should then ask about elevation of mood in the form of euphoria, irritability and overactivity. There should be a question as to the possibility of psychotic features as well as actively asking about suicidal ideation.

It is important to explore medication history and medical history, and briefly look for the presence of comorbidities; in particular, anxiety disorders and alcohol.

PROBLEM SOLVING

The main point of this station is that the candidate is presented with a highly atypical presentation. This is always an indication to review the diagnosis.

There is a lot to do in a short space of time. The candidate may need to make provision for this at the beginning of the interview by informing the patient that they may have to hurry them along at times due to time constraints but that they should feel free to ask any questions as they go along.

ADDITIONAL POINTS

The candidate may gain marks for delineating a clear history with an exploration of potential triggers. Additionally an exploration for the shifts in mood should be explored. They should ask about physical health, including thyroid disease, antidepressant-induced switching, suboptimal medication regimes, the effects of lithium withdrawal, and erratic compliance.

Note that at this stage it is difficult to say definitively what is wrong so this section should be approached with caution. The candidate may indicate that it would be useful to obtain information from a close relative.

FURTHER READING

National Institute for Health and Clinical Excellence (2006) *Bipolar disorder: the management of bipolar disorder in adults, children and adolescents, in primary and secondary care.* NICE clinical guideline 38. London: NICE.

World Health Organization (2003) *The ICD 10 classification of mental and behavioural disorders: diagnostic criteria for research.* Geneva: World Health Organization.

1b: Bipolar management

KEY POINTS

Clear delineation of the issues
Clear outline of potential risks; namely relapse if poor compliance, risk of self-
    harm whilst hypomanic or depressed
Need for investigations
Drug management (acute phase and long term)
Biopsychosocial approach

INTRODUCE YOURSELF

SET THE SCENE

The candidate may wish to start with a concise statement of their entire management strategy.

'In terms of management of this patient, I would consider investigations and treatment. Treatment would involve managing the acute phase and then prophylaxis.'

COMPLETING THE TASKS

Investigations

Take a full history and mental state, perform a physical examination, perform a full blood screen (including thyroid function), perform a urine drug screen, take collateral/informant history and obtain the old notes.

'I would consider a rating scale (such as the Young Mania Rating Scale) given the variation of her symptoms, allowing a more accurate recording of fluctuation, and perhaps identify a pattern (including any potential triggers). I would consider a magnetic resonance imaging (MRI) brain scan if this has not been done already.'

Treatment

'I would want to take her off her antidepressant in the first instance. It may be appropriate to observe for a period as this in itself may restore the balance in mood. My preferred setting would be regular outpatient reviews, although the decision would involve the patient, considering the home environment and issues of risk.'

Immediate: management would include the initiation of an antipsychotic with proven efficacy in mania such as olanzapine or risperidone as well as a benzodiazepine if necessary.

Medium and long term: 'I would also consider a mood stabilizer. She is of child-bearing age, so I would want to discuss the implications of this fully with her. There is a risk of relapse if she is poorly compliant with her medication. I would explore her capacity to make a decision relating to this treatment choice.'

'In order to aid adherence I would provide psychoeducation in the first instance, stressing the need to maintain her medication.'

'I would also refer her for cognitive behavioural therapy which may have a range of benefits in the form of medication adherence, help with identification of triggers, treatment of mood symptoms (in particular her depression), and help with stress and lifestyle management.'

'I would want her to be assigned to a key worker (which may be me). I think it would be helpful in this case to discuss this lady with the multi-disciplinary team (MDT) and decide if she would also benefit from help from a community psychiatric nurse (CPN). As part of her care agreement, I would want her characteristic symptoms of depressive or hypomanic episodes documented together with the early intervention strategies which the patient and her treatment team are to enact when faced with these symptoms.'

PROBLEM SOLVING

Some candidates are unsure whether to mention the term 'biopsychosocial' in a patient's management. The author suggests that what may be more important is to make it clear to the examiner which of the three 'phases' of treatment you are dealing with when addressing treatment.

ADDITIONAL POINTS

Although not included here, examiners often attempt to differentiate the high-achieving candidates by asking about an individual's prognosis. Have a clear list of prognoses for the common psychiatric disorders likely to present in the exam: depression, schizophrenia, personality disorder.

FURTHER READING
Frangou, S. (2005) Advancing the pharmacological treatment of bipolar depression. *Advances in Psychiatric Treatment, 11,* 28–37.

STATION 2

2a: Mood history

KEY POINTS
Clarification of diagnosis
Use of open and closed questioning
Sensitivity and empathy
Psychosocial factors
Risk assessment

INTRODUCE YOURSELF

SET THE SCENE

This patient has been depressed for 3 years. She lost her job as she was not performing. She has a partner who is not supportive and who drinks heavily. He has been both verbally and physically abusive in the past.

The candidate will find that this lady does in fact have an atypical depression, namely mood reactivity, variability of mood, tension, overeating, oversleeping, fatigue.

Clarify the patient's understanding of the purpose of the meeting, namely, given the long duration of her symptoms, to see if there is more that can be done to help her mood.

COMPLETING THE TASKS

The task says that you should take a mood history and past psychiatric history. Start with open questions about her mood and then ask about low mood, poor energy levels and anhedonia followed by associated symptoms as listed in ICD-10 or DSM-IV.

PROBLEM SOLVING

Some candidates may fail to identify this as a case of depression but atypical depression is an important diagnosis given that it is said to be associated with increased distress, suicidal ideation and disability compared with 'typical' depression. Despite this, they should be able to highlight the psychosocial stressors that are having an impact on her mood. The differential includes dysthymia and mixed anxiety and depression. One should make an effort to exclude these as possibilities.

Owing to limited time, it will be difficult to cover her past psychiatric history comprehensively. It is sufficient to ask about when she first became depressed and the reasons for this (the patient in the station will maintain that she has been depressed constantly since then), the number of times (roughly) she has been admitted to hospital and whether they were formal or informal admissions. As always at this stage, whether she has tried to harm herself needs to be clarified. Finally, a medication review (still considered past psychiatric history) would include which medications she had taken for her mood and whether she felt any of them helped. One would also need to enquire into how long she took these medications and if she had problems tolerating any of them.

ADDITIONAL POINTS

A common failing in this situation is that candidates are unclear about the symptoms (which many argue are arbitrary) to differentiate moderate from major depression. For a clear understanding of this, one should read the ICD-10 diagnostic criteria.

The candidate will gain extra marks for taking the history in a structured way. They should, however, not be afraid to further explore the information provided by the patient, as a simple tick-list approach to symptoms will not be rewarded.

FURTHER READING

American Psychiatric Association (1994) *Diagnostic and Statistical Manual of Mental Disorders*, 4th edn. Washington, DC: American Psychiatric Association.

Brown, G.W. & Harris, T.O. (eds) (1978) *Social Origins of Depression. A Study of Psychiatric Disorder in Women*, 5th edn. London: Routledge.

Brown, G.W., Harris, T.O. & Hepworth, C. (1995) Loss, humiliation and entrapment among women developing depression: a patient and non-patient comparison. *Psychological Medicine*, 25, 7–21.

Kendler, K.S., Hettema, J.M., Butera, F., Gardner, C.O. & Prescott, C.A. (2003) Life event dimensions of loss, humiliation, entrapment, and danger in the prediction of onsets of major depression and generalized anxiety. *Archives of General Psychiatry*, 60, 789–96.

2b: Atypical depression

> **KEY POINTS**
> Management strategy pertinent to the patient's care
> Addressing psychosocial issues
> Consideration of patient's wishes (avoidance of paternalistic approach)
> Evidence basis for the treatment of depression
> Social services role in children's care

INTRODUCE YOURSELF

SET THE SCENE

The candidate may wish to outline the main issue pertinent to this case scenario early on. This will demonstrate to the examiner that they are aware of the real issue in this situation and hopefully ensure a pass. They may wish to say something along the lines of: 'This situation is really about the management of a patient in the context of psychosocial adversity. The main issue is how to manage the depression in the context of these psychosocial stressors and the risks present to herself and others.'

COMPLETING THE TASKS

'The major issue is the management of her depressive illness and her risk of suicide. I would therefore want to perform a full risk assessment.'

One needs to consider whether she needs inpatient care. Is her home situation currently safe? Does she need a mental health assessment, or would she do well with home treatment? Is she living in a home situation where home treatment would be possible or desirable or could she be treated as an outpatient? Could she go to stay with a relative? Alternatively, in some Trusts there are 'women's houses' that may be more suitable than a general adult ward.

'If we decide we can manage her as an outpatient (i.e. we can manage the risk and can contract her safety), my treatments would consist of biological and psychosocial interventions.'

'I note that this lady is on amitriptyline. I would want to know the reasons for such a choice. I would then want to explore if it had been of benefit. It does have sedative properties and may not be the treatment of choice as she is sleeping more than usual and has ideas of self-harm, which might include overdosing.'

'The social interventions in this individual will be of particular importance. I would refer her to the social worker within our team to look into her current financial situation and ensure her basic needs are being met (for example, is she on benefits? does she have any money? is she eating?). She may need a review of her housing. She may also need a referral to other services such as Relate, if she requires support for her marriage.'

PROBLEM SOLVING

This is a management station. When addressing risk the candidate should avoid the temptation to start outlining in detail their risk history. They should mention the salient points.

ADDITIONAL POINTS

Good candidates might make reference to Barbui and Hotopf's (2001) meta-analysis indicating the possibility of increased effectiveness of amitriptyline in comparison to alternative antidepressants but a lower level of tolerability. Although monoamine oxidase inhibitors (MAOIs) have largely fallen out of favour, they may also wish to indicate knowledge of the literature suggesting that phenelzine has some efficacy in atypical depression.

FURTHER READING

Barbui, C. & Hotopf, M. (2001) Amitriptyline vs the rest: still the leading antidepressant after 40 years of randomised controlled trials. *British Journal of Psychiatry*, *178*, 129–44.

Stewart, J.W., Tricamo, E., McGrath, P.J. & Quitkin, F.M. (1997) Prophylactic efficacy of phenelzine and imipramine in chronic atypical depression: likelihood of recurrence on discontinuation after 6 months' remission. *American Journal of Psychiatry*, *154*, 31–6.

STATION 3

3a: First-onset psychosis

KEY POINTS
Awareness of first-onset psychotic episode
Implications of this experience for future care and engagement
Importance of medication in the early phase
Psychosis history
Exploration of aetiological factors
Adherence to specified timeframe

INTRODUCE YOURSELF

SET THE SCENE

Explain to the consultant that you have not seen that patient as yet, but this is a critical time for this individual as the most likely diagnosis seems to be first-onset psychosis.

Explain that the decision to admit was presumably based on his preference and potential risks. 'I have not been provided with information as to whether this is to be a formal or informal admission. I want to clarify the reasons for this preference.'

COMPLETING THE TASKS

'In terms of a differential, I would consider:

- a pre-psychotic state or prodrome, psychotic episode, or transient psychotic experience;
- a depressive episode with psychotic features;
- schizoaffective state;
- manic episode;

- an anxiety disorder due to the clear high levels of distress;
- personality disorder – e.g. schizotypal, paranoid;
- drug-induced psychosis – intoxication or withdrawal;
- organic illness, including neurological disorders (tumour, temporal lobe epilepsy) and autoimmune conditions.'

Management would consist of investigations and treatment.

Investigations

'I would want to investigate for important comorbidities such as substance misuse. Physical investigations would include a full blood screen, glucose, liver and thyroid function and lipids. I would also want baseline physical observations.'

Full history, mental state and detailed physical examination. 'I would pay attention to biological, psychological and social vulnerabilities and possible precipitants. I would want to continue monitoring of his mood to pick up on any potential signs of hopelessness, depression and suicidal ideation. My investigations may involve a period of watchful waiting on the ward if this psychotic episode is a new phenomenon.'

Treatment

'If, however, he has clear-cut first rank symptoms and these psychotic experiences have been occurring for some time, I would start an antipsychotic immediately. I would also bear in mind (although this would not delay instigation of treatment) that both ICD-10 and DSM-IV require a 4-week history of symptoms to diagnose schizophrenia. I would prescribe him a benzodiazepine to alleviate any significant distress or anxiety.'

'The early assignment of a keyworker is particularly important in an individual to facilitate engagement and provide psychoeducation. My preference would be to provide feedback to him and the family together if he was happy with this.'

PROBLEM SOLVING

First contact with mental health services is important as it may influence engagement and counter the individual's and their relatives' prejudices and issues of stigma. This should be reflected throughout the management of this scenario.

Essentially the candidate should deal with three main issues in the acute setting: treating the psychotic symptoms, treating factors associated with their development such as anxiety and addressing a patient's confusion concerning their symptoms. A bio-psychosocial means to address this should be taken.

ADDITIONAL POINTS
Consider the specific and more global risks:
- risks associated with his high level of distress;
- the risk of lack of engagement which may have long-term implications for his contact with services;
- the risk of damage to his social network and reputation which may worsen the longer he stays untreated;
- risk of labelling as 'schizophrenic' at too early a stage.

The good candidate will have an awareness of the National Service Framework and its suggestion of the need for early intervention and treatment to reduce levels of morbidity.

FURTHER READING

Department of Health (1999) *A National Service Framework for Mental Health: Modern Standards and Service Models*. London: Department of Health.

Marshall, M. & Rathbone, J. (2006) Early intervention for psychosis. *Cochrane Database of Systematic Reviews*, Issue 3. Art. No.: CD004718. DOI: 10.1002/14651858.CD004718.pub2.

National Institute of Clinical Excellence (2002) *Schizophrenia: Core Interventions in the Treatment and Management of Schizophrenia in Primary and Secondary Care*. London: NICE.

3b: Discussion with relative

KEY POINTS
Issues relating to son's consent
Rapport
Dealing with anger
Explanation of condition and its management in lay terms
Answering her enquiries about bipolar affective disorder (BAD)

INTRODUCE YOURSELF

SET THE SCENE
'Thanks for coming to see me today. I know this must be a very worrying time for you, and you have some questions about your son.'

COMPLETING THE TASKS

Management in the least restrictive setting. Awareness of likely differential diagnosis, diagnostic uncertainty and how it can help to 'wait and see'. This, however, should not be the case for management. After a period of observation (if deemed appropriate), a low-dose antipsychotic should be instigated with careful review after 2–3 weeks with a low threshold to change antipsychotic if there have been no signs of improvement.

Engagement is an independent predictor of treatment retention rates.

Try to address the patient's perception of the usefulness of professional help, any negative stereotypes of mental illness and fears of mental health services.

You may be prompted with: 'What medication would you start this patient on if he remains psychotic?' Advice would be to consider aspects of his presentation but to consider a tablet such as risperidone, amisulpride or olanzapine at a low dose in the first instance, checking for signs of at least initial response from 2–3 weeks. The choice of medication would be discussed with the patient so he could make an informed collaborative decision.

How would you deal with denial?

Long term:

Investigation of how he is doing at university, associated stressors and any drug or alcohol misuse.

Whether he needs a doctor's note in support of problems he may be having.

Suggestion of referral to OT.

Referral to MIND or other voluntary associations.

Further discussion on early-onset treatment and the debate between efficacy vs. effectiveness.

There should be a clear idea in the candidate's mind of the resources available to this individual by way of a home treatment team, crisis resolution teams, day hospital or referral to specialist services.

Before he left, an attempt would be made to make an advance directive and distribute it to all concerned. It has been suggested that service users may benefit from writing an account of their experience in the notes. Care would be arranged via the Care Programme Approach.

A return to university will depend on his progress. A discussion with the university will be needed. If he responds well to treatment he should be able to return with support. A switch to a less demanding course is sometimes beneficial.

PROBLEM SOLVING

You will have to mention that although your colleagues have seen her son, you have not, but will do so immediately after this meeting. This may inflame her further, but at least you have been straight with her from the start.

Advise that if it is indeed schizophrenia, he would be likely to remain on medication for at least 1–2 years. Be prepared to discuss the difference between bipolar affective disorder and schizophrenia.

ADDITIONAL POINTS

Explore their viewpoint on what might have contributed to this current state. Use predisposing, precipitating and maintaining factors rather than arguing on a purely biological basis. A blame-free approach is particularly important.

Address practical issues such as what home life is like and whether in this situation it would be appropriate to send this patient home – adequate exploration of the risks.

Where does he live – would his care have to be transferred to another CMHT?

Be prepared to discuss the following: family work, social recovery work, training schemes, assertive outreach.

STATION 4

4a: Hoarding

> **KEY POINTS**
> Understanding the definition of obsessive acts and compulsive rituals in eliciting the psychopathology
> Exploration of the implications of this psychopathology
> The differentials of hoarding
> Emotional attachment to objects hoarded
> Clear communication
> Demonstration of empathy and sensitivity

INTRODUCE YOURSELF

SET THE SCENE

'Hello Dr Jones, I'm Dr_____. I wonder if I might ask you some questions? How have you been feeling? What problems have you been experiencing of late?' 'I couldn't help but notice that you seem to have lots of things stored here and it looks like they have been here for some time. Is there a particular reason for this?'

COMPLETING THE TASKS

This gentleman collects items that he finds in his day-to-day life and subsequent thoughts of removing them generate distress (i.e. where to put them, whether they are needed). He avoids such problems by setting them aside.

The candidate is advised to start with an open question on the patient's welfare, i.e. his presenting complaint, but narrow it down very quickly to the task in hand.

Direct questions about possible symptoms:

- Do you wash or clean a lot?
- Do you check things a lot?
- Are there particular thoughts that keep bothering you that you'd like to get rid of but can't?
- Do your daily activities take a long time to finish?
- Are you concerned about putting things in a special order?
- Do these problems trouble you?
- What use are these items to you?
- Does it make living here more difficult? Do you find it difficult to move around?
- Physically are you well?

Concerning cognition, it is not necessary given the time constraints to do a full cognitive assessment. A few questions on orientation and then the delayed recall task (which is thought to be the most sensitive indicator of cognitive impairment) should suffice. With respect to possible learning disability, it is already volunteered in the vignette that he is a doctor (what sort?). One could ask a single question on academic performance.

PROBLEM SOLVING

The task really rests on the differential diagnosis so it is important to be as systematic in this approach as possible. This could be written out during your preparation/reading time.

The request is quite clear, specifically asking for an exploration of diagnosis. The candidate need not therefore go into a full psychiatric history (e.g. forensic history etc.) concerning hoarding, aside from aspects that aid the question in hand.

It may seem that there are too many diagnoses to try to exclude, but the candidate should in many ways be led by the patient's responses. Attempts to formally ascertain a diagnosis specific to hoarding and OCD-related symptoms will in itself separate the diagnosis from a range of other differentials.

ADDITIONAL POINTS

The range of differentials given the non-aetiological definition of hoarding includes:

a. obsessive compulsive disorders;

b. depression – either with obsessional thoughts related to the low mood, or squalor secondary to retardation and anergia;

c. psychosis – with the squalor directly related to psychotic beliefs or due to the 'negative' symptoms e.g. psychomotor slowing, underactivity;

d. bereavement reaction;

e. impulse control disorder;

f. Diogenes syndrome;

g. organic: alcohol abuse, dementia, brain injury, temporal lobe epilepsy, post-encephalopathic complications, Tourette's syndrome;

h. personality disorder: schizotypal, obsessive–compulsive personality disorder (OCPD);

i. learning disability.

Some demonstration of a school of thought regarding OCD as a neuropsychiatric condition as demonstrated by some questions related to associated neurological problems e.g. tics and abnormal involuntary actions.

A history like this is most probably indicative of a chronic disorder. The patient may show little resistance to the compulsions. A good candidate asks for a time when previously the subject resisted rituals (rather than taking the patient's response at face value), e.g. 'I understand that now you don't resist these things but was there ever a time when you did?'

Exploration of covert as well as overt rituals as these are equally important in terms of treatment.

FURTHER READING

Gelder, M., Lopez-Ibor, J. & Andreasen, N. (2001) *New Oxford Textbook of Psychiatry*. Oxford: Oxford University Press.

Loewenstein, D.A., Barker, W.W., Harwood, D.G., Luis, C., Acevedo, A., Rodriguez, I. & Duara, R. (2000) Utility of a modified Mini-Mental State Examination with extended delayed recall in screening for mild cognitive impairment and dementia among community dwelling elders. *International Journal of Geriatric Psychiatry*, *15*, 434–40.

Maier, T. (2004) On phenomenology and classification of hoarding: A review. *Acta Psychiatrica Scandinavica*, *110*, 323–37.

National Institute for Health and Clinical Excellence (2005). *Treating obsessive-compulsive disorder (OCD) and body dysmorphic disorder (BDD) in adults, children and young people. Understanding NICE guidance – information for people with OCD or BDD, their families and carers, and the public.* NICE clinical guideline 31. Available at http://www.nice.gov.uk/cg31.

Steketee, G. & Frost, R. (2003) Compulsive hoarding: current status of the research. *Clinical Psychology Review, 23,* 905–27.

4b: Hoarding management

> **KEY POINTS**
> Risks adequately explored
> Treatment options
> Pros and cons of an admission
> Need for multi-agency involvement (including GP and Social Services, psychology)
> Dealing with a professional colleague

INTRODUCE YOURSELF
'Hello, I'm Dr_____. Could I discuss Dr Jones with you?'

SET THE SCENE
You could summarize your findings here and also the areas of main concern.

COMPLETING THE TASKS
'The treatment for this condition involves a stepped care approach. The literature suggests that hoarding is particularly difficult to treat. It is clear from the case presented that this is a severe situation that potentially poses a range of risks; nevertheless, I would hope that the choice of intervention would be as therapeutic as possible. It may be that a brief admission may be necessary as the council wishes to make the living conditions more habitable/safe. It may be that the patient would be willing to engage in treatment that would involve gradual removal of the refuse in his house.'

'In terms of investigations, I would want to exclude any physical illness or disability that may be contributing to this presentation. The range of investigations would be guided by the clinical assessment of full history, mental state and physical examination.'

'I would refer him to an experienced psychologist who would instigate a programme of cognitive behavioural therapy (CBT) (including exposure to obsessive thoughts and response prevention of mental rituals and neutralizing strategies).'

'I would refer him to occupational therapy to more accurately assess his living conditions and functioning within his household. I would want to liaise closely with you (social worker) in terms of an acceptable plan as to how to deal with this clean-up.'

This gentleman will need a lot of input and is likely to need a community psychiatric nurse to visit him regularly at home, perhaps as a joint keyworker.

It is important to emphasize engagement. This may be an issue particularly in someone who may be reclusive. One of the concerns is that hoarders generally lack insight into the risk that there may be to themselves, their environment and their neighbours.

'I would also consider:

- the risk of severe self-neglect, fire, falling (especially elderly people), poor sanitation;
- the fact that beliefs can be so strongly held that they threaten those who try to intervene;
- that the outcomes of hoarding can lead to the building being condemned and the occupant evicted.'

PROBLEM SOLVING

It may be tempting for the candidate to very quickly go down the route of engaging in a discussion as to the National Assistance Act or Public Health Act. The use of such measures is in fact relatively rare and is likely to be guided by social services.

Concerning medication, there needs to be an acknowledgement that the evidence base of efficacy in this group is poor. One needs to clarify what aspect of the presentation is being treated, i.e. is there a significant anxiety component associated with the condition? One could discuss this as a possibility in a collaborative way with the patient, but the mainstay of treatment is likely to be a talking therapy.

ADDITIONAL POINTS

Bear in mind his interest in psychodynamic analysis; this could be explored further. Has he had it before, for instance? The evidence base supports CBT but that wouldn't necessarily exclude the long-term possibility of psychodynamic therapy, especially as Diogenes syndrome (which remains on the differential) is said to be associated with personality disorders.

- Recognition that this is difficult to treat, with high dropout rates (engagement, treatment failure and poor outcome).
- Awareness of psychodynamic theory on OCD – early aggressive sexual trauma with maladaptive use of defence mechanisms (e.g. reaction formation and magical undoing). Early psychoanalysts likened hoarding behaviour to purposeful internal retainment of one's faeces and reasoned a fixation at the anal-erotic stage of development as its cause.
- The CBT theory of OCD is centred on an enduring tendency of sufferers to interpret their own mental activity as indicating personal 'responsibility' with a secondary pattern of discomfort and subsequent attempts to neutralize their anxiety. There are more specific models for hoarding.
- A brief mention of Diogenes syndrome but note that this does not have operationalized criteria, and is multi-aetiological in origin. The literature suggests an absence of insight and distress by such activities as opposed to an obsessive compulsive disorder.
- If asked about OCPD, it does not have the degree of functional impairment characteristic of OCD and it is egosyntonic.

FURTHER READING

Freud, S. (1908) Character and anal eroticism. In J. Strachey (ed.) *Collected Papers* [English trans.]. London: Hogarth Press.

Maier, T. (2004) On phenomenology and classification of hoarding: A review. *Acta Psychiatrica Scandinavica*, *110*, 323–37.

National Institute for Health and Clinical Excellence (2005). *Treating obsessive-compulsive disorder (OCD) and body dysmorphic disorder (BDD) in adults, children and young people. Understanding NICE guidance – information for people with OCD or BDD, their families and carers, and the public.* NICE clinical guideline 31. Available at http://www.nice.org.uk/cg31.

Steketee, G. & Frost, R. (2003) Compulsive hoarding: current status of the research. *Clinical Psychology Review*, *23*, 905–27.

STATION 5: Post-traumatic stress disorder (PTSD)

INTRODUCE YOURSELF

SET THE SCENE

KEY POINTS
Empathy and rapport
Demonstration of the psychological implications of this illness
Features salient to the potential diagnosis
Risks adequately explored
Treatment options
Clear, concise communication and management style

'I heard a little about what happened to you last month. It sounds very distressing. I'm sorry if it upsets you, but are you able to tell me a little more about what happened?'

COMPLETING THE TASKS

This is a likely case of post-traumatic stress disorder.

In the differential consider:

- an anxiety disorder that has begun (or was pre-existing);
- a depressive disorder that had begun (or was pre-existing);
- an adjustment disorder – although this trauma is clearly of a more severe nature than would be expected for this category;
- a psychotic illness perhaps with an affective component.

Consider also comorbidities known to be associated with this condition, for example panic attacks, alcohol/substance misuse or deliberate self-harm.

To manage the situation, gather further information about the trauma and its personal relevance to the patient. In particular, explore the cognitions relevant to the event, as they have a bearing on management.

Did he know the person who was shot? Did he know the attacker? Was he also supposed to be targeted or was he the main target? Is his life currently in danger? What happened after the event? What was the involvement of the police? Was the attacker apprehended?

Explore the mental state and look for evidence of the preferred differential. Include a risk assessment given the potential risks associated with comorbidities and indeed given the high level of risk from the presenting complaint.

Does this man now have:

- depression (the features of which are...)?
- an anxiety disorder (the features of which are...)?
- PTSD? Look for three broad categories of symptoms:
  reliving (in the form of flashbacks, recurring dreams);
  avoidance of situations similar to the stressor (which may also be associated with difficulty remembering and thinking about the trauma);
  arousal manifest as an exaggerated startle reflex, irritability and problems sleeping.

The choice of treatment is medication (usually selective serotonin reuptake inhibitors (SSRIs)), trauma-focused CBT or eye-movement desensitization and reprocessing (EMDR).

Before referral for psychological intervention (and in view of a potential waiting list), simple measures of psychoeducation are helpful and may include details of the types of symptoms that are common after trauma (e.g. reliving, problems sleeping), and reassurance that these symptoms need not necessarily spiral (as many fear that they will go mad or lose control).

Additionally, it is important to explore ideas of guilt and shame (for instance rape victims feeling they had led on their attacker or in this case perhaps a belief that he should have helped the individual), as many patients with PTSD hold themselves responsible in some way. By the nature of the cognitions, they may have not revealed this to anyone thus far.

PROBLEM SOLVING

It is important once again to explore the risks, as not only may this gentleman perceive himself to be in danger but this may in fact be true. This needs to be contrasted by raised expectations and perceived increased likelihood of danger secondary to the illness.

ADDITIONAL POINTS

In these individuals, comorbidity is common. It is therefore important to stress, even if you confirm a diagnosis of PTSD, that you have assessed for evidence of comorbidity.

Many candidates are unable to describe EMDR. Its most unique aspect is the component of bilateral stimulation of the brain using eye movements, bilateral sound, or bilateral tactile stimulation coupled with cognitions, visualized images and body sensation. EMDR also employs dual attention (stimulus discrimination in CBT) to allow the individual to vacillate between the traumatic material and the safety of the present moment. It clearly has a cognitive restructuring component, but a recent study found the procedure to be less effective if the eye movements are removed.

FURTHER READING

Lee, C.W. & Drummond, P.D. (2008) Effects of eye movement versus therapist instructions on the processing of distressing memories. *Journal of Anxiety Disorders, 22,* 801–8.

STATION 6: Treatment-resistant schizophrenia

INTRODUCE YOURSELF

KEY POINTS
Dealing with a senior colleague
Management of treatment resistance
Bio-psychosocial options
Consideration of risks
Consideration of husband's current involvement

SET THE SCENE

This is an unusual, seemingly psychotic presentation. Consider the issues relevant to her care, an idea of differentials, risks and finally management.

COMPLETING THE TASKS

'I would want to clarify the nature of the urgency of the assessment and reasons for this. Is there a risk posed in terms of her husband no longer being able to cope and becoming frustrated with her? Similarly, does she pose a risk to others in her current state? We know she is agitated and confused. Are there, for instance, children at home who may suffer as a result of her illness (including psychological damage)? Does she pose a direct risk to them?'

'I would want to check her medication history in terms of dosage, duration and adherence. I would want to review the diagnosis, especially due to the atypical nature of her symptoms. Although previously excluded, I would want to consider organic contributions to her presentation and also consider the potential effect of comorbidity.'

'I would consider an admission for this lady. There is evidence of depleted family resources, with her husband expressing an inability to cope. Additionally, she may be a suitable candidate for initiation of clozapine.'

'I would explore whether she would be happy to come in on a voluntary basis or whether we need recourse to the Mental Health Act. I would still discuss the option of home treatment to see if this was a viable alternative.'

On admission, management would consist of investigations and treatment.

'I would review the history, previous notes and medications. I would take a history of current symptoms, perform a mental state and physical examination. My investigations would be guided by these findings but in preparation for instigation of clozapine, I would also perform a full blood screen and baseline physical observations, including an ECG and her weight. I would want to ensure that there were no contraindications presented by the history, namely a history of seizures, blood disorders or cardiac problems.'

'During this time, I would explain in detail to the patient and her family about clozapine, its potential benefits and side effects. I would want to start the medication in as collaborative a fashion as possible. I would explain the need for ongoing blood tests and the fact that this medication needs to be taken regularly.'

'Concerning the psychosocial aspect of her care, I would want to understand the husband's previous concerns that led to discharge. I would explore what effect her illness has had on the family and whether there was evidence of high levels of expressed emotion at home. I think in this case, to facilitate compliance and engagement with the team, it would be important to try to come to a shared conceptualization of this lady's illness. I would still convey the diagnosis, but it may be easier for them to understand schizophrenia in the context of their perception of the impact of the psychosocial stressors.'

'If the patient was still unwell after 4 months, I would ensure first that she was taking the medication regularly and would request plasma tests for this. It may be an option to increase the dose to bring her levels up to around 0.35mg/L, although I recognize there is little relationship between plasma levels and clinical response. There is still a further response between 3 and 6 months so it may be reasonable to continue with monotherapy.'

'Augmentation with agents such as amisulpride, omega-3 triglycerides (EPA) or lamotrigine is used. If this failed, I would consider placing her back on the antipsychotic that she had most success with and really pushing the psychosocial interventions such as CBT for psychosis and support at home.'

PROBLEM SOLVING

Try to think what you would be considering in your own clinic in the management of this individual. There is a lot to cover, so it is important not to get bogged down in too much detail, for example listing a raft of blood tests one may do to investigate potential organic differentials.

ADDITIONAL POINTS

Basic knowledge of clozapine, its adverse effects, initiation and monitoring is expected. Recognition that the evidence for augmentation with clozapine is relatively sparse, consisting of case series and open trials in the main.

Given the acute onset, remitting course and symptom polymorphism, the possibility of a cycloid psychosis could be considered. The differential would include schizophrenia, atypical psychosis, schizoaffective psychosis, bouffée délirante or puerperal psychosis.

FURTHER READING

Leonhard, K. (1961) Cycloid psychoses-endogenous psychoses which are neither schizophrenic nor manic-depressive. *Journal of Mental Science*, 107, 632–48.

Taylor, D., Paton, C. & Kerwin, R. (2005) *The 2005–2006 Maudsley Prescribing Guidelines*, 8th edn. London: Taylor & Francis.

STATION 7: Folie à deux

KEY POINTS
Outline of the issues relevant to the situation
Awareness of potential risks
Differential diagnosis
Management of two separate individuals
Immediate and long-term management

INTRODUCE YOURSELF

SET THE SCENE

'This sounds like a case of folie à deux (or induced delusional disorder in ICD-10). My understanding is that it usually happens to two people who live together. The index case tends to be the more dominant of the individuals, often with a pre-existing psychotic illness, and the psychosis is induced in the other person. The inductee may be in some form of vulnerable state with either a mental or physical disability.'

COMPLETING THE TASKS

'In terms of a differential, these would include the usual differentials for psychosis in the index case. For the second individual these may be the same but may include factors that reflect a potential vulnerability such as a learning disability or a dependent personality. Then there are the variations applicable to folie à deux, so it is possible that both individuals may have a history of psychosis and one may simply have added the delusions of their associate. Alternatively, but less likely, they may have become psychotic at the same time, especially as they are twins and may share a genetic link.'

'The differential for a psychotic person would be the same for any psychotic person. I would want to exclude organic causes, acute confusional states, metabolic derangement, early-onset dementia or late-onset schizophrenia.'

'I would also want to consider the possibility that these two are not isolated cases. There is mention in the literature of several cases of induced psychosis (folie à trois, or folie en famille, etc...) but the differential in this case is unlikely to be of a belief developed in the context of two people simply living in close proximity (i.e. a subcultural belief).'

'From the GPs I would need to know any past psychiatric history, past medical history and in particular if there was any past relevant family history. One of the twins has recently moved back in and I would want to investigate the cause for this. Additionally I would ensure that she is registered in the area.'

'I think in this case it may be less likely that this couple is going to come to an outpatient appointment. It may also prove useful to see the home environment. I therefore think the best approach is a domiciliary visit. I would go along with a member of my own team as well as someone who knows them (this may be the GP). This may alleviate any potential suspiciousness. I would need to think about my safety and the safety of others as we are unsure what level of risk this involves.'

'My history taking would involve assessing for the features in my differential. I would therefore take a full history (including a developmental history) from both ladies. The other possibility is to get one of my colleagues to take a collateral history. I would be looking for the features of my differential.'

'Management involves separation of the two and treatment of the index case. Given that these individuals live together, this is likely to involve an admission. We may need to do further investigations such as IQ testing and imaging.'

'The long-term management would involve consideration of whether these two individuals could live together again. I would want to assess their capacity (namely their ability to understand, appreciate, reason and express a choice about their living arrangements) to make this decision as there may be a possibility that once back in the same household they would relapse. I would also consider how they were coping in the house together and whether alternative accommodation would be more suitable for them. They may, for instance, be agreeable to the suggestion of sheltered accommodation, perhaps in the same area.'

PROBLEM SOLVING

This is a station where some may find difficulty applying a broad structure as it is so unusual. There is much in the literature as to rare differentials and even rarer variations of this illness. A large knowledge base about the condition is not necessary to gain marks in this station.

For the candidate it may be easier to outline what they know about this condition very early on and then to apply this with a view to addressing management. They need to still include reference to (1) the main issues of the case, (2) risks, (3) assessment and (4) management.

ADDITIONAL POINTS

When asked about long-term management one could also mention consideration of referral to a psychiatrist with a research interest in schizophrenia and genetics for a second opinion. This would be if the psychosis proved longstanding or treatment resistant.

FURTHER READING

Sims, A. (1995) *Symptoms in the Mind*, 2nd edn. London: W.B. Saunders.

Chapter 2

Old age psychiatry

Dr Justin Sauer

O LINKED STATION 1

1a.

This 74-year-old depressed patient has failed to respond to therapeutic doses of lofepramine, sertraline and more recently a combination of venlafaxine and mirtazapine. A worsening of mood and the emergence of psychotic features led to a compulsory admission to hospital under the Mental Health Act (MHA) (1983). He has been seen by the ward psychologist but is too depressed currently to engage with cognitive behavioural therapy. The staff are concerned about his dietary intake which has declined since his admission. Over the last week fluid intake has also reduced and blood samples now show deranged urea and electrolytes (U&Es) consistent with dehydration. His wife wonders if he should be transferred to a medical ward. In the absence of senior colleagues you see this gentleman on the ward.

Explain to this gentleman how you wish to manage him further and what this is likely to involve.

1b.

You meet with his wife who is concerned about her husband's further deterioration since admission to hospital. You inform her that the team believe that electro-convulsive therapy (ECT) should now be considered in view of his worsening condition.

His wife has heard only negative things about ECT and wants more information.

O LINKED STATION 2

2a.

You are about to see a patient in your clinic. Below is the referral letter.

Dear Psychogeriatrician

Re: Prof. Michael Baugh – 15.06.32. Weston Hill Rise, Southwark, London

Thank you for seeing this retired sociologist who lives alone. He has reported worsening of his memory and I wonder if he has a dementing illness. He has a history of hypertension. No major surgical procedures. I have given him an antibiotic for a recent UTI.

Current Medication: Trimethoprim 200mg b.d.
Simvastatin 20mg
Aspirin 75mg
Enalapril 20mg

He has one daughter, Mrs Carol Davies. She works but is happy to speak to you.

Sincerely
Dr Byron Moore

Take a history of memory loss and explain how you intend to manage him.

Do not perform a cognitive assessment.

2b.

You meet with Prof. Baugh again in your clinic. Following a full initial assessment and the results of investigations, you diagnosed this gentleman with Alzheimer's-type dementia and initiated anticholinesterase inhibitor treatment. You meet with him for a review, which he attends with his daughter. She tells you in confidence that his personality has changed significantly. She finds him to be difficult and embarrassing, and on several occasions he has exposed himself. This is completely out of character and predates the new medication. You explain that you will assess him further.

Assess his frontal, temporal and parietal lobe function.

SINGLE STATIONS

3.

This elderly woman with vascular dementia was taken to hospital by the police after she was found wandering the streets in the early hours of the morning barefoot and dressed only in her nightclothes. She was confused and afraid.

She has been assessed in Accident and Emergency and they have ruled out a physical aetiology. The casualty doctor informs you that she was seen in hospital a year ago by the neurologists after she had a transient ischaemic attack. She denies drinking alcohol but is a smoker. She scored 7 out of 10 on an abbreviated mental test score today and is now asking to return home.

Assess if this patient is safe to go home. Do not carry out a cognitive assessment.

4.

You have been asked by a solicitor to assess this elderly woman. Her son has concerns that his mother has suddenly changed her will. He believes that his sister is plotting against him to have him excluded from any inheritance.

Assess this woman to see if she has testamentary capacity.

5.

This 67-year-old civil engineer has noticed that his memory has deteriorated. He has felt less 'sharp' at work and although he has no concerns about his ability to do the job, he has found grasping new information quite difficult. He has a history of dyslipidaemia and hypertension for which he is prescribed medication. He has seen his general practitioner (GP) and clinical examination is reported as unremarkable. There is no past psychiatric history. The GP has concerns that the presentation represents a likely dementing process, although this has not been discussed with the patient.

Carry out a cognitive assessment.

6.

This is Mr Shaw. Your team have been seeing his mother at a nursing home since her admission there 2 months ago. She has Alzheimer's disease and had been irritable, aggressive and wandering whilst living in her own home. At that time she was assessed and prescribed olanzapine. She settled initially, but has since become irritable again and the GP increased the dose.

Today the son has asked to see you. He is angry and upset that his mother has been prescribed an antipsychotic and thinks she is over-sedated. He has also read an article about the 'dangers' of these medications in dementia.

Manage this situation and advise him on alternative approaches to behavioural change in dementia.

STATION 1

1a: Depression – treatment resistance

KEY POINTS
Communication and rapport
Explaining concerns
Medical issues
Pharmacological approach
ECT
Risk

INTRODUCE YOURSELF

'Hello, my name is Dr_____, I'm one of the psychiatrists.'

SET THE SCENE

Explain that you are one of the doctors looking after him and that you want to find out how he is feeling. Ask him why he is eating and drinking less and explain to him the results of his blood tests. Discuss the concerns of the team and explain that you wanted to talk about what you should do next.

COMPLETING THE TASKS

Explain to this gentleman how you intend to manage him further and what this is likely to involve.

Explain to the patient that he has been on two antidepressants to which he did not respond and now a combination of antidepressants, and still he remains depressed (we assume that the previous drugs were taken at therapeutic doses and for adequate time periods).

Treatment options

Medical

Explain your concerns about his hydration status and that you want to do some repeat blood testing today. If he remains dehydrated or has deteriorated further, he is likely to need intravenous (IV) rehydration. Remind him that the nursing staff are monitoring his food and fluid intake and that you will be asking them to continue to do this as well as monitor his blood pressure. Ask if the staff have been offering him drinks or build-ups on a regular basis.

Psychological

This has been attempted but he has been assessed as currently unsuitable. You could ask what happened when he met with the psychologist.

Pharmacological

Options include:

> Lithium – augmentation with lithium is supported by a good evidence base. The concern in this case would be his poor fluid intake which would make toxicity more likely.

Tri-iodothyronine – there is evidence to suggest augmenting with T3 can be of benefit and is well tolerated. He would need to have his thyroid function monitored.

Other second choice medication in refractory depression includes lamotrigine, pindolol, monoamine oxidase inhibitors (MAOIs) and tryptophan, but these are supported by less robust research evidence.

ECT

In light of the following:

- severely depressed;
- resistant to drug treatment;
- too unwell to undergo CBT;
- concern re food and fluid intake;

discuss ECT as a treatment option. Ask whether he knows anything about ECT.

Explain process:

Preparation e.g. consent process, physical examination, investigations, ensuring he is fit for anaesthesia (note his current dehydration).

The ECT itself includes anaesthesia, electrode placement, induced seizure, recovery. A course of treatment involves typically 6–12 treatments in total (twice per week).

Potential benefits of treatment:

Expect clinical improvement to start after 2–3 treatments.

Approximately 70 per cent likelihood of it being successful.

Adverse effects:

Short-term: headache, muscle aches, nausea, disorientation with memory loss (short term, pre ECT).

Longer-term: about a third of people who have ECT complain of persistent gaps in autobiographical memory – often for the time around their depression. Normally able to learn new material and perform normally on cognitive testing.

RISK

The main risk issues here relate to this patient's further deterioration if he continues to deteriorate physically. Appropriate treatment of his depression will hopefully lead to improved mental state and a return to more normal eating and drinking. He may none the less need fluid rehydration which will require transfer to a medical ward. He is depressed and as part of your assessment you should ask about suicidal thoughts.

Risk of death following ECT is approximately 1 in 100,000 treatments (due to anaesthetic risk).

PROBLEM SOLVING

You are likely to be confronted by a very withdrawn and depressed individual, which is likely to slow you down. Do not be seen to rush through unsympathetically. Take time to explain the issues.

It would be important to ask him if he is taking and swallowing the medication. Physical causes of depression should have already been excluded (e.g. thyroid dysfunction) and other physical medication that can cause depression should be reviewed (e.g. diuretics and antihypertensives).

ADDITIONAL POINTS

If time were not an issue it would be important to confirm the diagnosis of depression. Examining his mental state and reviewing his psychiatric history and medical records would be useful.

This gentleman is currently admitted under a treatment section of the MHA. If he refuses to have ECT and has capacity then he cannot be treated unless it is deemed necessary as urgent treatment in order to save his life. ECT may only be given to an incapacitated patient where it does not conflict with any advance directive, decision of a donee or deputy or decision of the Court of Protection.

FURTHER READING

Taylor, D., Paton, C. & Kerwin, R. (2007) *The Maudsley Prescribing Guidelines*, 9th edn. London: Informa Healthcare.

1b: ECT

KEY POINTS
Communication
Empathy
Rationale for treatment approach
Explanation of ECT
Risks
Answering other questions

INTRODUCE YOURSELF

Hello, my name is Dr_____, I'm one of the psychiatrists.'

SET THE SCENE

Thank his wife for meeting you and share your genuine concerns about her husband's condition. Mention that you have just met with him and have discussed the possibilities in terms of further treatment. Explain that ECT does have a bad press, but that it is extremely effective in depression and that you would be happy to answer any questions she might have.

COMPLETING THE TASKS

His wife has heard only negative things about ECT and wants more information.

Start by asking her what she already knows about ECT. Your conversation is likely to cover a number of the following issues.

Rationale

Explain that her husband has been treated with two different antidepressants and now a combination of treatments without any improvement. The psychologists are not able to engage with him and whilst you could add in some additional medications, his poor fluid and food intake make his condition more serious. ECT, whilst remaining unpopular in the media and among some patient groups, is usually reserved for just such serious cases.

The procedure

ECT involves the use of electricity which induces a 'fit' or 'seizure' whilst the patient is asleep. The patient is given a very short anaesthetic and muscle relaxant (minutes), so they are only aware of going to sleep. At all times the anaesthetist, psychiatrist and ECT nurses will be present.

ECT pads which deliver the treatment are placed on the head. The anaesthetic means people are sleeping and are not aware of the treatment procedure.

ECT can either be given to one side of the head (unilateral) or to both sides (bilateral). Bilateral ECT seems to work more effectively and more rapidly than unilateral ECT, but may also induce greater short-term memory loss. You can start with unilateral ECT and then switch to bilateral ECT if there is no significant improvement.

Treatment length

A usual course of treatment is between 6 and 12 sessions and given twice a week.

Benefits

Likelihood of treatment response: increases treatment response from 2/3 with antidepressants alone to 4/5 with ECT. It is one of the most effective treatments for depression. It is generally considered safe and there is no evidence base to date showing that ECT harms the brain.

Adverse effects

Short-term:

> Common side effects include headache and drowsiness immediately after ECT which usually settles within a few hours.

> Sometimes people do complain of short-term memory loss, but this is usually temporary and only involves recent things, for example what you had done just before the treatment.

> Unilateral treatment can reduce the effects on memory.

Long-term: Some individuals describe longer-term memory problems.

How it works

We are not sure how ECT works but believe that the treatment causes a release of neurotransmitters or 'natural brain chemicals' whose imbalance is thought to underlie depression. This artificially induced release of 'feel-good chemicals' may be how it works.

RISK

Whilst ECT is associated with some risks, there are also risks of not having treatment, which include further delay in recovery from depression and deterioration in physical health which could lead to death if not eating or drinking sufficiently. Risk of death following ECT is approximately 1 in 100,000 treatments (due to anaesthetic risk).

PROBLEM SOLVING

There are those that consider ECT to be ineffective, inhumane and degrading and that it belongs to a different era. Concerns also relate to its side effects and that it might permanently damage the brain. His wife has concerns and a negative view of ECT. It is important to be balanced in your discussion and that you do not down-play the adverse effects.

ADDITIONAL POINTS

Unilateral ECT: Electrode is placed on the non-dominant side, 4 cm above the midpoint between the external angle of the eye and the auditory meatus. The other electrode is placed 10 cm above the first, above and in line with the meatus on the same side.

Bilateral: On each side electrodes are placed 4 cm above the midpoint of the line between the external auditory meatus and the lateral angle of the eye.

Some of the neurochemical changes following ECT include increased noradrenaline, dopamine, serotonin and reduced acetylcholine.

ECT can also be useful in mania, lethal catatonia, Parkinson's disease and neuroleptic malignant syndrome (NMS).

Adequate seizure length is thought to be around 25 seconds (on EEG tracing) or $\geq$ 15 seconds (peripheral observation).

Investigations prior to ECT/anaesthetic include: full [blood] count (FBC), U&E, electrocardiogram (ECG), chest X-ray (CXR).

Sickle cell screening is important for African–Caribbean and Mediterranean people.

FURTHER READING

National Institute for Health and Clinical Excellence (NICE) (2005) *Electroconvulsive therapy (ECT): the clinical effectiveness and cost effectiveness of electroconvulsive therapy (ECT) for depressive illness, schizophrenia, catatonia and mania.*
http://www.nice.org.uk/guidance/TA59.

STATION 2

2a: Memory loss

KEY POINTS
Communication and rapport
Empathy
History of memory loss
Likely diagnosis
Further management
Risk issues

INTRODUCE YOURSELF

'Hello, my name is Dr_____, I'm one of the psychiatrists.'

SET THE SCENE

'Your GP has written to me with concerns about your memory, is that correct?' 'Could you tell me what's been happening?'

COMPLETING THE TASKS

1. History of memory loss

Your interview will involve taking the patient through the development of memory impairment and how this has affected the different facets of his life.

Presenting complaint

Your history taking should incorporate some of the common causes for memory loss.

Differential:

> Dementia has a slow insidious course whereas delirium is usually more rapid.
>
> Depression can present with poor attention, concentration and bradyphrenia.
>
> Depression can occur following life events and physical ill health. Often there are subjective complaints of memory loss in depression, unlike dementia where people will frequently hide or compensate for deficits.
>
> In amnestic disorder there is memory impairment rather than global cognitive decline.
>
> Also consider alcohol and substance misuse, schizophrenia and malingering.

Dementia:

> What memory problems has he noticed?
>
> Memories for recent events, learning new information or remote memories (personal or impersonal)?
>
> Enquire about aphasia (e.g. nominal), agnosia, apraxia (e.g. dressing) and executive functioning (planning, organizing, sequencing and abstract ability).

Duration and time course of the memory loss (e.g. gradual, step-wise).

Insidious onset, recent memory affected, remote memory fairly well preserved (Alzheimer's disease (AD)).

More abrupt onset, stepwise decline, fluctuating course, nocturnal confusion, personality relatively spared (vascular dementia).

Fluctuations in cognitive function, visual hallucinations, spontaneous features of parkinsonism (dementia with Lewy bodies (DLB)).

What memory problems have other people noticed?

Has anyone commented on his personality changing in any way? (frontotemporal dementia (FTD)).

Premorbid functioning e.g. job, education level.

Medical history

Currently he has a urinary tract infection (UTI). Has this caused an acute confusional state?

This patient has cardiovascular risk factors including hypertension and hypercholesterolaemia. Ask how long he has been treated for these. Ask about smoking, diabetes and alcohol consumption. Ask why he takes aspirin and whether he has any problems with his heart. Has he ever had transient ischaemic attacks or a cerebro-vascular accident (CVA)? Ask whether the GP has arranged for him to have further blood tests or an ECG and whether he has had a magnetic resonance imaging (MRI) brain scan. If not, explain that you would be looking to arrange this to rule out some other causes of memory problems.

Social functioning

Ask what impact any deficits have on his day-to-day functioning.

Any support he is receiving.

Any difficulties with basic self-care: washing, dressing, feeding.

Ability to manage at home with cooking, cleaning, washing.

Ability to deal with finances, driving, shopping.

Collateral history

Ask his permission to speak to his daughter to obtain collateral history.

2. Management

First you will need to make a diagnosis and this is based on your clinical assessment, physical examination and investigations which include memory tests, blood tests and brain imaging.

The actor will ask you what you think is wrong with him and what you will do should he have dementia.

Most likely diagnoses in this scenario: Alzheimer's or vascular dementia. Recent worsening due to a delirium, secondary to urinary tract infection. Consider management under bio, psycho, social headings. Management will depend on the degree of cognitive and functional impairment.

Biological

Optimizing vascular risk factors e.g. hypertension, dyslipidaemia, diabetes, atrial fibrillation, smoking cessation (if present).

Additional medication for untreated physical risk factors.

Possible role for acetyl cholinesterase inhibitors in AD (± memantine) – be aware of recent NICE guidelines.

Possible benefit from anti-inflammatory drugs and gingko biloba (some evidence).

Treat any psychiatric comorbidity e.g. antidepressants.

Advice re alcohol if drinking heavily.

Psychological

Cognitive stimulation; memory training, CBT for depression.

Reality orientation, validation therapy, reminiscence therapy.

Social

Ensuring adequate social support e.g. carer/home help/meals on wheels/day centre.

Compliance aids for medication (if still self-medicating).

OT assessment and adaptations for the home environment e.g. memory prompts, devices.

Alzheimer's Society – information resource and carer's assessment.

Support for daughter e.g. carer's group.

RISK

It is important to ask about situations where he has put himself at risk and how often this has happened e.g. getting locked out of the house due to forgetting keys, getting lost, driving or leaving the cooker on.

PROBLEM SOLVING

Although the professor is already being treated for a urinary tact infection it is important to consider delirium in your differential diagnosis. Features include:

- impaired consciousness and attention;
- rapid onset;
- psychotic symptoms; usually visual hallucinations, transient delusions;
- disturbance of the sleep–wake cycle;
- emotional disturbance; depression, anxiety, perplexity;
- disturbance of motor activity; both under- and over-activity.

ADDITIONAL POINTS

When considering anti-dementia treatment, remember to take into account the NICE guidelines, any arrhythmias and a history of dyspepsia or gastric ulceration. It is important to explain that the drugs are not a cure, that benefits are modest, but they can delay the course of the illness for some people.

Three acetylcholinesterase inhibitors (donepezil, galantamine and rivastigmine) are currently available. They are all similar in their clinical effect on memory and improved attention and motivation. Usually if no improvement is apparent after 3–4 months treatment is stopped. Common side effects include headache, nausea, vomiting, anorexia, weight loss and diarrhoea.

Although licensed for treating moderate to severe Alzheimer's disease, memantine is not currently supported by the NICE guidelines. Memantine is an N-methyl-D-aspartate (NMDA) receptor antagonist that affects glutamate transmission.

FURTHER READING

Bullock, R. (2002) New drugs for Alzheimer's disease and other dementias. *British Journal of Psychiatry, 180*, 135–9.

2b: Frontal/temporal/parietal lobes

KEY POINTS
Effective communication
Putting patient at ease
Explaining rationale for tests
Frontal lobe
Temporal lobe
Parietal lobe

INTRODUCE YOURSELF

Reintroduce yourself to Prof. Baugh. Ask if he remembers your last meeting.

SET THE SCENE

Asking him how he has been getting on with the new medication would be a good way to lead in to the station. Explain that you've spoken to his daughter and that you'd like to do some more tests to see how the different parts of his brain are working. Inform him that you ask these questions of many people you see and that he should not worry if he makes a few mistakes as some of the questions are more difficult than others.

COMPLETING THE TASKS

1. Frontal lobes

Personality:	'Have you changed in yourself in any way?' 'In what way?'
Motor sequencing (Luria's test):	Demonstrate the hand sequence – 'fist, edge, palm' five times and then ask the patient to repeat with both hands. 30 seconds each side.
Verbal fluency:	Ask the patient to generate as many words as possible (not names or places) for the letters 'F, A and S'. One minute each and record all responses. (Depending upon time available, one minute for just one letter would be adequate.)
Category fluency:	Ask the patient to name e.g. as many animals with four legs in one minute as they can. Record all responses.
Abstract reasoning (proverb interpretation):	Ask the patient to interpret what a proverb might mean: 'Too many cooks spoil the broth' (or similar).
Cognitive estimates:	'How many camels are there in Holland?' 'How tall is the Post Office Tower?'
Abstract similarities:	Ask the patient in what way the following are similar. 'An apple and a banana?' 'A table and chair?'
Primitive reflexes:	Grasp reflex Rooting reflex Palmomental reflex

2. Temporal lobes

Dominant lobe
Receptive dysphasia:

Alexia	Ask the patient to read something.
Agraphia	Ask the patient to write something.

Impaired learning and retention of verbal material:

Ask the patient to repeat an address, 42 West Register Street, and to recall it after 5 minutes.

Non-dominant lobe
Visuospatial difficulties:

Anomia	Ask the patient to name a wrist watch, strap and buckle.
Prosopagnosia	Ask if he recognizes the 'Queen' on a £5 note.
Hemisomatopagnosia	Belief that a limb is absent when it is not.

Impaired learning and retention of non-verbal material such as music or drawings:

Ask the patient to copy a simple drawing and to repeat from memory 5 minutes later.

Bilateral lesions

Amnesic syndromes (Korsakoff's amnesia, Kluver Bucy syndrome). Assess short- and long-term memories.

3. Parietal lobes

	Function	Task
Dominant lobe		
Dysphasia:	receptive dysphasia	obvious from conversation
Gerstmann's syndrome:	finger agnosia	'point to left ring finger with right index finger'
dyscalculia	simple arithmetic	
right–left disorientation		'touch left ear with right hand'
agraphia		ask the patient to draw something
Non-dominant lobe		
Neglect (inattention):	Neglects one side	Ask him to draw a clock face with dials and numbers
Prosopagnosia:	Failure to recognize faces (as above)	
Anosognosia:	Failure to recognize disabled body part	
Constructional apraxia:	Unable to copy visually presented drawing	Copy interlocking pentagons
Topographical disorientation:	Difficult finding way especially in new environment.	Ask if he gets lost or confused in new places
Bilateral lobe		
Astereognosia:	Inability to identify object through touch alone	Ask him to identify key/coin with his eyes closed
Agraphagnosia:	Failure to identify letters drawn onthe palm	Ask him to identify H or W drawn with top of pen on his palm, with his eyes closed

RISK

It would be prudent to sensitively mention reports of his having exposed himself and briefly assess the risk issues. Can he remember this happening, where and when did this happen? Was anyone the target of this behaviour and was it related to cognitive decline or of a sexual nature?

PROBLEM SOLVING

The patient is likely either to become fed up with your continuous testing or to be offended by your mentioning his having exposed himself. This is a potential source of conflict and the style in which you ask your questions makes all the difference. For example: 'You exposed yourself in front of other people. Why did you do this?' is clumsier and less considerate than, 'Some people I see who have had problems with their memory do things out of character, such as exposing themselves. Has anything like this happened to you?'

ADDITIONAL POINTS

Features of frontal lobe dysfunction:

Disinhibition, distractibility

Lack of drive

Errors of judgement

Failure to anticipate

Perseveration

Poor adaptation to change

Over-familiarity

Sexual indiscretion

Consequences of neurological damage to temporal lobes structures:

Changes in behaviour/personality

Increased aggression, agitation or instability (limbic system)

Contralateral homonymous upper quadrantanopia (assess visual fields)

Depersonalization

Disturbance of sexual function

Epileptic phenomena

Psychotic disturbances akin to schizophrenia

Potential neurological consequences of parietal lobe damage:

Homonymous lower quadrantanopia (optic radiation)

Astereognosis, reduced discrimination (sensory cortex)

FURTHER READING

Lishman, W.A. (1998) *Organic psychiatry*, 3rd edn. Oxford: Blackwell Science.

STATION 3: Wandering

KEY POINTS

Communication and rapport

History of events

Risk assessment

Mental state assessment

Personal circumstances

Management plan

INTRODUCE YOURSELF

'Hello, my name is Dr_____, I'm one of the psychiatrists.'

SET THE SCENE

Ask what happened this morning, can she remember any details?

COMPLETING THE TASKS

Assess if this patient is safe to go home

This woman has put herself in an extremely vulnerable situation and management will involve an assessment of risk and of her current mental state. It will also depend on her current social circumstances and whether there are any family members or close friends who will be able to provide support, should she return home today.

Risk assessment

Can she remember what happened? If so take her through the events.

Why did she leave the property?

Can she remember her home address?

Does she live alone? (You would want to speak to anyone living at home with her, neighbours or warden if in supported accommodation – how has she been managing?)

Does she have any next of kin or friends who you would be able to talk to?

Are there any healthcare professionals (or allied) involved? (Community mental health team (CMHT) for older adults, community psychiatric nurse (CPN), social worker, occupational therapist, day centre.)

Has anything like this happened before? (You would want to corroborate this from A&E, police and family doctor.)

It is important to find out about her living conditions (food, hygiene, gas/electricity).

Is she looking after herself appropriately?

Important to note her current level of personal care (unkempt/undernourished).

History of alcohol or substance misuse?

History of falling?

Likelihood of repeating episodes? (Any old medical records in A&E?)

History of harming self or others?

History of behavioural disturbances? (In public or at home.)

Is she prescribed any regular medication? (Acetylcholinesterase inhibitors/antipsychotics/antidepressants, is she taking them appropriately?)

Has she been started on any new medication (e.g. diuretics, digoxin)?

Capacity assessment

Demonstrating capacity with regard to the event and associated risks would be somewhat reassuring if considering a return home. Capacity is defined as follows:

The person must be able to understand and retain the information long enough to make a judgement. They should be able to weigh up the pros and cons of their choice. The person should be able to communicate the decision made.

Current mental state

Excluding functional illness is important and will affect your management. Ask relevant questions to rule out:

Psychosis (presence of abnormal perceptions/delusions – paranoid/persecutory/command?)

Affective illness (mania/severe depression)

Neurotic, stress related and somatoform disorder (dissociative fugue)

Behavioural syndromes (somnambulism).

Further management

Respite or hospital admission

Admitting the patient would depend upon the information gathered during the interview. Even if cognitively impaired, the patient should be part of the process and continually updated. Admitting an elderly patient with dementia can be extremely distressing and you would want to provide them with appropriate reassurance. Rather than hospital admission, it might be that a period of time in a residential or nursing home would be more appropriate.

CMHT follow-up

If not already known to mental health services, she would benefit from an assessment and follow-up. The multi-disciplinary team (MDT) will almost certainly have a role in looking at her medication, considering her cardiovascular risk factors, nursing input to monitor her mental state, and OT to look at her accommodation and any modifications, particularly in view of her wandering behaviour.

Care package

She might benefit from more support depending on her social circumstances and ability to care for herself and her home environment. The social worker or care manager will be able to advise on financial matters and moving to more supported accommodation where appropriate.

RISK

Consider the following:

In the household: gas, appliance use, smoking, fire, flooding, poor heating in winter

Financial: managing bills, access to money, pension

Diet: doing the shopping, preparing meals, malnutrition

Falls: At home and outside. What adaptations might be needed?

Abuse: Financial (family, friends, tradesmen, opportunists), emotional

Security: wandering, locking up (theft, burglary).

PROBLEM SOLVING

The actor will put you under pressure to make a decision to let her go home. If you have performed a full risk assessment and key aspects of the mental state examination you would still need to talk to family members and professionals that might be involved before arriving at a decision. If she has capacity and no evidence of mental illness then she would be within her rights to leave, but you should try to persuade her to stay a little longer until you have spoken to the relevant people that are involved in her care.

ADDITIONAL POINTS

Cognitive assessment: Although not asked to assess cognitive function, ordinarily you would be looking to do the mini mental state examination or similar in such circumstances.

Assisted technology: Devices can be installed in the home that alert a centre to an individual's activities. This can, for example, alert one to the fact that the front door has been opened at night. Similarly, the use of mobile phones or other devices attached to coats can allow people to be tracked if they put themselves at risk from wandering.

Further medical assessment: She has been cleared medically and for the purposes of the exam you would assume that to be the case. However, in reality you want to know the details of what examinations and tests have been performed. Is there any evidence of a fall or head injury? She should have had a full neurological assessment and, if not, you would want to do this. What were the results of blood tests and urinalysis? Does her presentation represent an acute confusional state (delirium)? Ideally she should have had brain imaging (CT/MRI) in view of the history of transient ischaemic attack (TIA).

FURTHER READING

Ballard, C., O'Brien, J., James, I. & Swann, A. (2001) *Dementia: Management of behavioural and psychological symptoms.* Oxford: Oxford University Press.

STATION 4: Testamentary capacity

KEY POINTS
Communication
Rapport
Explanation of the process
Testamentary capacity assessment
Relevant mental state examination
Answering other questions

INTRODUCE YOURSELF

'Hello, my name is Dr_____, I'm one of the psychiatrists.'

SET THE SCENE

You need to explain who has requested the assessment and why. You should inform her that the interview will form the basis of a report that will be sent to her son's solicitor and that it could also be used as evidence in court.

COMPLETING THE TASKS

Assess this woman to see if she has testamentary capacity

Testamentary capacity (TC) is the ability to make a valid will. When there is doubt as to TC a doctor, usually a psychiatrist, is often asked for an opinion. Mental impairment can be grounds for a legal challenge, as can undue influence on the individual in making or changing a will.

The specific components of TC can be assessed by asking about their understanding of a will and its purpose. A general estimate of their property and its value is essential. Ask about the potential heirs and their wishes with respect to each. Reasons to include or exclude individuals should be explored. Ask about previous wills and whether they have a copy to show you.

Requirements for testamentary capacity:

1. The person must understand the nature of the act and its effects. The individual understands that they are giving their property to one or more objects of their regard.
2. The person must know the extent of his/her property. An exact knowledge is not expected but they should be able to give an idea of what property they have and its extent.
3. The person must know the legal heirs, those included and excluded and how the will distributes the property.
4. The person has no mental disorder affecting 1–3 above. If a mental disorder is present, any legal challenge will depend upon demonstrating its impact on the ability to complete a will as set out in the criteria for TC as shown above.
5. The person must not be subject to undue influence by one or more third parties.

In assessing testamentary capacity it should be determined:

- whether there is/was a major psychiatric disorder;
- whether this psychiatric disorder impairs the ability to know she was making a will;
- whether delusions are present that involve the estate or heirs;
- whether this disorder impairs her ability to know the nature and value of the estate;
- whether this disorder impairs her ability to identify the heirs that would usually be considered;
- whether the individual is vulnerable to undue influence.

Clinical assessment is very important as a number of conditions can interfere with valid will completion. Major psychiatric illness such as schizophrenia and organic disease such as dementia are common examples. Their presence, however, does not always mean that the individual lacks TC. Someone with a psychotic illness who believes the FBI has bugged their apartment, for example, may know very well the size of their estate, their children and how it should be divided between them. Psychosis/delusions that would invalidate a person's capacity to make a will often involve their heirs in a negative way. If dementia is suspected you would need to perform a test of cognitive function (e.g. mini mental state examination (MMSE)).

RISK

As in all scenarios in the exam, where there is an opportunity to demonstrate you are a safe trainee, do so. A screening question as part of your mental state examination (MSE) on suicide/self-harm would do.

PROBLEM SOLVING

The solicitor will expect you to assess TC specifically in relation to the criteria as set out above.

Elderly people are often advised by lawyers to have an evaluation of testamentary capacity at the time a will is executed.

Video taping is increasingly used at the time of will execution, which can later be used in court.

ADDITIONAL POINTS

Ordinarily, all relevant medical and psychiatric records would be available and also an estimate of the value and nature of the estate. This information would be sent to you by the solicitor. The criteria for TC date back to 1870 and the case of Banks v Goodfellow.

FURTHER READING

Banks v Goodfellow (1870) LR 5 QB 549.

STATION 5: Cognitive assessment

KEY POINTS
Communication
Empathy and rapport
Cognitive assessment
Further lobar assessment
Explanation of results
Answering other questions

INTRODUCE YOURSELF

'Hello, my name is Dr_____, I'm one of the psychiatrists.'

SET THE SCENE

'I've had some correspondence from your GP who says you've had some concerns about your memory. Is that correct? Would you tell me what's been happening?'

COMPLETING THE TASKS

Ask if you can test his memory. Try to develop rapport. Tell him that you'll be asking him some things which seem easy and some which are more difficult. Tell him not to worry if he makes mistakes.

You will be expected to use the mini mental state examination and should memorize it. You should complete this assessment with time to spare.

		Score
Orientation:	What is the:	
	Year?	1
	Season?	1
	Month?	1
	Date?	1
	Day of the week?	1
	Where are we:	
	Country?	1
	County?	1
	Town/village?	1
	Hospital/street?	1
	Ward/House number?	1
Registration:		
Name three objects	(apple, table, penny)	3
Attention:	Spell WORLD backwards (or subtracting serial sevens)	5
Recall:	Ask for the three objects learned in registration	3
Language:	Point to a pencil and a watch and have the patient name them	2
Repeating:	Repeat, 'No ifs ands or buts'	1
Three-stage command:	'take this piece of paper in your right hand, fold it in half, and put it on the floor'	3
Reading:	Please read this and do as this says. Write down on a piece of paper 'PLEASE CLOSE YOUR EYES'.	1
Writing:	Please write a sentence of your choice. (It must make sense and be grammatical)	1
Copying:	Copy this design	1
	Angles, no. of lines and overlap must be correct to score	

You should produce an MMSE score at the end. Writing the results down as you go along is therefore important. You will then be able to explain any areas of concern and what this means. Giving feedback to the patient is important, as is reassurance.

If appropriate and time allows, move on to frontal lobes. It is also useful to ask questions relating to remote memory, personal (wedding date, children's birthdays – although you will not be able to validate this) and impersonal (historical events).

RISK

A discussion concerning the risk of developing dementia might ensue:

- older age;
- strong family history;
- cardiovascular disease;
- hypertension, diabetes, hypercholesterolaemia, atrial fibrillation;
- head trauma.

PROBLEM SOLVING

In such scenarios people often express a concern about risks to their children. Explain that we are all at risk of developing AD if we live long enough. The risk can only be approximated in the broadest terms. On balance the risk to first degree relatives of patients with AD who develop the disorder at any time up to the age of 85 years is slightly increased. The risk to the children of an affected individual is in the region of 1 in 5 to 1 in 6.

ADDITIONAL POINTS

Clock drawing is increasingly used in cognitive assessment. It is easy to do and is a useful way of demonstrating disease progression with time.

'This is a clock face. Please fill the numbers and then set the time to 10 past 11.'

- Sensitive to deterioration
- Repeat 3–6 monthly

It assesses:

- comprehension;
- abstract thinking;
- planning;
- visual memory;
- visuo-spatial abilities;
- motivation;
- concentration.

FURTHER READING

Folstein, M.F., Folstein, S.E. & McHugh, P.R. (1975) 'Mini-mental state': a practical method for grading the cognitive state of patients for the clinician. *Journal of Psychiatric Research*, 12, 189.

STATION 6: Behavioural and psychological symptoms of dementia (BPSD)

KEY POINTS
Communication
Dealing with an angry relative
Addressing concerns
Explanation of treatment rationale and the evidence
Alternative treatment options
Risk issues

INTRODUCE YOURSELF

'Hello, my name is Dr____, I'm one of the psychiatrists.'

SET THE SCENE

'Thanks for coming to see me today. We've been involved in your mother's care for the last few months and I understand you have some questions about her treatment. Please tell me your concerns and I'll try my best to help.'

COMPLETING THE TASKS

Managing the situation

Express concern about his mother being over-sedated and that you will be reviewing her immediately after your discussion. Answer his questions about the use of medication in dementia and the rationale. Demonstrating some knowledge in this area and providing options should also help diffuse his anger.

Explain that BPSD is often due to our inability to understand the needs of the person with dementia. Many patients respond well to sensory stimulation, activities and social interaction. Simple interventions such as frequent toileting, good lighting, quality communication, fresh air and time in the open can make a difference. Hearing aids and analgesia for pain can make significant differences, where appropriate. A historical account of their likes and dislikes can assist the nursing home, for example their dietary preferences.

Use of antipsychotics

Cochrane review (Ballard 2006): 'Olanzapine and risperidone are useful in reducing aggression and risperidone reduces psychosis, but both are associated with serious adverse cerebrovascular events and EPSE. Despite the modest efficacy, the significant increase in adverse events confirms that neither risperidone nor olanzapine should be routinely used to treat dementia patients with aggression or psychosis unless there is severe distress or risk of physical harm to those living and working with the patient.'

Some recommendations are that risperidone and olanzapine should not be used for behavioural symptoms of dementia. Certainly the possibility of cerebrovascular events should be considered carefully before treating any patient with a history of stroke or transient ischaemic attack; risk factors for cardiovascular disease (CVD) (hypertension (HT), diabetes mellitus (DM), smoking, and atrial fibrillation (AF)) should also be considered.

Other atypical antipsychotics, such as quetiapine and amisulpride, are now used in place of risperidone or olanzapine, but the cardiovascular events are possibly a class effect.

The NICE–SCIE dementia guideline (2006) gives recommendations for good practice. They state that those with mild–moderate non-cognitive symptoms should not be prescribed antipsychotics and those with severe non-cognitive symptoms may be offered treatment with an antipsychotic drug after certain procedures have been followed and conditions met.

Other pharmacological approaches

Treating an affective component (antidepressants)

Anticholinesterase inhibitors (recent studies suggest limited value in behavioural disturbance)

Memantine (licensed for behavioural component, but not in the NICE guidance)

Mood stabilisers (anticonvulsants) can also be used for agitation.

Non pharmacological approaches

Aromatherapy and massage

Music therapy and white noise (masking other sounds)

Bright light therapy (related to melatonin)

Psychology – looking for triggers or management advice to carers or staff including:

Structured interventions: using prompts e.g. encouraging them to reminisce about important or enjoyable events that can help the person maintain an activity

Stimulated presence therapy: where a video or audio recording is made by friends or family recalling events in the life. It can help to calm people or encourage their participation.

RISK

The Alzheimer's Society have released statements stating that antipsychotics are inappropriately and over prescribed to people with dementia. They estimate that around 100,000 people with dementia in the UK are prescribed an antipsychotic.

BPSD can be extremely difficult for carers to handle. In nursing homes, staff should be trained to manage this with simple non-pharmacological approaches in the first instance. However, medication is often needed when such approaches have failed, particularly where carers are subjected to ongoing physical and verbal aggression, night-time disturbance and sexual disinhibition.

PROBLEM SOLVING

The son is upset and your success in this station will depend upon demonstrating knowledge and understanding of the issues. Providing the possibility of an alternative tailored management plan will also help.

ADDITIONAL POINTS

BPSD include:

Motor behaviour: agitation, aggression, restlessness

Social interactions: withdrawn, inappropriateness, disinhibition

Speech: increased or reduced, mumbling, shouting

Mood/Anxiety: anger, lability, anxiety, fear

Thoughts: delusions, paranoia, depression

Perceptions: visual and auditory hallucinations

Biological: sleep disturbance, incontinence, reduced appetite.

FURTHER READING

Ballard, C.G., Waite, J. & Birks, J. (2006) Atypical antipsychotics for aggression and psychosis in Alzheimer's disease. *Cochrane Database of Systematic Reviews.*

NICE–SCIE (2006) *Dementia: The NICE-SCIE guideline on supporting people with dementia and their carers in health and social care.* London: The British Psychological Society and the Royal College of Psychiatrists.

Chapter 3

Neuropsychiatry

Dr Derek Tracy

O LINKED STATION 1

1a.

An orthopaedic specialist registrar (SpR), Dr Arun, wants to discuss one of his inpatients who was admitted 10 days ago following a serious road traffic accident. The patient underwent external fixation of fractures in both femurs and required suturing for multiple superficial injuries.

Over the past few days this 20-year-old man has been behaving 'strangely' on the ward, for example trying to climb out of his bed and walk despite his leg injuries and nursing requests to remain in bed. Your colleague advises you that all blood tests have been within normal limits for several days, though a magnetic resonance image (MRI) of the patient's head taken yesterday shows frontal lobe contusions.

Dr Arun would like your opinion on what might, from a neuropsychiatric point of view, be causing this behaviour, and advice on management.

Discuss the differential diagnoses you are considering and how you might confirm or refute these. In general terms discuss treatment options available.

1b.

The orthopaedic SpR is grateful for your advice, though he admits he is not confident that he has given an adequate history and requests a review of this 20-year-old man.

You are given the most recent set of blood tests, which include full blood count (FBC), urea and electrolytes (U&Es), and liver function tests (LFTs) – all of which are normal – and a copy of the radiologist's report noting frontal lobe contusions on his MRI scan.

The patient says he cannot recall much about the accident but believes his memory since his operations has been fine – something corroborated by the nursing staff. He felt well in himself in the preceding weeks: he denies ever suffering with any mental health problems, describing himself as a 'chirpy, happy sort of guy'. He denies illicit drug use and says he rarely drinks alcohol.

He admits that his mother has said he's acting 'a bit weird' since the accident – she complained that he cursed frequently and told sexually explicit jokes in her presence – something she says he'd never normally do. The only change he has noticed is that he can't operate his mobile phone properly because 'there are too many buttons and controls to work out'.

In light of the neuroimaging results and the patient's comments, assess the relevant cognitive domains. Explain your findings to the patient, Mr Quixano.

O LINKED STATION 2

2a.

You are asked to see a 19-year-old female college student, Ms Finnegan, who has been admitted by the neurologists for further assessment of seizures. She has been having fits for over 2 years, and recalls having her first episode in school prior to an examination. Anticonvulsants over the past 2 years have not been helpful and video-telemetry during this admission has failed to show any epileptiform activity on electroencephalogram (EEG) during bouts of fitting.

In light of the telemetry findings, take a neuropsychiatric history from the patient.

2b.

The investigations and history are strongly suggestive of dissociative seizures. The patient is quite upset both by being referred to psychiatry and by the facts that her brain scan and blood tests were normal and no epileptiform activity has been found on video-telemetry. Since your last review she has repeatedly been telling staff that her mother thinks she's 'making it up'. She has asked for you to talk to her mother about dissociative seizures.

Discuss with the patient's mother what the findings mean, what treatment(s) are available and what the prognosis is for non-epileptic seizures.

O LINKED STATION 3

3a.

You have been referred a 68-year-old man with Parkinson's disease who, during an admission for management of worsening tremor, has been difficult to manage on the ward. He has appeared agitated at times and has been frequently noted to lie naked and fully exposed on his bed. A neuropsychiatric assessment is requested.

Take a relevant history from the patient, Mr Whitman, and consider what may be causing the recent difficulties.

3b.

Your assessment of Mr Whitman shows that he has been suffering with fleeting visual hallucinations of 'ghosts' that distract and irritate him and have led to much of his agitation on the ward. He was somewhat disorientated, thinking he was at home with his daughter Kay, but besides intermittent agitation, his affect seemed generally euthymic. The symptoms have been there for some time, though his wife feels they've worsened since starting his new medication with this admission.

Mrs Whitman wants to know what you can do to help her husband. Discuss with her in lay terms what might be happening and how you might be able to help.

SINGLE STATIONS

4.

A general practitioner (GP) refers a 20-year-old woman who has been complaining of frequent grimacing and clearing her throat. She attends your outpatient clinic with her friend as she reports feeling very embarrassed and fed up with this problem.

Take a history from this patient, Sunita, and discuss differential diagnoses and treatment options with her.

5.

A junior colleague, Dr Dedalus, currently in his first psychiatry post, asks for advice about one of his outpatients. The patient is a 46-year-old man with a 25-year history of paranoid schizophrenia. After a period of poor adherence to a previous medication, your colleague has recently commenced a different antipsychotic. The patient is in the next room with his mother, who is complaining that he isn't 'moving properly' at the moment. Dr Dedalus is aware that antipsychotics can cause movement problems, but he doesn't want to start opening books in front of the patient and his irate mother.

Discuss what might be happening, how this might be clarified by the history and give advice on further management.

6.

The neurology team have admitted a 35-year-old man, Mr Bloom, for a full work-up and investigations on the background of 15 years of full body pain and generalized weakness which have never been successfully managed. This admission has included an MRI of the patient's head, an EEG, an autoantibody screen including rheumatoid markers and routine bloods and physical examination – all of which have been unremarkable, in keeping with past findings. Prescribed analgesia and a trial with a transcutaneous electrical nerve stimulator (TENS) machine have been unsuccessful at treating his pain. The neurology SpR requests a neuropsychiatric review, advising you that their team feel 'it's all in his head'. They have advised him of the negative findings, the fact that they've no further investigations planned and that they aim to discharge him shortly.

Take a *brief* symptom history from this patient, who admits that he is surprised at being referred to a psychiatrist as he's never had to see one before.

Focus on possible psychiatric diagnoses and feed back a suitable model for his symptoms.

7.

Dr Clov, a consultant neurologist, requests a ward review of Ms Hamm, a 48-year-old woman with a 10-year history of multiple sclerosis. Whilst an inpatient for assessment and management of a relapse of her multiple sclerosis (MS), she has become quite tearful and low in mood, saying that she doesn't wish to carry on any more.

Take a history from the patient and discuss treatment options with her.

STATION 1

1a: Assessment of a head injury

KEY POINTS
Clarity of communication
Differential diagnoses
History of accident
Investigations and results
History of 'strange behaviour'
Management options

INTRODUCE YOURSELF

SET THE SCENE

'Thank you for referring this very interesting patient; I'm Dr_____, the neuropsychiatry SpR. I'd like to clarify some issues you previously mentioned...'

COMPLETING THE TASKS

The differential diagnosis is large, so it is important to be as structured as possible when discussing this. Organic causes include an acute brain injury and delirium with multiple potential causes. There might be withdrawal from alcohol or drugs, medication-induced confusion and mental illness, including depression and psychosis. The history, examination and investigations to date will help shed light on the likelihood of each of these differentials.

It's important to clarify the circumstances surrounding the road traffic accident (RTA): is there any evidence of the crash being intentional or of the patient having consumed drugs or alcohol prior to the accident?

Although not expected to be an expert in orthopaedics, the neuropsychiatric SpR should get a brief description of the nature of the initial injuries and subsequent surgery – the timeframe and how complicated the procedure(s) was/were. Was there initial loss of consciousness, and if so, how long did this last – comas lasting over a few days have a poor prognosis. Is there any evidence of post-traumatic amnesia? Did the patient have any seizures? Peri-operative confusion might well be expected, particularly in a traumatic emergency case. The candidate will need to be satisfied that physical examination and investigations are both thorough and recent. Is there evidence that the patient's behaviour is related to physical changes in his health? Were there any abnormalities on examination – especially neurologically? How is the patient being physically managed at present?

'Strange behaviour' is quite vague; it's necessary to expand on this. Check the timeframe – are the symptoms changeable; is there confusion or disorientation; is the patient agitated; is there evidence of withdrawal from any substances?

The candidate is looking for evidence of delirium, which would be suggested by a fluctuating pattern of abnormal behaviour in the context of disorientation. This might be caused by post-operative haematological abnormalities, withdrawal from drugs or alcohol, medication-induced or a concussion injury. Neuroimaging suggests frontal lobe damage: enquire about symptoms of disinhibition and apathy.

As well as physical causes for apparently unusual behaviour, it is vital to ask about the mental state: could the patient be suicidal and trying to harm himself intentionally? Is there any evidence of psychotic symptoms? Is there any past psychiatric history? Psychiatric symptoms could either precede the injury or be caused (or exacerbated) by them. Post brain injury psychosis is not common, but depression occurs in about a quarter.

Management will depend upon identifying the cause of the behaviour: for example, rectifying electrolyte imbalances, treating alcohol withdrawal and reducing (where practicable) opiate analgesia.

Environmental management of a distressed or confused patient should not be underestimated, and simple measures such as ensuring adequate lighting and provision of location and time cues (e.g. a board with the ward name, day and date) can be invaluable.

Sedation could be considered, taking into account the fact that additional medications may in fact worsen confusion. Options might include a benzodiazepine such as lorazepam. Of course, should a mental illness be identified, this would need to be treated appropriately.

PROBLEM SOLVING

This station may present as daunting owing to the number of differential diagnoses involved. It's important to remain as structured as possible, and run through the history, investigations and management in the hierarchical manner which candidates should do in all cases: namely organic illness, secondary to drugs, and functional mental illnesses.

ADDITIONAL POINTS

An understanding of the potential for drugs (whether illicit, licit such as alcohol, or prescribed) to cause confusion is essential. It would look impressive to delineate drugs into the categories above, and to display awareness of how both initiation of and withdrawal from many substances can alter the mental state. Drugs to enquire about specifically include alcohol, opiates and benzodiazepines.

Management of confused hospital inpatients is a common neuropsychiatric problem. Medication is frequently less helpful than clear communication with the patient and staff. The introduction of simple procedures, such as ensuring that staff always identify themselves to the patient, and environmental cues, such as good lighting, can be hugely helpful.

FURTHER READING

Fleminger, S. (2008) Long-term psychiatric disorders after traumatic brain injury. *European Journal of Anaesthesiology, Suppl 42*, 123–30.

Fleminger, S., Greenwood, R.J. & Oliver, D.L. (2003) Pharmacological management for agitation and aggression in people with acquired brain injury. *Cochrane Database of Systematic Reviews.*

Mitchell, A.J. (2004) *Neuropsychiatry and behavioural neurology explained.* Edinburgh: Saunders Publishers.

Silver, J.M. et al. (2001) The association between head injuries and psychiatric disorders: findings from the New Haven NIMH Epidemiological Catchment Area Study, 935–45.

1b: Assessment of a head injury

> **KEY POINTS**
> General communication and empathy
> Explanation of tests
> Knowledge of tests
> Clarity of testing
> Explanation of results

INTRODUCE YOURSELF

SET THE SCENE

'Thank you for seeing me. I'm sorry to hear about the accident. It seems as if you may be having some difficulties that you didn't have before: I'd like to do a few tests with you to check this in more detail if I may – they're not too difficult, and I'll explain each one before we do it, but don't worry if you make mistakes.'

COMPLETING THE TASKS

The history and investigations suggest frontal lobe impairment. The frontal lobes are involved in higher cognitive and executive functioning, though assessing a so-called dysexecutive syndrome is clinically difficult without extensive neuropsychological batteries.

However, 'bedside testing' can explore established subdomains of frontal lobe function such as abstract reasoning; mental flexibility; executive motor programming; interference resistance; inhibitory control and autonomy.

The order of the following tests is not particularly important once all domains are covered.

1. *Abstract reasoning*. Neuropsychologists employ complex card-sorting tasks to assess abstract reasoning, but at the bedside either proverb interpretation or categorization/conceptualization tasks can be utilized. Proverb interpretation involves getting the subject to explain the metaphorical meaning of a well-known proverb such as 'people in glasshouses shouldn't throw stones'. Categorization/ conceptualization tasks involve asking subjects to state how two objects are similar to each other, and how they differ from one another, for example:
   'I know this might sound like an unusual thing to do, but I'd like you to tell me, as best you can, how you think a "car" is *similar* to a "train".' After allowing the patient time to give their response, follow up with 'Thank you, and now can you tell me how a "car" is *different* from a "train"'?'
   Frontal lobe dysfunction may lead to impaired abstract reasoning with resulting concrete interpretations of proverbs and categories: for example, 'throwing stones will break the glass' or 'trains and cars are both red'.
2. *Mental flexibility*. The subject is challenged to list as many words (barring the names of people and places) beginning with a given letter (traditionally 'f', 'a' or 's') or by a given category (e.g. 'animals') as possible in one minute. This tests the subject's ability to design a cognitive strategy: 'normal' functioning depends on the scale utilized, but a healthy individual should be able to name more than 20 words or animals.

'Now I'm going to time you doing this next task. In one minute, I'd like you to tell me as many words as you can that begin with the letter "f". They can be any words except the names of people or places. Is that clear? Ok, we'll start the minute NOW.'

3. *Motor sequencing.* Copying and continuing a complex multistage motor sequence, such as the Luria series of 'fist, palm, and edge'. Frontal lobe impairment can lead to difficulty learning or executing the demonstrated sequence.

4. *Interference resistance.* The Stroop test involves subjects naming the colours of printed words whilst ignoring what the word actually says. At the bedside a finger-tap test can be employed. When the examiner taps their finger once, the subject should tap theirs twice; when the examiner taps twice, the subject should tap once. This test explores the subject's ability to override competing stimuli.

'We're going to do a "tapping" test next. When I tap my finger <u>once</u>, like this, I'd like you to tap your finger <u>twice</u>: let's try that. Ok, and when I tap my finger <u>twice</u>, like this, I'd like you to tap your finger <u>once</u>: let's try that. Is that clear?

5. *Inhibitory control.* This is a 'go/no-go' variation of the finger-tap test above. In this version the subject taps twice when the examiner taps once, but does nothing when the examiner taps twice. Impairment can lead to loss of inhibitory control, with subjects continuing to tap even when they shouldn't.

'The next test is another "tapping" test, but the rules are slightly different. When I tap my finger <u>once</u>, you tap your finger <u>twice</u>, like the last time: let's try that. Now when I tap my finger <u>twice</u>, you <u>do nothing</u> – don't tap at all: let's try that. Is that clear?

6. *Autonomy.* This is the subject's independence from environmental cues. It can be assessed by telling the subject to do exactly what you command, then placing your hands on the subject's palms and telling them 'do not grab my hands'. Lack of environmental independence will result in the subject grabbing the examiner's hands.

'In this last test, I'd like you to listen very carefully to what I say, and do what I tell you. Could you place your hands on your lap with your palms facing upwards like I'm doing? Great, now DO NOT GRAB MY HANDS.'

Explaining the results of all investigations requires tact and delicacy, especially when results are suboptimal. The reasons for getting candidates to explain results include assessing this communication skill, as well as checking their knowledge of what the test assesses and their ability to record performance.

In this example, the candidate can remind the subject that the brain scan showed some 'bruising' on the front parts of the brain after the accident, and that this might explain some of the difficulties the patient and his mother had noted. The tests were a good way of looking at this further, and measuring any difficulties so that any necessary help can be given, and future improvements noted.

PROBLEM SOLVING

As mentioned, the order of testing is not important, once the major subdomains are reviewed. However, the candidate should have their own structured method for examining the frontal lobes: this will allow the candidate to look more professional in testing, as well as reducing the chance of omitting a test.

In the abstract reasoning task, categorization/conceptualization is usually a preferable test to proverb interpretation. This is because proverb interpretation is culturally, linguistically and educationally biased: many subjects will not have heard a given proverb before. If this task is utilized, one should ask the subject 'have you heard the phrase......before?', and only ask for its interpretation if the subject says yes.

Time is obviously short and precious in examinations: a single trial of each test will probably suffice, although ambiguous performance on any given test may warrant a second example. In a similar vein, it should prove possible to abort a verbal fluency task after less than 30 seconds: in an examination the point is to demonstrate familiarity and competence with the test – I would add the caveat that if the candidate does end the task early, they should identify that they are doing so for reasons of time, and explain how ordinarily one should continue for the full minute.

ADDITIONAL POINTS

It is usually easy to tell candidates who have just a theoretical knowledge of frontal lobe tests apart from those who have actually clinically administered them. The tests are beguilingly simple, but can be difficult to explain to others (and indeed difficult to perform – try explaining what 'A rolling stone gathers no moss' means to someone!). Practise these tests, especially on 'non-medical' friends – it's all too easy to think one knows them and can therefore explain them.

Whilst not essential, use of a recognized scale such as the Frontal Assessment Battery demonstrates structure (and aids recollection) as well as allowing scored measurement using a validated tool and affording the opportunity to retest and monitor change.

FURTHER READING

Dubois, B. et al. (2000) The FAB: A frontal assessment battery at bedside. *Neurology, 55,* 1621–6.

Hodges, J. (2007) *Cognitive assessment for clinicians.* Oxford: Oxford University Press.

STATION 2

2a: Assessment of non-epileptic seizures

KEY POINTS
Sympathetic communication
History of seizures
Exploration of other psychological factors
Consideration of alcohol, drugs
Patient's understanding of results

INTRODUCE YOURSELF

SET THE SCENE

'Hello Ms Finnegan, I'm Dr_____, one of the psychiatrists in this hospital. My colleague has asked me to have a chat with you about the seizures you've been having. Were you aware that the video-telemetry hasn't shown any epileptic activity during your fits? I'd like to explore other avenues to see if we can find out what's causing your seizures.'

COMPLETING THE TASKS

Good initial engagement is essential. Patients with non-epileptic seizures are frequently very resistant and guarded about seeing psychiatrists, suspecting that this means they're either 'mad' or feigning illness. It's important to start gently but with the facts. Careful consideration needs to be given to the precise phraseology used: it can be helpful to follow the patient's lead in how they describe their seizures – for example 'fits', 'episodes', 'turns' or 'shaking' – being careful, however, not to use the word 'epilepsy'.

A good history of the seizures is required, even if the information has already been relayed to you by the neurologists – they will be looking for, and giving salience to, different aspects of the history from neuropsychiatrists. How long have the fits been occurring, how frequently do they occur, are there any obvious precipitating factors, and how do they resolve? Have others described the nature of the seizures; for example the pattern of movement, and any variation? Is the pattern changing over time?

There are no pathognomonic features of dissociative seizures. However, factors that might make one more suspicious of dissociative seizures include retained consciousness, violent or thrashing movements, shutting of eyes (including resistance to opening), lack of tongue biting and urinary incontinence, and a general lack of physical injuries due to 'controlled' falling. Dissociative seizures are more likely to have a gradual onset and fluctuating course. It is also extremely pertinent to explore psychological factors such as exacerbation of seizure frequency in the face of increased distress and conversely a noted decrease when more relaxed. Whilst the patient may be unaware of this or deny it, a general sense of the pressure they're under and their overall mood is important. Seizures may also occur more frequently in emotionally salient environments, for example only in front of friends but not at home.

Although video-telemetry failed to show epileptic activity during filmed seizures, it's important to remember that dissociative seizures are more common in those who have, and who have had, epilepsy. Check for possible organic causes such as head injuries, and ask about alcohol and illicit drug use. Was there any history in the past of epilepsy or seizures: were there any positive findings such as an abnormal EEG?

Family history is similarly important: there is an increased risk of dissociative seizures where there is someone to model on, albeit subconsciously. This also extends to friends with epilepsy.

It is important to assess the patient's understanding of the results: unfortunately, on many occasions patients have rather brusquely been told 'you don't have epilepsy', with no further explanation.

PROBLEM SOLVING

Candidates may find patient engagement and building a rapport a difficult component of this station. This can be due both to patient hostility to a psychiatric review and to the doctor's concern about offending the patient or choosing the 'wrong' term to explain what's happening.

Openness and honesty are essential. It has been the author's experience that it can be very helpful to talk about how common seizures are, and to note that some are caused by abnormal firing of brain cells (epilepsy) but that some are not, without giving weight or primacy to either.

Finally, whilst the station is leading towards a diagnosis of dissociative seizures, the possibility of an alternative undiagnosed psychiatric illness, whether aetiological (panic attacks may in particular mimic the 'aura' of a seizure) or comorbid, must be considered.

ADDITIONAL POINTS

Non-epileptic seizures, pseudo-seizures and dissociative seizures are mistakenly used as interchangeable synonyms, though they are in fact not identical. The different terminology is confusing both for patients and doctors: pick a term and stick with it. Many people find terms such as hysterical or pseudo-seizures a pejorative one, with the implicit meaning that the seizures are 'fake'. Furthermore, non-epileptic seizures include provoked seizures caused by various conditions such as arteriovenous malformations, cerebro-vascular accidents, drug intoxication and withdrawal, and head injury. ICD-10 uses the diagnosis of dissociative seizures and, from a neuropsychiatric viewpoint, this is probably the most sensible term to use.

FURTHER READING

Brown, R. & Trimble, M. (2000) Dissociative psychopathology, non-epileptic seizures, and neurology. *Journal of Neurology, Neurosurgery and Psychiatry*, 69, 285–91.

Mellers, J. (2005) The approach to patients with 'non-epileptic seizures'. *Postgraduate Medical Journal*, 81, 498–504.

2b: Assessment of non-epileptic seizures

KEY POINTS
Sympathetic engagement
Clear explanation of video-telemetry
Explanation of different seizure types
Treatment options
Prognosis

INTRODUCE YOURSELF

SET THE SCENE

'Hello Mrs Finnegan, I'm Dr_____, one of the psychiatrists in the hospital. As you know, I met with your daughter recently and she'd like me to explain to you what we've discussed and where we might proceed from here. Of course I'm very happy to do so and please feel free to interrupt me if I use any terminology or phrases you're not sure of. Before I start, are there any major questions you'd like answered?'

COMPLETING THE TASKS

A sensitive approach to a potentially upset and confused relative is required. Affording time at the start for the mother to voice the major areas of concern may help build a relationship, show you're interested in her particular worries, and allow you to point out areas that must be covered. Adequate explanation of any terminology used is essential. A suggested approach to the relative follows:

A seizure or fit is caused by abnormal brain functioning, and can result in unusual movements, behaviour and changes in consciousness. Different things can cause such fits, and it's important to identify the cause so that the correct treatment can be started.

'A common cause of fits, and one that many people are aware of, is epilepsy. Epilepsy is caused by abnormal excessive firing of brain cells, and is treated with anticonvulsant medications that work by reducing this increased activity. Epilepsy can be measured by an electroencephalogram, or EEG. This is a simple, painless and relatively quick test where electrodes are placed on the head, and the underlying activity is monitored.

'A problem with EEGs is that they are frequently normal or inconclusive between fits, and it can be hard to prove that epileptic changes are occurring. In some cases, as occurred with your daughter, the doctors set up an EEG to run over 24 or 48 hours whilst simultaneously videoing the patient. That way they can see on the video footage when the fit occurred, and look for the relevant part of the EEG. With this information they can decide whether or not it is epilepsy that is causing the fits.

'In your daughter's case, no epileptic activity was detected during her fits, and so epilepsy is not the cause of her problem. Also, the blood tests and brain scan she had were normal, which is good news, and that ruled out some other serious potential causes of seizures, such as infections, multiple sclerosis and problems with the brain's blood supply.

'A common cause of non-epileptic seizures is what is known as dissociative seizures. Whilst this isn't yet fully understood, it seems that some individuals are prone to "break off" or "dissociate" subconsciously from everyday life in light of distress, though they may not be able to identify this distress clearly. This can manifest in different ways, including, as appears to be the case with your daughter, having seizures or fits.

'Dissociative seizures are involuntary and outside the patient's control: they are not "faking" or "making up" symptoms. However, identifying that the *cause* is psychological allows appropriate psychological *treatment*. The current treatment of choice is known as cognitive behavioural therapy, or CBT. This explores the thoughts and feelings an individual experiences in various settings, and how they can interplay to affect behaviour. The aim in your daughter's case would be to look at what might be happening psychologically around the time of her fits, and how altering this might lessen the number and severity of her fits.

'The good news is that this is a treatment that doesn't require any drugs, and that people undergoing CBT for dissociative seizures tend to do reasonably well: indeed there's evidence that just knowing that the cause is psychological can of itself improve the symptoms.'

PROBLEM SOLVING

Dissociative seizures are more common in those who've had epilepsy in the past, and about a fifth of those with dissociative seizures will have current comorbid epilepsy. Given these facts and the frequent desire for a 'medical' cause, patients and relatives may challenge the diagnosis, citing for example ambiguous EEGs (and remember that non-specific EEG abnormalities are seen in about one-sixth of healthy individuals) or the concept that the EEG might have 'missed' some fits. Such arguments are impossible to refute, and usually best avoided. If directly challenged, the clinician should not become defensive; instead, he or she should accept the raised points, but try to move the discussion past this. For example, in such a situation, it would be correct to note that the seizures filmed were non-epileptic, and therefore the treatments offered should reflect this. Symptoms and investigations can always, and should be, revisited.

ADDITIONAL POINTS

The issue of whether or not symptoms could be feigned for psychological gain (a factitious disorder) or fraudulent gain (malingering) may be at the back of the clinician's mind. Clearly this is an extremely sensitive area to explore, and guidelines on this topic cannot be prescriptive. Dissociative seizures are, by definition, considered unconscious and it is worth bearing in mind that dissociative seizures are frequently quite dissimilar to epileptic seizures and most patients admitted for video-telemetry have a fit in an environment where they know they're being closely scrutinized – factors that mitigate against intentional deception.

It is worth remembering that dissociative seizures are a subtype of non-epileptic seizure, and the clinician needs to satisfy themself that other causes have been ruled out.

FURTHER READING

http://www.epilepsy.org.uk/info/nonep.html
http://www.patient.co.uk/showdoc/40026034/

STATION 3

3a: Unusual behaviour in PD

KEY POINTS
Clear history of events
Collateral information
Awareness of differentials
Review of medications
Basic cognitive assessment

INTRODUCE YOURSELF

SET THE SCENE

'Hello Mr Whitman, I'm Dr____, one of the neuropsychiatrists in this hospital. I've been asked by my colleagues to have a chat with you about how you've been getting on in hospital. Some of what I'm going to ask you may seem a little personal, but it's important information for me to obtain, so I hope you'll bear with me.'

COMPLETING THE TASKS

There is a lot of ground to cover in this station, so it is essential to be as focused and structured as possible. A leading introductory question is likely to be required to quickly open the area for discussion.

'I understand from some of the staff on the ward that at times you haven't seemed yourself recently. For example, there was some concern that perhaps you've been feeling a bit irritated or fed up recently, and sometimes you haven't been taking care of your personal dress as well as you might. Does this ring a bell with you?'

This rapidly establishes what you want to talk about and the patient and his wife will respond directly to it. An immediate observation should be the patient's level of insight: is he aware there's a problem?

The differentials are large, so the candidate must remain structured to keep a grip on the station. From even this most brief of introductory vignettes the candidate should be thinking of the following:

- Part of the pathology of Parkinson's, for example:
  Cognitive impairment (dementia)
  Delirium
  Psychosis
  Depression
  Anxiety
  Personality changes including apathy and emotional lability

- Medication induced
  Drug (dopamine)-induced delirium
  Drug-induced psychosis
  Drug-induced personality changes such as disinhibition and hypersexuality

- A comorbid psychiatric illness, such as depression.

Whilst a reasonably large list for a timed exam (and it's not exhaustive – for example, it presumes the behaviour is truly pathological), it allows for suitable probes to be asked: what is the timeframe of such behaviour; is it related to any medication changes; what have the patient's mood and anxiety levels been like; is the memory as good as it has been; has the patient seen or heard things that no one else does, or seem to have any new and unusual ideas; have friends and family noticed any differences, or thought that the patient is not quite the same person as before?

PROBLEM SOLVING

It is important not to be seduced by 'finding' the diagnosis. Even if early questioning heavily points to, for example, a depressive disorder, it is essential to continue to screen for other causes and comorbidity, for example coexisting cognitive decline.

Time is likely to militate against a full cognitive examination so the candidate needs to show awareness of the importance of this task and highlight that it is an area to return to:

'You feel your memory isn't what it once was. When I've more time, I'd like to examine this in some depth. For the moment, would you mind if I asked you a few quick memory questions? Could you tell me:

- what date it is today?
- what your date of birth is?
- whereabouts we are at the moment?'

In practice it is seldom possible to confidently state that low mood is 'comorbid' or 'psychological' as opposed to a neuropsychiatric complication of a Parkinsonian picture (see additional points). However, the candidate should look for a past psychiatric history, including prior to diagnosis with Parkinson's, and get a sense from the patient about his beliefs surrounding any low mood.

Even if he doesn't attribute any salience to the Parkinsonian medication, it is helpful to establish what the patient is taking, and in clinical practice it is important to ask specific questions around disinhibitory hypersexuality and gambling.

ADDITIONAL POINTS

Parkinson's, like multiple sclerosis, has a higher than expected rate of affective disorders when the overall disability of the disease is taken into account. The Global Parkinson's Disease Survey (2002) showed 50 per cent prevalence for depression of at least mild severity. However, it is rarely possible to accurately determine if a mood or anxiety disorder is directly 'caused' by Parkinson's pathology or is psychologically secondary or independent of it, though some authors have argued that thoughts of self-harm are less frequent when it is part of the neurological disease.

A diagnostic difficulty is the fact that several overlapping symptoms with different causes may coexist. For example, apparent psychomotor retardation may be part of a depressive disorder or simply part of the Parkinson's disease. Similarly, apathy and mild cognitive impairment might falsely suggest depression.

FURTHER READING

Findley, L. (2002) Global Parkinson's Disease Steering Committee. Factors impacting on quality of life in Parkinson's disease: results from an international survey. *Movement Disorders*, *17*, 60–7.

Leentjens, A., Driessen, G., Weber, W., Drukker, M. & van Os, J. (2008) Mental health care use in Parkinson's disease: a record linkage study. *Neuroepidemiology*, *30*, 71–5.

Weintraub, D. (2008) Parkinson's disease – Part 3: Neuropsychiatric symptoms. *American Journal of Managed Care*, *14*, s59–s69.

3b: Unusual behaviour in PD

KEY POINTS
Clear non-technical explanations
Structured differentials
Logical management plan
Non-pharmacological interventions
Awareness of medication interactions
Awareness of limitations of treatment

INTRODUCE YOURSELF

SET THE SCENE

'Hello Mrs Whitman, my name is Dr____, I'm one of the psychiatrists. I understand you wanted to talk about what we can do to help your husband. I think it's important to state that at this point I am not completely certain about the exact cause of your husband's symptoms, but we can talk about possible treatment options which we'll tailor as our understanding of what's happening improves, and of course depending on your husband's response.'

COMPLETING THE TASKS

The candidate hasn't been let off the diagnostic hook following the first part of this station! More information is available, narrowing the likely differentials, but now these must be explicitly stated, with the added requirements of tact and avoidance of overly technical medical terminology. A major mood or anxiety disorder has largely been excluded, but there's evidence of disorientation and hallucinations that have been exacerbated by recent medication changes. At this stage there's insufficient information to state a diagnosis, and thus management plan, with confidence. However, the station design allows the candidate to demonstrate their logical thought processes to the examiner. A further benefit (to the candidate) of this particular station is that by asking for explanations in lay terms, it avoids the need to mention some specifics such as medication doses etc.

The disorientation may be a delirium or a dementia, and both may manifest with hallucinations and other psychotic phenomena. Of course, the delirium may be an acute problem over a chronic dementia. To further complicate things, the psychotic symptom(s) may be independent of the cognitive impairment. Clarifying questions are required, and aetiology and management options will follow from the answers.

'When I asked your husband some memory questions recently, he got some answers wrong. I wonder if this is something that has been happening for a while. Does this change from day to day or has it been stable? Have the medications made this part worse?'

'Has he been having other memory problems before he came in: perhaps problems with names or faces, or getting lost when out?'

'I want to ask some questions about the "ghosts" he's been seeing. Have they only been there since he came into hospital? Has he had any other problems seeing or hearing things that no one else seems able to see or hear? I know these questions may seem unusual, but have you noted that he's been having unusual ideas recently, and/or any concerns about anyone trying to harm him, or control him or his thoughts in any way?'

Although the candidate will still not have sufficient information, nevertheless one must proceed through possible differential diagnoses and hence management options.

The suggestion is of a delirium, whether or not on top of pre-existing dementia, and apparently caused or exacerbated by medication.

'Some of the problems Mr Whitman seems to be having with his memory look like it might be what we call a "delirium". That's to say it's a sudden change in the ability to focus attention or remember or think clearly. It can vary, sometimes dramatically, from hour to hour and day to day, and it can have many causes. We'll have to arrange some further tests to see if, for example, there are any underlying infective or metabolic problems that might be causing this. Treatment will depend on what we find.'

Simple environmental causes must be addressed:

'Often simple things such as keeping lights on, and reminding staff and visitors to keep things simple and repeat themselves frequently, can be very useful.'

Medication as a *cause* of the delirium needs to be addressed, given the fact that the vignette mentions this directly. However, reducing medication can bring about its own problems by exacerbating the Parkinson's. The candidate needs to exercise tact by accepting that the problem could be iatrogenic without attributing blame, and by discussing possible medication changes without promising something they cannot necessarily deliver:

'It is possible that the new medication, or indeed interactions with other medications, could be causing some of these symptoms. However, the medications are obviously very important, and we'll have to think carefully and consult colleagues in the pharmacy department and the neurologists before making any changes, and any changes will probably be done quite gradually.'

Treating psychotic symptoms in PD is difficult and the point of such a station is to allow the candidate to demonstrate their knowledge of these problems, and suggest possible treatment options with reference to them. A step-wise rationale is required, with awareness of and active seeking for any side effects of treatment:

- If thought likely to be secondary to a delirium, no active treatment for the hallucinations, besides management of the underlying delirium, may be required.
- Similarly, in cases where hallucinations are not unduly troublesome, watchful waiting may be sufficient.
- Medications with anticholinergic side effects should be reduced or stopped *where possible*.
- The dose of any dopaminergic drugs may need to be reduced. This should be done gradually to watch for evidence that it's effective in reducing symptoms as well as worsening of PD.
- An antipsychotic may be added. Typical antipsychotics must be avoided owing to the high propensity to cause extra-pyramidal side effects (EPSE). Choose an atypical: there is some evidence for quetiapine having fewer motor side effects than other atypicals.
- In severe cases other options such as electro-convulsive therapy (ECT) and clozapine can be considered.

PROBLEM SOLVING

Good clinical practice leads one to aim to establish a good rapport with patients and relatives, especially prior to tackling difficult or sensitive areas, and also not to unduly promise or reassure about diagnoses or treatments in the light of inadequate information. However, timed clinical examinations depart from actual practice in several aspects and force the candidate to adopt a manner and practice different to the 'real world'. This station is forcing the candidate's hand somewhat: there is little to say to console the candidate on this matter except to note that exams and exam styles must be dealt with. It is far better to deal with the exam topic directly than to lose marks through avoidance and worrying about the implications of direct advice or a poor rapport – remember you're dealing with actors, not patients! Statements along the lines of 'of course if I'd more time I'd like to do/check/find out about', 'whilst I can't make any firm decisions now, the lines we're thinking along include' and 'I know this must be a very sensitive topic, so please forgive me for being so personal so quickly but it's important that I check if' may make the candidate feel more at ease.

A temptation in a station such as this is to get caught up in pharmacological management, whether by adding or removing medications; however, good environmental management is as important in delirium and dementing processes. Simple examples in a hospital environment include adequate lighting, cues such as clocks, calendars and photos from home, assigning regular members of staff to look after the patient who can repeat information in non-technical terms as required. Finally, don't forget that psychotic symptoms are not necessarily caused by dopaminergic treatments – dyskinesias are more common as side effects to such drugs – and psychotic symptoms may be part of a progressive neurodegenerative disease.

ADDITIONAL POINTS

Mitchell has proposed a classification system of psychosis in Parkinson's disease: type I – pure psychosis, type II – delirium and type III – degenerative psychosis, each of which can be further subcategorized into a) caused by the pathophysiology of the disease and b) drug induced.

Dementia and psychosis frequently coexist and the presence of one increases the risk of developing the other.

Ten of the 25 most commonly prescribed medications in the elderly are associated with delirium. Polypharmacy and poor physical health are general risk factors, and watch in particular for medications with anticholinergic properties.

FURTHER READING

Meagher, D. (2001) Delirium: optimising management. *British Medical Journal, 322,* 144–9.

Mitchell, A. (2004) *Neuropsychiatry and behavioural neurology explained.* Edinburgh: Saunders Publishers.

Taylor, D., Paton, C. & Kerwin, R. (2007) *The Maudsley Prescribing Guidelines,* 9th edn.

STATION 4: Assessment of tics

KEY POINTS
Engagement with embarrassed patient
Tourette's diagnostic criteria
Consideration of differential diagnoses
Conveying diagnoses to patient
Understanding of management options

INTRODUCE YOURSELF

SET THE SCENE

'Thank you for coming to see me today. Can I call you Sunita? I'm Dr____, one of the psychiatrists. As you know, your GP has asked me to have a chat with you about some throat clearing and face movements which I understand have been bothering you – is that correct?'

Always consider confidentiality issues. It is worth clarifying here whether she is happy for her friend to be present throughout, as you will need to discuss personal and medical matters.

COMPLETING THE TASKS

You have been prompted that this is a patient ill at ease, and it's important to rapidly establish a good rapport. Allow the patient some time to give her version of the complaint.

You must be able to define what a tic is (and is not): a voluntary (though see below), rapid, recurrent, non-rhythmic *motor* movement or *vocal* (also known as phonic) production of sudden onset with no apparent purpose. They may be *simple* (e.g. a blink or uttering a word) or *complex* (e.g. pulling at clothes or repeating whole sentences). Subtle motor tics may not be visible to an observer, though felt by the sufferer.

Tics are not involuntary – unlike most other movement disorders, they are suppressible though to the sufferer they feel very difficult to resist, and a sense of an irresistible build-up of pressure before tic onset is frequently described. Ask about attempts to suppress the tics.

Look for factors that exacerbate and relieve the tics: as might be expected, they tend to increase during excitation and periods of stress, and are lessened by relaxation and distraction techniques. Get a history of the duration and severity of the tics.

Although this station has prompted information about two apparently simple motor tics, it is important to ask explicitly about other types – for diagnostic reasons as well as the fact that tics are frequently embarrassing and thus information may not be offered freely. This is particularly true of complex phonic or vocal tics, which can include utterance of socially unacceptable words or phrases (coprolalia), repetition of previously uttered sentences (palilalia) or copying the speech of others (echolalia).

The history will need to explore current and past psychiatric problems. Unusual movements or actions might be part of an obsessional-compulsive disorder, and a depressive or anxiety disorder might be the precipitating factor in the production of the tics. Furthermore, autism and attention-deficit/hyperactivity disorder (ADHD) are strongly associated with tic production.

The differential diagnosis for tics is large, and management will obviously depend upon the aetiology. The full range of causes of tics is beyond the scope of this vignette, except to remark that it includes many chromosomal and developmental abnormalities, severe infections (especially encephalitis) and medication induced (including L-dopa and some anticonvulsants). ICD-10 has a section (F95) on tic disorders and it includes the subcategories of transient tic disorder, chronic motor or vocal tic disorder and combined vocal and multiple motor tic disorder (Tourette's). Tourette's syndrome diagnostically requires at least two motor tics *and* at least one vocal tic, though they don't need to have all occurred at the same time. It usually starts in childhood, though this is not necessary for diagnosis.

Management can be pharmacological and psychological. Haloperidol remains the drug of choice (though interestingly haloperidol can *cause* tics) but other antipsychotics, including newer atypicals with fewer movement side effects, are also being increasingly used. There is less evidence for other drug classes, though antidepressants have been used with varying efficacy, particularly when comorbid obsessive–compulsive disorder (OCD) or depression is diagnosed.

Psychological interventions can vary from support, reassurance and psychoeducation through teaching relaxation and biofeedback techniques to lessen the frequency of occurrence. Habit reversal training (HRT) is a CBT-styled treatment that builds up awareness of tic onset and attempts to replace this with a competing urge.

PROBLEM SOLVING

Sensitivity is required with an embarrassed patient who has potentially socially unacceptable symptoms. A thoughtful approach is necessary both in eliciting the symptoms and also in talking about possible diagnoses, which can have pejorative connotations. However, false reassurance should not be given.

The obvious diagnosis is Tourette's syndrome: most candidates will know this without being clear on the diagnostic criteria. A good candidate will show phenomenological awareness of what a tic is, which groups occur (motor and vocal) and the existence of both simple and complex varieties. It is impossible to cover all the possible causes of tics in an objective structured clinical exam (OSCE) station, but a sensible approach would be to show awareness of these possibilities by briefly asking about personal and family developmental and genetic problems, as well as checking for any co-temporal medication initiation or changes.

ADDITIONAL POINTS

Be aware of the differences between tics and other motor problems. Fasciculations are involuntary movements of muscle fibres but not whole muscles, and typically occur peri-ocularly. Dyskinesia is a generic name for a variety of involuntary movements. Tardive dyskinesia (TD) is not infrequently seen in psychiatric practice as a side effect of chronic antipsychotic use, and tends to manifest as stereotyped involuntary facial muscle movements. Chorea is a dyskinesia seen in Huntington's disease and Sydenham's chorea, and is characterized by non-repetitive, irregular rapid movements of hands or feet which can look like 'dancing' or piano playing. A dystonia is a sustained muscle contraction and can have many causes.

FURTHER READING

http://www.tsa.org.uk

Ghanizadeh, A. & Mosallaei, S. (2008) Psychiatric disorders and behavioural problems in children and adolescents with Tourette syndrome. *Brain and Development*, in press.

Riddle, M. & Carlson. J. (2001) Clinical psychopharmacology for Tourette syndrome and associated disorders. *Advances in Neurology*, 85, 343–54.

STATION 5: Movement disorder in schizophrenia

> **KEY POINTS**
> Clarification of history
> Specific EPSE questions
> Consideration of NMS and catatonia
> Clear advice
> Awareness of treatments
> Supporting a colleague

INTRODUCE YOURSELF

SET THE SCENE

'It sounds like your patient is having some problems. I'm happy to come in to review the patient with you, but perhaps you can clarify his complaint a little.'

COMPLETING THE TASKS

This is a purposefully open and vague vignette designed to test the candidate's ability to work logically through movement problems in schizophrenia. The main areas to explore are extra-pyramidal side effects, negative symptoms of schizophrenia, neuroleptic malignant syndrome and schizophrenic catatonia. Finally, consideration must be given to the possibility that the movement abnormalities are part of positive symptomatology, for example delusionally driven.

The brief history initially given hints at medication change, and this in conjunction with the potential seriousness of *neuromuscular malignant syndrome* (NMS) means that this diagnosis should be tackled first. NMS is caused by dopaminergic antagonism leading to sympathetic over-activity. It is associated with all antipsychotic drugs, though with increased prevalence in older typical antipsychotics, as well as with changes in antipsychotics and (especially rapid) dose increases. It's characterized by fever, rigidity and delirium, and diagnosed by this clinical presentation in conjunction with raised serum creatine kinase, a raised white cell count and autonomic instability. It's a medical emergency requiring hospital admission, though the treatment is largely supportive.

You will need to question Dr Dedalus to assess if this could be the case, advising him of its presentation, seriousness and management:

'My first concern, on the information I have so far, is that your patient may have neuromuscular malignant syndrome, or NMS, as this is a medical emergency. It's caused by, amongst other things, antipsychotic medications, and I understand you've recently commenced a new drug. Sufferers present with confusion and rigidity, with fluctuating levels of consciousness and fever. If we've any concerns that this is the case, we'll need to organize a medical admission for assessment and monitoring, including blood pressure and heart rate, and have CK levels taken: is there any evidence of such a picture with him at this time? In particular, does he appear delirious with a confused and fluctuating mental state?'

Having safely ruled out the most important differential, the candidate can work through EPSE. Again considering the information of the recent drug change, it's worth tackling the EPSE logically by time to onset: namely acute dystonias, akathesia, Parkinsonism and Tardive dyskinesias.

'I'm pleased that it doesn't sound like NMS, though you should organize routine bloods including a white cell count and CPK levels. The largest, and most common, group of movement disorders seen in schizophrenia are the extra-pyramidal side effects, or EPSE, which are caused by dopamine blockade in the nigrostriatal pathway. They're far less common with newer atypical antipsychotics.'

The four EPSE seen are:

1. *Acute dystonic reactions*: rapid occurrence, usually in treatment-naïve patients. More common in young men, and manifests with torticollis (head and neck twisted to the side) and oculogyric crises (eyes rolled up to the side). Treatment is with an intramuscular (i.m.) or intravenous (i.v.) anticholinergic agent (the patient may not be able to swallow).
2. *Akathisia*: usually occurs within the first week or so of commencement of treatment. It is described as an irresistible sense or urge to move, or an inner restlessness, usually affecting the lower limbs most. Sufferers describe it as hugely frustrating, and it commonly leads to non-compliance with treatment. It can be quite difficult to treat, though the symptom usually abates with time. Practical steps include reducing the dose of the antipsychotic and changing to a newer atypical with a lower side-effect profile, such as quetiapine. Benzodiazepines, the anti-hypertensive agent clonidine and propranolol and antimuscarinic drugs have been used, though with far from convincing results.
3. *Parkinsonism*: usually manifests with a triad of bradykinesia, resting tremor and cog-wheel rigidity, and occurs in about one-fifth of classical/typical antipsychotics over a period of months to years. Treatment can be tricky, and obviously anti-Parkinsonian medication should not be used owing to the risks of psychosis. Dose reduction can be tried, but if taking a typical antipsychotic, this should be changed to an atypical.
4. *Tardive dyskinesia*: a long-term problem of stereotyped movements, usually of the face and hands, such as lip smacking and tongue protrusion, which can be very difficult to treat. Counter-intuitively it is worsened by drug reduction or stoppage, as it is caused by dopamine receptor up-regulation in response to chronic iatrogenic dopaminergic (DA) blockade. Some studies suggest that only half of those affected will respond to treatment. The major therapeutic option is switching to an atypical if not already on one, and on to clozapine if this fails. Although far less likely to occur on atypicals, TD has been reported with their use.

Having considered the emergency presentation of NMS, and the EPSE, focus turns to movement problems that are functional parts of schizophrenia, whether positive or negative symptoms. Although rare, catatonic schizophrenia should be ruled out. Catatonia is a descriptive syndrome with a 'classic' (though not always seen together) triad of symptoms of akinesia, mutism and waxy flexibility, and it can have a large number of causes, including organic as well as functional: 'catatonia' is not synonymous with 'catatonic schizophrenia'! There is a large list of other symptoms reported, such as automatic obedience, stereotypies, posturing and so forth, but initial efforts should be focused on this triad. Presentation of catatonic symptoms 25 years after initial diagnosis would be unusual, but if proven, treatment would consist of benzodiazepines, usually lorazepam, which can be titrated to high doses, with recourse to ECT should this fail.

PROBLEM SOLVING

A danger with this station is presuming to see 'what it's asking' – in this case about EPSE – and forgetting about everything else. It would be hugely remiss to fail to consider both positive and negative symptoms of schizophrenia, especially in a patient with such a longstanding illness, and potentially catastrophic to leave out NMS.

Stations with this design (explaining diagnoses, investigations, results to patients, families, colleagues, etc.) are quite open, and often require the candidate to do most of the talking – an uncomfortable examination experience at times. It's all the more important in such stations to remain as structured as possible, with guidance from the patient/colleague/family member's cues.

ADDITIONAL POINTS

Whilst not essential, it would look impressive to mention scales that could be used. These allow quantitative analysis of the symptoms and afford the ability to measure changes with time. Scales which might be used include:

- Akathisia: Barnes Akathisia Scale
- Parkinsonism: Simpson–Angus Rating Scale, Hoehn and Yahr Staging of Parkinson's Disease, Unified Parkinson Disease Rating Scale (UPDRS)
- Tardive dyskinesia: Abnormal Involuntary Movement Scale (AIMS)
- Symptom of illness, viz. a negative or positive symptom of schizophrenia: Positive and Negative Symptoms of Schizophrenia Scale (PANSS), Brief Psychiatric Rating Scale (BPRS).

FURTHER READING

Soares-Weiser, K. & Rathbone, J. (2006) Neuroleptic reduction and/or cessation and neuroleptics as specific treatments for tardive dyskinesia. *Cochrane Database of Systematic Reviews*, 2006; CD000459

Taylor, D., Paton, C. & Kerwin, R. (2007) *The Maudsley Prescribing Guidelines*, 9th edn. London: Informa Healthcare.

STATION 6: Medically unexplained symptoms

KEY POINTS
Sympathetic, understanding manner
Clear, concise history taking
Screen for primary mental illness
Medically unexplained symptoms (MUS) differentials
Suitable explanation to patient

INTRODUCE YOURSELF

SET THE SCENE

'Hello Mr Bloom, my name is Dr_____, a psychiatrist. I'd like to have a chat with you about some of the problems you've been having. Would that be okay?'

COMPLETING THE TASKS

Good time management is essential – the past history is undoubtedly long and complex and it will be impossible to obtain as full a history as one would like. The aim, rather, is to get a brief overview of the main symptoms whilst keeping possible psychiatric diagnoses in mind. One conceptual model for medically unexplained symptoms is:

1. Possible organic illness, but not fully understood, and with evidence of a psychological component. Examples include fibromyalgia, irritable bowel syndrome (IBS), chronic fatigue and neurasthenia. An important point is that whilst the pathology might be poorly understood, and at times controversial, there's good evidence that psychological interventions help *regardless* of the aetiology.
2. A primary psychiatric illness, in particular depression, anxiety and OCD. Patients might be alexithymic, have poor insight into their mental state, or have cultural difficulties talking about feelings.
3. Somatoform disorders, including somatization disorder and hypochondriacal disorder, and dissociative disorders.
4. Factitious and malingering disorders whereby the patient is consciously feigning symptoms for psychological or external gain respectively.

With this in mind, a brief history can be taken. A useful way to begin would be to ask the patient's opinion of what might be causing the symptoms, and why investigations have been negative and treatments ineffective. Precipitants, exacerbants and relieving factors, especially psychological ones, should be looked for. The first category above should be obvious in that it is likely that such a patient would suggest it, or have had it suggested in the past. Similarly, although not common, dissociative disorders (with the exception of dissociative seizures) are usually obvious by their physiological improbability combined with a psychogenic aetiology and frequent lack of concern (*la belle indifference*).

Candidates can have difficulty differentiating somatoform disorders – perhaps the most likely diagnosis in this case from the brief information given – something exacerbated by ICD-10's multiple sub-categories, eponymous syndromes and nebulous terms such as 'Briquet's', 'Da Costa's syndrome', 'psychasthenia' and 'neurocirculatory asthenia'! The most important categories, and ones diagnostically sufficient for membership candidates, are somatization disorder and hypochondriacal disorder. In broad terms, whilst both have medically unexplained symptoms, individuals with somatization disorder will have longstanding multi-system *complaints*, which frequently cannot be physiologically reconciled, for which they seek *treatment*. Conversely, again in crude terms, individuals with hypochondriasis tend to seek *investigations* to rule out *illnesses* (classically tumours) with an undue focus and misinterpretation of normal body signals. Therefore, it is essential to quickly explore the patient's understanding and concerns about their symptoms: have they been reassured by negative investigations, or do they need 'one more scan'?

It is important to explore any obvious psychopathology of depression, anxiety and OCD (and if suggested, albeit rarely, psychosis) both as a possible primary diagnosis but also as a secondary exacerbating phenomenon. Patients may be reluctant to talk about such feelings for fear of being labelled 'psychiatric', so sensitivity is required. One might normalize the situation, for example noting how 'things frequently appear worse when we feel a bit down; for example, we might find that pain felt worse when we were more tired. Have you ever noticed this?' or 'given the amount you've been through, it wouldn't be surprising to get a bit fed up or blue about things – has this happened?' A few quick questions on mood, anxiety and obsessional and compulsive symptoms can follow, though be careful with biological symptoms of depression – these could be manifestations of either a depressive or a somatoform disorder.

This broaching of the psychological leads on to the final part of the station – discussing possible psychological causes, and through this psychological management. This is a sensitive area and one needs to be careful to avoid the patient assuming that the implication is that the symptoms aren't real. A general, non-judgemental opening statement along the lines of:

'We talked about how the psychological can affect the physical – for example, how you can feel "butterflies in your stomach" when nervous, or how a stubbed toe feels worse in cold weather – and how common this is for all of us. Given all the negative findings to date, I wonder if it's possible that there could be a psychological component to some of your symptoms – could, for example, stress have made you pay more attention to your body's signals? I know these symptoms are real and uncomfortable when you feel them.'

A follow-up to this, considering treatment, avoids the need for direct confrontation at this early stage of engagement:

'Your doctors have mentioned how treatments to date have unfortunately been unsuccessful. We commonly find that psychological help can be really valuable, regardless of the cause of the illness. For example, managing pain in arthritis, or helping people manage illnesses we poorly understand, like IBS. I think this might be something really useful in helping you, and one of the great things about psychological treatment is that it doesn't have side effects like medications can. How would you feel about this?'

PROBLEM SOLVING

Sensitivity and tact are needed. In this station, the idea of somatoform or hypochondriacal illnesses can be raised but the patient need not be directly challenged – something unlikely to occur on a first assessment in clinical practice. Ultimately, a time may occur in treatment where the patient will need to be confronted and told that further investigations should not occur, and that the diagnosis is a psychological one, but this could be catastrophic at a first appointment. Rather, the candidate's role is to introduce the idea of body–mind interactions, and how the psychological can both instigate and treat such symptoms.

Watch out for stations asking for feedback – it's all too easy in the stress of an examination to get caught up in history taking and only remember the feedback section as the final bell goes!

ADDITIONAL POINTS

The term 'psychosomatic' has become common parlance and should be avoided lest it be misinterpreted as 'making it up'. If asked for a diagnosis directly, an honest and direct approach must be adhered to, no matter how uncomfortable this may feel. 'Somatoform disorder' is an overarching diagnostic umbrella that might help explain how the mind and body can interact in the first instance. Assessment of medically unexplained symptoms is a common scenario in both liaison and neuropsychiatry.

FURTHER READING

Creed, F. & Barsky, A. (2004) A systematic review of the epidemiology of somatisation disorder and hypochondriasis. *Journal of Psychosomatic Research*, *56*, 391–408.

Hatcher, S. & Arroll, B. (2008) Assessment and management of medically unexplained symptoms. *British Medical Journal*, *336*, 1124–28.

STATION 7: Low mood in MS

KEY POINTS
Sympathetic history taking
Awareness of MS impairment
Medication issues
Risk assessment
Psychological treatment
Ability to convey findings clearly

INTRODUCE YOURSELF

SET THE SCENE

'Hello Ms Hamm, I'm Dr____, a psychiatrist in this hospital. Your doctor has asked me to have a chat with you about how you've been feeling recently, is that okay?'

COMPLETING THE TASKS

Depressive criteria will need to be assessed, including a brief risk history, but psychosocial and organic precipitants for the patient's current affect will require careful consideration. The fact that the patient is currently in hospital implies an MS relapse – what has happened, and what is the degree of disability at this time? Is the patient's low mood based around this relapse, or fear of her ability to cope in the future? What support – from family and friends, professionals and charitable organizations – is in place after discharge? Does this need to be re-evaluated during this admission, for example with a home occupational therapist (OT) or physiotherapy visit? Have there been any recent changes or additions to the patient's medications, particularly steroids or β-interferon?

Cognitive impairment occurs in up to half of all MS sufferers and it can both cause and exacerbate other psychological symptoms: ask about problems with memory, apathy, paying attention, and ability to carry out day-to-day activities (not due to physical impairment, but rather motivational and higher executive dysfunction).

The past psychiatric history needs to be explored, looking at previous episodes of depression, if any, and the effectiveness of any treatment given. It is important to check for evidence of previous periods of euphoria, anxiety or psychosis – all neuropsychiatric complications of MS.

Treatment options will depend on the history taken. Concern about iatrogenic low mood secondary to steroids or β-interferon use must be tackled cautiously – one might be wrong and also create damage in the patient's relationship with the treating neurologist. However, if the patient has noted recent changes, then it is important to recognize (and be seen to recognize) this fact:

'All medications can have side effects, and some people have become lower in mood due to steroids or β-interferon. However, we must consider the possible benefits you're getting from these medications, the risks of stopping them, and the fact that the low mood may not be due to them. I know this is quite a complex business, so perhaps we can have a joint discussion with your neurologist present where we can weigh up the pros and cons of changing these drugs.'

Should depression be diagnosed then it's perfectly reasonable to discuss antidepressant medication – just make sure that there's no current or past history of elation. **Check to see if the patient is already on an antidepressant – this may be prescribed for other reasons such as tricyclic antidepressants (TCAs) for pain or bladder control.** Previous response, if any, to antidepressants will guide prescribing, but in general selective serotonin reuptake inhibitors (SSRIs) are considered first-line treatment as TCAs can be poorly tolerated in MS.

Psychological support should be considered, especially CBT. Other psychosocial routes might include local support groups, the Multiple Sclerosis Society, appropriate home help and OT. This will be guided by the patient's concerns.

Mood stabilizers can be used during periods of elation, though lithium should be prescribed with care because of its propensity to cause polyuria, which can be devastating if there is a problem with continence.

The literature on the treatment of psychotic symptoms is smaller, though there is evidence for the use of atypical antipsychotics. Cognitive impairment is a difficult symptom to treat – there has been some research looking at acetylcholinesterase inhibitors – though advice can be given about practical measures such as keeping a diary, writing down important information, etc. Remember that cognitive impairment may be due to low mood or a side effect of medication.

PROBLEM SOLVING

Remember to ask about current and past symptoms of elation. Pathological laughter and crying (PLC) is a syndrome occurring in about one in ten MS sufferers, particularly in late stage disease. Psychotic symptoms seldom if ever progress to a full schizophrenia-like picture: just because the patient does not present as 'obviously psychotic', don't fail to ask about hallucinations, which occur in about 20 per cent of patients. There is unlikely to be time to do a formal cognitive assessment; the usual 'trick' of asking about poor memory, concentration and mentioning how one would like to revisit this domain for 'more formal and thorough testing' at a later time should suffice to demonstrate that the candidate is aware of, and understands the significance of, these symptoms.

ADDITIONAL POINTS

All chronic illnesses are associated with higher than average rates of depression. Multiple sclerosis has a higher rate than expected for degree of disability, suggesting at least a partial organic basis. Whilst there is evidence for β-interferon causing low mood, the significance of this may have been overstated.

FURTHER READING

Patten, S., Beck, C.A., Williams, J.V.A., Barbui, C. & Metz, L.M. (2003) Major depression in multiple sclerosis: a population based perspective. *Neurology, 61,* 1524–7.

Thomas, P.W., Thomas, S., Hillier, C., Galvin, K. & Baker, R. (2006) Psychological interventions for multiple sclerosis. *Cochrane Database of Systematic Reviews.*

http://www.mssociety.org.uk

Zephir, H., De Seze, J., Stojkovic, T., Delisse, B., Ferriby, D., Cabaret, M. & Vermersch, P. (2003) Multiple sclerosis and depression: influence of interferon beta therapy. *Multiple Sclerosis, 9,* 284–8.

Chapter 4   Drs Armin Raznahan and Dennis Ougrin
Child and adolescent psychiatry

○ LINKED STATION 1

1a.

Sacha Gurani is an 11-year-old girl who was referred by her GP to Child and Adolescent Mental Health Services (CAMHS). Her mother is very concerned about persistent school refusal which started 3 months ago. Sacha had refused to go to school in the past but her mother had been able to make her go using a variety of coercive strategies that no longer work.

Take a history from Sacha's mother (Mrs Gurani) and establish a differential diagnosis.

1b.

After completing your initial assessment of the young person you reach a working diagnosis of separation anxiety disorder of childhood (SAD).

Briefly explain what SAD is to Sacha's father.

Propose investigations and management for a preliminary diagnosis of separation anxiety disorder of childhood and give the prognosis.

○ LINKED STATION 2

2a.

You are assessing Richard Chip, a white British 17-year-old referred to a day patient unit from a local community team. He presented with a period of deterioration of his school performance and increasingly uncharacteristic behaviour, with social withdrawal, loss of usual interests and irritability. He reports feelings of people laughing at him and he sometimes has 'a horrible feeling' as if he were a 'puppet'.

Take a relevant history. In the next station you will meet his mother.

2b.

Following your assessment, you have diagnosed a moderate to severe depressive episode. You have already discussed the diagnosis with Richard and his family.

Explain to Richard's mother the treatment plan and prognosis. (Assume that Richard gave his consent for you to share this information.)

○ LINKED STATION 3

3a.

Nadia Burrell, a 16-year-old girl, presented to A&E at 2 a.m. this morning with an overdose of 16 paracetamol tablets. She is accompanied by her mother, Mrs Burrell. Nadia was at a friend's home when she took the overdose after a fight. She was admitted overnight and is now medically cleared. Nadia has already been seen by a social worker who expressed no immediate concerns. She is medically fit for discharge.

Assess the risk of suicide and violence.

Conclude by making a brief risk summary and formulation to the examiner.

3b.

You have now interviewed both Nadia and her mother and you consider Nadia to be fit for discharge with urgent community follow-up. However, her mother indicates that she is in two minds about the need for community follow-up as things now appear to be OK and the family are ready to move on. Nadia is also ambivalent and she gave her consent for you to discuss her treatment plan with Mrs Burrell. She stated that she will only attend follow-up appointments if accompanied by her mother.

Assess Mrs Burrell's views and explore the importance of community follow-up with her.

SINGLE STATIONS

4.

This 17-year-old has been exposing herself to young children at a local school. Several parents have become concerned and have notified the police and the school's head teacher.

The young woman has a history of learning disability and attends a special school. She has shown sexually inappropriate behaviour which has improved somewhat over the years. Her foster parents report ongoing challenging behaviour and have reported a history of self-harm.

She attends a special school where she boards for 3 days a week and you have been asked to assess her there by staff at the school. Parental consent has been obtained. You first arrange an interview with a member of staff at the young woman's residential placement.

Take a behaviour history.

Establish the possible aetiology and perpetuating factors.

5.

You are at work and have been approached by a receptionist who informs you that a local journalist is at reception. They are writing a piece on a local child with autism who has been excluded from one of the schools. As part of the article they would like an expert opinion on autism.

Your consultant is not available, and having discussed this with the Trust public relations department you agree to meet the journalist briefly to make a comment.

Talk to the journalist and give an overview of the condition. The journalist wants general advice on what parents concerned about a child should do.

6.

Sarah is a 9-year-old girl who was admitted via A&E complaining of a sudden loss of sensation and movement in both her legs.

She has been fully investigated over the past week by the paediatricians and no clear medical cause for her symptoms could be identified. She was discussed with your consultant in liaison psychiatry who wondered if she might have a conversion disorder. A joint meeting has been arranged for two weeks' time when this will be discussed with Sarah, her family and the paediatricians. Your consultant is currently on leave.

The receptionist informs you that Sarah's father is in the department. He is very angry and is saying that his child is not mad or faking it.

Take a history from the father and answer his questions.

Discuss the next steps with him.

7.

GP Referral Letter

Dear Doctor

Re: Simon Harrington, 8 years old. 17 Evershaw Road, SE19, London

I would be grateful for your opinion on this child who has become increasingly difficult for his mother to manage.

Past Medical History: Otitis media, Gastroenteritis, Fracture fibula, right.

Medication: none.

His mother is asking for a psychiatric opinion. I have examined him today and he appears a physically fit and healthy child. Of note, he smelt of cigarettes, but denied smoking. I do not believe he has access to illicit substances such as cannabis. Your advice would be appreciated.

Yours sincerely

Dr Jane Michaels

Simon refused to come for his appointment today and has locked himself in his bedroom.

Take a history from his mother.

Discuss the investigations you would like to perform.

Explain your likely diagnosis.

STATION 1

1a: School refusal

> **KEY POINTS**
> Communication and empathy
> Explain professional role, purpose of this meeting and the boundaries of confidentiality
> History of presenting complaint
> Differential diagnoses
> Disorders associated with school refusal
> Risk assessment

INTRODUCE YOURSELF

'Hello, I'm Dr_____, I'm one of the child psychiatrists.'

SET THE SCENE

'I've been asked to see you today as your GP was concerned about your daughter's school attendance.'

'Could you tell me if there is anything you are concerned about?'

COMPLETING THE TASKS

History of presenting complaint

Time of onset of the symptoms

Severity of the symptoms

Associated events (bullying, accidents, other life events)

Course of the symptoms

Factors exacerbating/factors ameliorating the symptoms

Number of days school was attended in the last month

Is school refusal pervasive or specific to certain subjects/days/teachers?

Reasons for refusal as perceived by the mother

Reasons for refusal as perceived by the young person, if known (mother's view)

Associated distress in young person and important others

Impact of the symptoms on school, friendships, family relationships and leisure

Ask specifically about symptoms of separation anxiety:

- worrying about: separation or being taken away, being alone or something unpleasant happening to the attachment figures;
- refusing to: go to school, sleep alone or sleep in a strange place due to the worries;
- checking if the attachment figures are OK at night;

- reporting: nightmares about separation, aches, pains, feeling sick and signs of distress on separation.

Establishing differential diagnosis

Screening for social phobia: Avoiding or fear of social situations (meeting other people or doing things in front of other people)

Screening for agoraphobia: Avoiding or fear of crowds, public places, travelling alone, being far from home

Screening for depression: Low mood, low energy and anhedonia

Differentiating from truancy: truancy is...

egosyntonic (Is Sacha upset about not attending school?)

wilful (Is Sacha free from pressure in her decision not to attend school?)

associated with other antisocial activity.

Parents may be unaware of truancy for some time

Differentiating from a physical illness:

Take a thorough medical history and note any symptoms of physical illness at present. Is there a link with school refusal?

Are the symptoms typical of school refusal (headaches, sore throat, stomach-aches)?

Do the symptoms arise at times of separation? When the child is at home? When the child settles at school?

Ask screening questions for disorders associated with school refusal

Consider the following:

- global or specific learning problems (persistent worries about school performance);
- depression (poor concentration, sleep difficulty, somatic complaints);
- autism spectrum disorder (ASD) (social awkwardness and withdrawal, social skills deficits, communication deficits, repetitive behaviours, adherence to routines);
- attention deficit hyperactivity disorder (ADHD) (restlessness, inattention and impulsivity);
- conduct disorder/oppositional defiant disorder.

Risk assessment

If your screening questions include any of those listed below, suggest a significant level of risk – this should prompt further questioning:

- Establish the nature of the coercive measures alluded to in the referral: 'Could you tell me a bit more about the way Sacha is disciplined at home?'
- Assess the nature of bullying at school: 'Have you ever been concerned about Sacha being bullied or picked on at school?'
- Assess the nature of family relationships: 'How does Sacha get on with other family members?'
- Assess the risk of self-harm and suicide: 'Has Sacha ever tried to harm herself or kill herself?'
- Assess the risk of violence to others: 'Has Sacha ever started fights?'
- Establish if there is a need for child protection (think: is this child at risk of significant harm?).

PROBLEM SOLVING

Sacha's mother may become defensive when asked about the way Sacha is disciplined. Candidates should show appropriate empathy and consideration whilst also gathering an adequate history.

ADDITIONAL POINTS

A good candidate will:

a. Start with open questions and use closed questions to clarify specific points.

b. Allow the mother to talk without interruption initially and provide an opportunity to ask questions.

c. Be courteous and polite.

d. Use summaries, reflections and clarifications.

e. Take a non-judgemental stance.

f. Demonstrate cultural sensitivity.

g. Seek consent to gather further information.

1b: Explaining a diagnosis

KEY POINTS

Communication and rapport

Explains a preliminary diagnosis of separation anxiety disorder to the father

Proposes further investigations

Seeks expertise from other members of the team

Outlines behavioural programme for separation anxiety disorder

Gives prognosis for separation anxiety disorder

INTRODUCE YOURSELF

SET THE SCENE

'On the basis of our discussion so far it appears that the most likely diagnosis is separation anxiety disorder of childhood. This is a preliminary diagnosis and it would be helpful to do some more investigations to make the final diagnosis. Before we continue, I'd like to ask you if you have heard of this condition before. What would you like to know about it by the time we finish this session?'

COMPLETING THE TASKS

Explaining SAD

SAD is a condition when fear of separation causes significantly more anxiety then would be expected in an average child. It begins in the early years of childhood. It is different from normal separation anxiety in that it is unusually severe or when it continues beyond the usual age period. It also causes significant problems in the child's activities, for example going to school.

Refusal to go to school often occurs at the time of change of school and after a period of legitimate absence from school (like holidays or illness). SAD is common and about 4 per cent of children have it. It is more common in girls than in boys (2:1). Many children cannot do their daily activities because of SAD.

Proposing further investigations

In this scenario you have not seen the young person yet, so of course the first thing to propose is an assessment of the young person.

Give some thought to the assessment setting, chaperone (usually a parent), colleagues that might accompany you and arranging a suitable time.

Biological

Arrange information gathering (with parental consent) and physical investigations.

Focus on the features of hyperthyroidism, migraine, asthma, seizures, lead intoxication, caffeinism (including from carbonated beverages).

Non-prescription drugs with side effects that may mimic anxiety include diet pills, antihistamines and cold medicines.

Document headaches and abdominal complaints to establish the baseline and to differentiate from side effects of medication if used in the future.

Developmental conditions associated with SAD include dyspraxia, sensory impairment and language disorders.

Prescription drugs with side effects that may mimic anxiety include antiasthmatics, sympathomimetics, steroids, selective serotonin reuptake inhibitors (SSRIs) and antipsychotics (akathisia, neuroleptic-induced SAD).

Psychological

Contact (with parental consent) the mental health professionals that the young person may have seen before.

Consider psychometric testing for global or specific learning problems.

Social

Contact school (teachers, SENCo (Special Educational Needs Co-ordinator), educational psychologist, mentors, learning support workers as applicable) with parental consent. Investigate learning profile (does she have a statement of Special Educational Needs?), quality of interpersonal relationships (including bullying), specific relationship problems and the features of emotional or disruptive disorders in the school setting.

Contact social services with parental consent. Look for previous contact with the family and evidence of child protection or child in need proceedings.

Outlining treatment options

Emphasize the importance of a collaborative approach – engage the child and the family and specifically comment on the multi-disciplinary nature of any treatment.

Establish the goals of the treatment. If the primary goal is dealing with school refusal, then a return to school at the earliest opportunity should be the stated target. In view of the relatively short duration of school refusal, a rapid reintroduction to school should be aimed for.

Two main therapeutic approaches used to treat school refusal underpinned by SAD are cognitive therapy and operant behavioural therapy. Both draw on functional analysis of the behaviour and make use of family resources. In practice, cognitive and behavioural techniques are frequently combined. Cognitive behavioural therapy (CBT) has been shown to be superior to the waiting list controls.

Treatment components are:

Psychoeducation for parents and teachers.

Help Sacha to return to school as quickly as possible. A graded (albeit very rapidly so) rather than abrupt reintroduction is the method most commonly used.

Reward Sacha with praise and tangible rewards for achieving the goals. The sorts of rewards used should be mutually agreed by parent and child in advance.

Pharmacological treatment
There have been small random allocation studies of SSRIs and imipramine showing some benefit and their use may be considered if CBT failed.

Home education
This could be considered in a tiny minority of patients with school refusal with refractory SAD.

Discussing the prognosis of SAD with the mother

The prognosis of SAD is good, with 80 per cent of children getting better within 18 months. Long-term consequences of SAD are not well established but it is possible that having SAD puts children at risk of developing anxiety and depressive disorders in adulthood.

PROBLEM SOLVING

Many parents of children with SAD feel disheartened, angry or guilty. These feelings might need to be acknowledged and hope instilled. Some parents might insist on the physical nature of the somatic symptoms. Candidates should not argue with the father about this but propose a co-operative approach – trying various treatment options and assessing outcomes together. That said, excessive medical investigations are usually unhelpful and may be traumatic for Sacha. These should be resisted.

ADDITIONAL POINTS

A good candidate will:

- take a whole system approach; engage a range of professionals and family members;
- be sensitive to the family culture, wishes and goals;
- be aware of the studies using SSRIs and imipramine in addition to psychological therapy;
- be aware of the options for intractable school refusal, including home education.

⇧ **FURTHER READING**

Kearney, C.A. (2008) School absenteeism and school refusal behaviour in youth: a contemporary review. *Clinical Psychology Review*, *28* (3), 451–71.

STATION 2

2a: Mood disturbance

KEY POINTS
Communication and rapport
History focused on mood disorders
Explores functional impairment
Differentiates the symptoms from psychosis
Explores comorbidity
Risk assessment

INTRODUCE YOURSELF

'Hello, I'm Dr_____, I'm one of the psychiatrists.'

SET THE SCENE

'I've been asked to see you today because your GP is concerned about your mood.' 'Could you tell me if there is anything you are concerned about?'

COMPLETING THE TASKS

Relevant history

Establish the following general aspects of the history of presenting complaint:

onset: what, when, how, why (precipitants);

course: fluctuations, alleviating and exacerbating factors, remedial action taken;

impact: on school (work), leisure, friendships, family;

distress: how distressed the young person is as a result of the symptoms.

Take a targeted history for recent symptoms of depression:

low mood;

loss of interest;

decreased energy;

loss of self-esteem;

excessive guilt;

suicidal thoughts/behaviour;

poor concentration;

agitation or retardation;

sleep disturbance;

change in appetite.

Take a targeted background history:

past psychiatric history;

age when disturbance first noted;

previous depressive symptoms;

history of psychiatric symptoms (especially depressive, psychotic or (hypo)manic), duration and treatment.

Developmental history:

developmental delays;

school attainment;

distress at separation from parents;

evidence of global or specific learning problems.

Medical history:

medical differential: hypothyroidism, mononucleosis, anaemia, malignancy, autoimmune diseases, head injury, hypoglycaemia, vitamin deficiency;

medication mimicking depression: stimulants, corticosteroids, clonidine, beta-blockers, diuretics, withdrawal of stimulants and benzodiazepines.

Family history:

psychiatric disorders (depression, suicidal behaviour, anxiety, psychosis and bipolar illness), criminality, substance abuse and medical illness;

perceived family relationship: discordant or supportive?

high expressed emotions;

history of intrafamilial abuse.

Social situation:

social adversity;

recent loss and other life events;

drugs and alcohol use;

interests and hopes;

criminality;

reciprocal social interactions, friendships, bullying;

romantic relationships and sexual orientation.

Exploring functional impairment

How much has your (symptoms you have elicited, for example sadness, irritability or loss of interest) upset or distressed you?

Has your sadness, irritability or loss of interest interfered with:

a. how well you get on with the rest of the family?
b. making and keeping friends?
c. learning or class work?
d. playing, hobbies, sports or other leisure activities?

Has your sadness, irritability or loss of interest made it harder for those around you (family, friends, teachers, etc.)?

Differentiating the symptoms from psychosis

Richard reports that other people are laughing at him. Such statements might represent:

a. an idea of reference;
b. an overvalued idea;
c. a paranoid delusion.

In order to qualify for being a delusion you need to show that his belief is:

• held beyond a shadow of doubt;
• not shared by others;
• preoccupying and of personal importance;
• held against evidence to the contrary.

Richard also reports feeling 'like a puppet'. It is important to determine if this indicates the presence of:

a. delusion of control;
b. derealization/depersonalization phenomena.

In order to qualify for depersonalization/derealization the following features must be present:

• feeling of unreality;
• unpleasant quality;
• non-delusional (see above);
• loss of affective response.

Exploring for comorbidities

Screening for anxiety disorders:

Are there symptoms of anxiety (biological, cognitive and behavioural)?

What situations do they arise in?

Are they distressing and impairing?

Screening for substance misuse:

Onset, nature, amount, frequency, context, features of dependency (psychological and physical), impact and distress.

Risk

Assess the:

• nature of family relationships;
• risk of self-harm and suicide;
• risk of violence to others;
• risk of non-engagement.

PROBLEM SOLVING

Richard may feel offended or upset by you trying to clarify the nature of the symptoms. This may be prevented by suggesting you are going to ask some questions that may seem strange or out of the ordinary. These questions are part of a usual psychiatric examination and you ask these of every person you see. If Richard is offended nonetheless (he may indicate this by saying 'Do you think I'm mad?'), you should not enter into arguments. A sensible way forward is to acknowledge that you asked the question in a way that offended Richard and re-frame it without backing down. 'Some young people have these experiences. Has it ever happened to you?'

ADDITIONAL POINTS

a. Start with open questions and use closed questions to clarify specific points.

b. Allow the patient to talk without interruption initially and provide an opportunity to ask questions.

c. Be courteous and polite.

d. Use summaries, reflections and clarifications.

e. Seek consent to gather further information.

f. Reassure the patient despite initial suspiciousness.

g. Elicit protective prognostic factors.

FURTHER READING

For suggested questions to establish the presence of low mood, please visit http://www.dawba.com for further information and more suggested questions.

2b: Explaining treatment and prognosis

KEY POINTS
Communication and rapport
Proposes collaborative approach with other professionals and family
Psychological therapies for depression
Pharmacological therapies for depression
Social interventions for depression
Prognosis for the first depressive episode

INTRODUCE YOURSELF

SET THE SCENE

'Thank you for agreeing to see me today. You met the team recently to discuss Richard's diagnosis and I think it's important over the next few minutes to discuss how we can treat his depression and what the future holds. Does that sound okay to you?'

COMPLETING THE TASKS

Establishing the goals and the framework of the treatment

Explore Mrs Chip's hopes and expectations.

Emphasize the importance of adopting a collaborative approach with other professionals, and engaging the young person and family (with the young person's consent) in all decision making.

Outlining the principles of psychological therapies for depression

The two most commonly used psychological therapies for depression are Cognitive Behavioural Therapy (CBT) and Interpersonal Therapy (IPT).

Ask if she knows anything about these treatments. If not, you should briefly discuss the principles, advantages and disadvantages of both.

'CBT is a "talking" treatment for depression. It is based on the idea that what happens to us is rarely either all good or all bad and we make it good or bad by having either good or bad thoughts about it. It may sound a bit confusing so let me give you an example. Say if a friend does not say hello to us we could think he doesn't like us or we could think he was too busy. Having a negative thought ("He doesn't like me") might make us feel sad. When we feel sad we my stop doing things we are good at. This could make our mood even worse and we could have even more bad thoughts about ourselves.

'During CBT we arrange weekly or two-weekly 1-hour sessions with a CBT therapist for at least 3 months. We then look at the kinds of thoughts that a young person has about themselves, other people or the world in general and see if these thoughts are helpful or not and if there may be a different way to see things. We also try to see if doing positive activities could help improve a young person's mood. We sometimes ask the young people to practise the skills they have learnt and keep a diary of their progress. However, CBT does not always work. In good studies about 50 per cent of young people who have CBT alone get better within the first few weeks of treatment. I could also give you information about useful websites and I could give you a leaflet explaining more about CBT.

'IPT is similar to CBT and is also a "talking treatment" with several 1-hour weekly or two-weekly sessions for at least 3 months. Unlike CBT, in IPT the therapist and the young person look mainly at the young person's relationships. This is because we know that most young people with depression could do with some help when it comes to their relationships. We also know that young people tend to get depressed at the time of relationship problems. During IPT the young person and the therapist look at the ways of improving the young person's relationships and dealing with some of the bad things that may have happened to the young person. Young people talk about their feelings and learn how to manage them. They also discover ways of communicating more effectively, solving problems and managing conflicts. During the treatment, other important people in the young person's life can participate (with the young person's consent). It is useful for young people to practise some of the skills at home and at school and to do role plays during the sessions. I could also give you information about useful websites and I could give you a leaflet explaining more about IPT.'

Outlining pharmacological therapies for depression

'Sometimes talking therapies may not work and this is when we start thinking about medication. There are many medicines available to treat depression but at present only one is recommended for treating depression in young people. It is called fluoxetine (e.g. Prozac). The way it works is not entirely clear but it increases the amount of a naturally occurring chemical called serotonin in our brain. We use fluoxetine to treat depression and sometimes other conditions. About two-thirds of young people with depression tend to get better. Fluoxetine takes about two to four weeks to work. As with any other medication, young people who take fluoxetine may have some side effects although most young people do not get any at all. Common side effects include headaches, upset stomach, feeling sick, feeling restless, poor appetite, fever and skin rash. Rare side effects include getting "high" in mood and very rarely having suicidal thoughts and self-harming. It should not be given to young people who are allergic to it or who are feeling "high" in their mood. If you take any other medication you need to let me know before starting fluoxetine. If fluoxetine does work we would recommend that you continued treatment for at least 6 months before stopping gradually. If it does not work, other medicines could be tried. About 50 per cent of young people will get better with a second medication. I would be happy to answer your questions about the medication treatment and I could also give you a leaflet with further information.'

Outlining social interventions for depression

'Social problems make young people more likely to have depression. These include poor housing, poverty, unemployment (either of a parent or of the young person), exposure to violence, discrimination on the basis of race and sexual orientation.

'Social interventions that can help in depression include educating family members and teachers about depression, dealing with bullying, establishing a healthy lifestyle with healthy food, sleep and exercise and helping the young person and the family improve their health and quality of life. In order for social interventions to be helpful we will need to involve other people like the family members, teachers and sometimes other health professionals and social workers.'

Prognosis

In the short term, most young people will recover from depression. Around 10 per cent of children and young people with depression recover within 3 months and 50 per cent by 12 months. By 24 months this figure is around 75 per cent. However, there is a high risk of depression recurring. It is about 30 per cent within 5 years and most young people are at risk of having another episode of depression in adulthood. Risk of suicide is estimated at around 3 per cent over a 10-year period. This is why greater understanding of depression and engagement with the multidisciplinary team is so important.

PROBLEM SOLVING

Mrs Chip may be alarmed by the reported increase in suicidality with SSRI treatment. The following facts need to be taken into account. There is evidence that treating young people with a drug like fluoxetine increases the risk of young people having suicidal thoughts and suicidal behaviour. There is no evidence that treating young people with a drug like fluoxetine increases the risk of suicide. The risk of developing suicidal thoughts and behaviour is very low with fluoxetine and the vast majority of young people do not develop this. There is evidence that the benefits of fluoxetine treatment outweigh the side effects. You should explain to Mrs Chip that regular and frequent monitoring of Richard's symptoms would be in place during the first few weeks of treatment (for example, once a week for the first four weeks). Mrs Chip could always give your team a call Monday to Friday 9 to 5 or contact a duty psychiatrist in the local A&E out of hours if she is concerned about any of the symptoms.

ADDITIONAL POINTS

Take a whole system approach; engage a range of professionals and family members in management.

Be sensitive to the family and the young person's wishes and goals.

Be aware of the latest studies in child depression (Treatment for Adolescents with Depression Study (TADS), Treatment of Resistant Depression in Adolescents (TORDIA)) and be familiar with their outcomes.

FURTHER READING

Zalsman, G. & Brent, D. (2006) *Child and Adolescent Psychiatric Clinics of North America. Depression.* Philadelphia: Saunders.

STATION 3

3a: Self-harm

KEY POINTS
Communication and rapport
Precursors and circumstances of the overdose
History of presenting problem
Explores substance use
Mental state examination
Risk summary and formulation

INTRODUCE YOURSELF

SET THE SCENE

COMPLETING THE TASKS

Exploring precursors and circumstances of the overdose

You need to have a good understanding of the following factors:

- Suicidal ideation (when, what, how severe)
- Method of self-harm
- Subjective and objective lethality
- Suicidal intent (assessment includes patients' belief about intent, preparation before the attempt, prevention of discovery and communication before and after the attempt)
- Precursors of the overdose: explore stressful life events: number, types, perceived degree of control over these events
- Explore interpersonal conflicts, losses (death, parental separation) and physical illness
- Precipitants of the overdose (frequently interpersonal problems)
- Associated features: use of drugs and alcohol self-harm paraphernalia)

- Reasons for the overdose (wanting to die, trying to escape from impossible situation, making others feel sorry, punish others, communicate distress)
- Reasons for living (future plans, responsibility to family, moral objections to suicide, fear of suicide).

Gathering history of presenting problem

Ask about historical/contextual factors that elevate the risk of suicide and self-harm:

- previous episodes of self-harm;
- previous suicidal attempts using violent methods;
- denial/minimizing of previous violence;
- use of prescribed medication (especially SSRIs and benzodiazepines);
- familial suicidal behaviour;
- familial psychopathology/substance misuse;
- family discord;
- history of emotional, physical or sexual abuse/exploitation;
- exposure to suicidal behaviour;
- exposure to violence;
- social isolation;
- history of delinquent and/or antisocial behaviour;
- history of impulsive behaviour;
- history of substance misuse;
- recent life events (especially loss);
- history of physical illness;
- recent discharge from services;
- family members expressing concern about suicide;
- gay, lesbian, bisexual orientation;
- history of psychiatric illness.

Ask about factors that elevate the risk of violence:;

- history of violent behaviour;
- history of non-violent antisocial behaviour;
- early onset of violence;
- denial/minimizing of previous violence;
- evidence of impulsive behaviour;
- disengaging from services;
- recent life events;
- substance misuse;
- familial violence/criminality/substance misuse;
- family members concerned about violence in the young person;
- exposure to violence;
- history of emotional, physical or sexual abuse/exploitation;
- history of self-harm/suicide attempts;
- poor school achievement;
- delinquent peer group;
- peer rejection;
- poor parenting;
- community disorganization;
- history of psychiatric illness.

Other historical factors associated with the risk of violence and suicide:

- history of accidental injuries;
- cultural isolation;
- history of self-neglect;

- social adversity;
- poor daily living skills.

Historical protective factors:

- good family relationships;
- problem-solving ability;
- peer support;
- pro-social behaviour;
- good social skills;
- good self-esteem;
- sense of control over life;
- positive school experiences;
- resilience to stress;
- positive attitude to treatment;
- positive attitude towards authority.

Screening for substance misuse

Enquire about substance misuse (refer to Additional Points).

Performing mental state examination

These features are of particular relevance to risk assessment:;

- signs of previous self-harm;
- evidence of self-neglect;
- psychomotor abnormalities (retardation or agitation);
- withdrawal, irritability, distractibility, apathy;
- poor eye contact, threatening body language, crying, tension;
- irritability, low or anxious mood;
- blunt or incongruous affect;
- hopelessness, self-blame, inappropriate guilt, helplessness, worthlessness and poor self-image;
- current attitude towards the overdose;
- current suicidal fantasies, thoughts or plans;
- current violent fantasies, thoughts or plans;
- high level of distress;
- feeling out of control;
- low empathy/remorse;
- evidence of paranoid delusions and passivity;
- evidence of hallucinations;
- poor concentration and distractibility;
- poor insight.

Risk summary and formulation

Make sure to leave 1 or 2 minutes at the end of the station for this. Rather than repeating every fact you elicited, it is important to show the examiner that you have a system for thinking about risk. One way of doing this is to intersect [risk to self, risk to others and risk from exploitation] with [protective factors, risk factors] whilst adding a time line [short-term and long-term risk].

For example, regarding risk to self – factors that increase risk of future deliberate self-harm (DSH) are a history of two attempts (including this one), alcohol use, the presence of marked family discord and a family history of self-harm. Protective factors are the presence of a network of supportive friends and the fact that all past acts of DSH have been impulsive, of low lethality and self-disclosed. (Use the same approach for risk to others and risk from exploitation.)

A concluding statement might follow the structure: 'In summary there is a mild/moderate/high short-term risk of self-harm/violence and mild/moderate/high long-term risk of self-harm/violence moderated by treatment engagement.'

PROBLEM SOLVING

Nadia may initially be reluctant to engage with the assessment. The following techniques could be employed to improve engagement:

- Give consideration to the positioning of the chairs and the room environment.
- Use open body language and thank Nadia for agreeing to see you.
- Acknowledge Nadia's feelings and empathize with her distress.
- Link her thoughts, emotions and behaviour.
- Avoid the 'Why?' questions and focus on 'What? When? and How?'

ADDITIONAL POINTS

These are suggested questions to screen for the presence of substance misuse based on Kiddie-Sads-Present and Lifetime Version (K-SADS-PL). Please visit http://www.wpic.pitt.edu/ksads/ksads-pl.pdf for further information.

How old were you when you had your first drink?

What's your favourite thing to drink?

Do you have a group of friends you usually drink with, or do you usually drink alone?

Where do you usually drink?

How old were you when you started to drink regularly, say two drinks or more per week?

In the past six months has there been at least one week in which you had at least two drinks?

Let me know if you have used any street drugs before, even if you have only tried them once. Which ones have you used?

In the past six months, what is the most you have used? Every day or almost every day for at least one week? Less? More? Was there a time when you used more?

FURTHER READING

Spirito, A. & Overholser, J. (2002) *Evaluating and treating adolescent suicide attempters: from research to practice (practical resources for the mental health professional)*. New York: Academic Press.

3b: Engaging a parent

KEY POINTS

Communication and rapport (including confidentiality limits and permission to contact others)

Clarifies the reasons and the procedure involved in community follow-up

Pros and cons of attending community follow-up

Uses co-operative stance

Makes practical arrangements to maximize the chances of attending follow-up

---

INTRODUCE YOURSELF

SET THE SCENE

COMPLETING THE TASKS

Clarify the reasons and process of community follow-up

The points to cover here are:

Being 16, Nadia is presumed to have capacity to make decisions about her treatment.

Nonetheless, it is good practice to involve family members in the decision making.

Parental support is one of the best predictors of engagement with follow-up.

British clinical guidelines require professionals to offer 7-day follow-up to all young people who have self-harmed.

The main reason for this is to monitor risk and to offer treatment to those young people who require it.

Establishing 'pros' and 'cons' of attending community follow-up

Start with the 'cons'. Explore in detail what are the negatives of attending community follow-up. Common reasons for reluctance to attend follow-up appointments include stigma, inconvenience, desire to put the episode behind the family and having had negative experience of contact with health professionals previously.

Then move on to 'pros'. Explore what are the good things about attending community follow-up. Common reasons for attending the follow-up appointments include a desire to understand the problematic behaviour, wish to improve relationships, reduce risk of further self-harm and a hope that the young person will learn new ways of dealing with problems.

Taking a co-operative stance

Avoid direct confrontation and arguments

Express empathy

Emphasize self-efficacy

Instil hope

Use open questions

Affirm positives

Provide reflections

Use summaries.

Enhancing parental motivation to attend follow-up

Several techniques may be used here. The example below is based on the motivational interviewing techniques (Rollnick & Miller, 2002).

On a scale of 0–10, with 0 having no motivation to attend follow-up and 10 having no doubts about attending, where are you right now?

Having obtained a summary score for the overall motivation, you can develop this part by exploring different elements of motivation.

Importance of attendance

How important is it that you and Nadia attend the follow-up appointments?

Not at all important | 0 | 1 | 2 | 3 | 4 | 5 | 6 | 7 | 8 | 9 | 10 | Very important

How come your score is not zero – tell me more about it. Why else? What would need to happen for you to move up one point?

You could use the same principles to ask:

How confident are you that you can attend the follow-up appointments?

How ready are you to attend the follow-up appointments?

The following practical factors increase the likelihood of attending the follow-up appointments:

- fixing the follow-up date and time at the initial assessment;
- arranging mutually convenient time where possible (take into account the young person's and other family members' commitments, like school, college or work);
- the assessor providing the follow-up personally;
- making a telephone call prior to the follow-up appointments;
- sending a letter prior to the follow-up appointments;
- explaining the reasons for the follow-up;
- explaining the possible treatment options beyond the initial follow-up session;
- thinking through the possible obstacles (transport, child care, ease of access).

PROBLEM SOLVING

The candidate may be faced with an ambivalent mother reluctant to attend the follow-up appointments primarily for stigma-related reasons.

The candidate should take a cooperative stance and stick to the facts rather than opinions. It may be helpful to dispel some myths. You could say that you see some young people who have mental illness but also young people who do not, but who could do better with psychological or social support. You could also say that most people could benefit from developing their potential in a supportive environment and that you work with other professionals who have a range of skills and expertise. Your team also works with other organizations that are not part of the mental health services, for example counselling services and educational advisors whose expertise may be called upon if required. All decisions about further treatment (if one is recommended) will be made in cooperation with the family members. You could also give Mrs Burrell written information about your service and leave some time to answer questions.

ADDITIONAL POINTS

Other factors that improve adherence to follow-up are:

- female sex;
- higher socioeconomic status;
- belonging to the dominant ethnic group;
- lower parental psychopathology;
- previous adherence to treatment;
- younger age;
- positive experience with previous healthcare contact;
- less severe psychopathology;
- supportive family members;
- therapeutic alliance with the assessor;
- belief that follow-up treatment will be useful and managable;
- follow up in non-clinical setting;
- using outreach services.

According to the Mental Capacity Act 2005, all people over 16 are presumed to be competent (this is a broader concept reflecting general maturity whereas capacity is frequently situation specific). In this instance you are dealing with a vulnerable young person who is ambivalent about engagement with the follow-up. Under these circumstances, engaging a parent (with the young person's consent) is especially important.

FURTHER READING

Rollnick, S. & Miller, W.R. (2002) *Motivational interviewing*, 2nd edn. New York: The Guilford Press.

STATION 4: Learning disability

KEY POINTS
Communication
Gathering details of the behaviours of concern
Assessing nature of learning disabilities
Assessing presence of possible mental/physical illness
Risk assessment
Quality of formulation

INTRODUCE YOURSELF

Introduce yourself to a member of staff. Ask the 17-year-old's name (referred to as 'P' below). Establish how long the informant has known her and how often they have had contact with her.

SET THE SCENE

Explain that you have been asked to find out a bit more about the nature of the difficult behaviours P displays. You will be asking a lot of questions and recognize that as they only see P in one setting they may not know how she is more generally.

COMPLETING THE TASKS

Gathering details of the behaviours of concern

Identify key problem behaviours.

> What is 'sexually inappropriate behaviour'?

> What is 'challenging behaviour'?

> What is 'self-harm' behaviour?

Get concrete examples of each.

Have these behaviours all become an issue over the same time? If not, what was the order in which they developed?

For each target behaviour establish:

> Time course – onset, progress since then

> Current frequency (e.g. monthly pattern linked to menstrual cycle)

> Antecedents e.g. change of carer, presence of a certain member of staff, certain time of day, sound

> Behaviour

> What does it look like?

> Any associated features e.g. appears to be in pain, epileptic phenomena

> Consequences

> Any possible positive (i.e. brings about something pleasant) or negative (i.e. takes away something unpleasant) reinforcers?

> How do others react?

> What has been tried so far – any good?

> Has it ever been a problem before?

With particular reference to sexual behaviours:

> What are the behaviours (self-exposure, touching, masturbation)?

> How do staff react to it now?

> Access to children in foster home

> How do these relate to past sexually inappropriate behaviours?

Is P ever unsupervised in such a way that she might be vulnerable to maltreatment by others?

With particular reference to self-harm:

Has this required medical attention?

Does it take a particular e.g. stereotyped form that may indicate a particular syndrome e.g. Lesh–Nyhan?

To what extent are these behaviours threatening the tenability of current foster and educational placements?

Why does P have foster carers?

Is there a documented history of sexual or physical abuse?

Aetiology

Is it known if P has mild/moderate or severe learning disabilities?

Is there a known cause for these learning disabilities (e.g. perinatal infection/neurogenetic syndrome)

Does P have functional expressive language?

To what extent can P understand language?

What are P's abilities with regards to activities of daily living, e.g. toileting, feeding, bathing, mobility?

Assess presence of possible mental/physical health problems:

Is P physically well?

Does she take any prescribed medications?

Have there been any altered physical symptoms recently (altered bowel habit, fever etc.)?

Is P behaving as if in pain?

Is P menstruating – when was her last menstrual period – pregnancy test?

Note: It is increasingly hard to confidently establish the presence of psychopathology as LD worsens, especially in non-verbal populations. However, LD is clearly associated with elevated rates of mental illness.

Ask about: withdrawal, altered sleep/appetite, tearfulness, activity levels, uncharacteristic behaviour.

Risk assessment

Risk of self-harm:

Is this self-injurious behaviour (SIB)? This tends to be stereotyped and most commonly skin picking, wrist biting, etc.

Is this better understood as purposeful, thought-out acts with the desire to end life (not incompatible with milder LD)?

Risk of exploitation:

Has P been maltreated?

Is she ever left unsupervised?

Is there any concern about those who supervise her?

Risk to others (of physical and/or sexual assault):

Frequency and severity of past behaviour

Are particular people targets of this behaviour?

To what extent can P understand the impact of her behaviour on others?

Are these behaviours planned and goal-directed, or for example is P hitting people unintentionally whilst resisting restraint?

Formulation of behavioural problems

An example might be:

- predisposing: severe LD, with chronic experience of physical and sexual abuse before entered care;
- precipitating: unidentified dental abscess, possible depressive illness and change of carer;
- perpetuating: ongoing pain from tooth, behaviour negatively reinforced by its resulting in P being 'calmed down' with provision of one-to-one attention and favourite food.

PROBLEM SOLVING

A helpful way to consider the formulation is to consider [Predisposing, Precipitating and Perpetuating] with [Bio-, psycho-, social] and form a 6 × 6 grid of potential contributors to P's problems. You are asked to 'establish the possible aetiology and perpetuating factors'. You will have gathered most of the information for this so far.

ADDITIONAL POINTS

Self-neglect is an important issue and relates to how much support P requires in order that her basic needs are secured (e.g. nutrition, access to health care). This is probably not essential to this station, however, and given the time constraints might be left out.

FURTHER READING

Xeniditis, K., Russell, A. & Murphy, D. (2001) Management of people with challenging behaviour. *Advances in Psychiatric Treatment*, 7, 109–16.

STATION 5: Autism spectrum disorder

KEY POINTS
Communicate in lay terms
Consider how your information will be used
Epidemiology and characteristics
Comorbidity and differential diagnoses
Aetiology
Screening and diagnosis
Treatment and prognosis

INTRODUCE YOURSELF

SET THE SCENE

Ask the journalist what in particular they would like to know about autism.

Ask where the information will go and state that you would like to see how you are being quoted before the article is printed. Be clear that whilst you are not an expert in this field you are happy to cover key aspects of autism. Refer the journalist to the National Autistic Society for further information.

COMPLETING THE TASKS

Epidemiology

Autism is one of a group of disorders characterized by early onset problems with social communication and a tendency to 'sameness' and repetitive behaviours.

Other 'autism spectrum disorders' are Asperger's syndrome and atypical autism.

Prevalence rates vary depending on whether one is talking about the whole spectrum or one sub-disorder.

All such estimates, however, have shown dramatic increases over the past decade. There are recent reports of 1 per cent prevalence in the UK for all ASDs.

Contrary to some concerns that this increase may be due to an environmental factor (e.g. MMR vaccination – now clearly disproved as a cause for ASD), the altered prevalence seems to reflect a change in how we diagnose the condition and the fact that children who would have been diagnosed with other disorders (e.g. learning disability, specific language problems) are now considered to have ASD.

Characteristics

Children with ASDs show early onset impairments in social reciprocity and communication as well as having a tendency towards repetitive behaviours and/or restricted interests.

Differences in development before age 3 and symptom profile determine if a child is thought to have autism, Asperger's syndrome or atypical autism.

ASDs are more prevalent in males (M:F 4:1 autism, 10:1 Asperger's syndrome).

Comorbidities and differential diagnosis

ASD is associated with learning disability (70 per cent autism, 30 to 40 per cent of all in spectrum), epilepsy (20 per cent), mental illness (elevated risk of anxiety, obsessive–compulsive disorder (OCD), psychosis and others).

Aetiology

In 10 to 15 per cent of cases ASD is seen in the context of a medical disorder thought to be causal (e.g. Tuberous Sclerosis, Phenylketonuria, Smith–Lemli–Opitz syndrome). The remaining 90 per cent are considered 'idiopathic'.

Idiopathic autism has the highest heritability estimate of all multifactorial psychiatric disorders (90 per cent). ASDs are familial and recurrence risk for ASD or related developmental condition in sibs is 10 per cent.

No clear environmental risks have been found. However, in identical twins that have the same DNA, one can have autism, and the other a different type of ASD. This suggests that environmental factors must play a role. The latest thinking regarding genetic risk is that in some instances lots of genetic factors are acting synergistically to generate risk for disorder, and in others an abnormality within a single larger stretch of DNA imparts risk.

Screening and diagnosis

Concerned carers of children should contact their GP or health visitor in the first instance.

The 'national plan for autism' recommends that if concerns remain after this, a general developmental assessment should be done by paediatricians, and if an ASD is still suspected then a specialist team should see the child. Special instruments exist to help screening (e.g. Childhood Autism Screening Test – CHAT).

Treatment and prognosis

Although there is no 'cure' for ASD, there is a lot of help available. General support is important for children and families e.g. access to voluntary agencies, provision of good information about ASD, making sure educational placement is right.

Some treatments try to support people with ASD in learning new skills or to directly teach them strategies for communication. It seems that the earlier these are begun the better, but there is not enough research yet to be clear what the 'active ingredient' in these 'psychoeducational' interventions is, or for whom they work best.

There is no evidence that dietary supplements or medication can be reliably used to improve the core features of ASD, although in some instances medicine can help with challenging behaviours which can be seen in ASD.

ASDs are lifelong. In the majority of cases, impairment persists and extra support is needed into adulthood.

PROBLEM SOLVING

It is important to be clear about what is *not* known and communicate this if necessary.

Direct the journalist towards other sources of information (e.g. http://www.nas.org.uk/).

Be clear that ASD is a heterogeneous group of conditions and that it is hard to generalize.

ADDITIONAL POINTS

It is important to distinguish ASD from deafness, generalized LD, specific developmental disorder of language, ADHD, attachment disorder, selective mutism, and schizotypal disorder.

The brain bases of ASD are poorly understood, but there is some evidence of early brain overgrowth and developing abnormalities in parts of the brain used when we have to interact with others or plan and control our behaviour.

Highly specialized tools such as the Autism Diagnostic Interview (ADI) tend to be used more in research but can sometimes be used clinically.

FURTHER READING

UK National Autism Plan: http://www.nas.org.uk/nas/jsp/polopoly.jsp?a=2178&d=368

Volkmar, F.R., Lord, C., Bailey, A., Schultz, R.T. & Klin, A. (2004) Autism and pervasive developmental disorders. *Journal of Child Psychology and Psychiatry*, *45* (1), 135–70.

STATION 6: Medically unexplained symptoms

KEY POINTS

Communication/calming father
Addressing father's concerns
History targeted towards somatoform and conversion disorders
Psychosocial history
Risk
Discussing next steps

INTRODUCE YOURSELF

SET THE SCENE

Be polite, respectful and calm.

Do not interrupt the father, who will be angry at first. Let him air his grievances.

Thank him for coming to see you. Demonstrate an understanding attitude [Nodding, 'I can see you are very upset', 'Of course this must be a concern for you']. Contextualize and qualify your meeting. Explain that your consultant is away, and that whilst you haven't been directly involved with Sarah's care, you are keen to help. Try to address the father's questions and concerns and plan next steps in preparation for the return of your consultant.

'Many thanks for clarifying things for me. In order to best help, I will need to ask you quite a few questions. As time is limited, please forgive me if I appear to be rushing you. We can always make an appointment to meet again in the near future.' This is a generally helpful line in CASC scenarios where tempers are high and there is a lot to cover.

COMPLETING THE TASKS

History targeted to somatoform and conversion disorders

Gather basic information about Sarah's symptoms:

Tempo of their onset – sudden/slow

Overall course since onset – worse/stable/improving

If they fluctuate – are there any factors that seem to be associated with improvement/worsening of symptoms?

Has she had ever them before? What happened then?

What do family think they are about?

Do they feel they are due to a physical disorder?

If so, is there one they are particularly worried about?

Are their concerns shaped by specific prior experiences of illness (e.g. affecting another relative)?

How does Sarah explain them?

Has she been preoccupied with the possibility that she has a named disease?

Has she ever expressed any bizarre/unusual beliefs in relation to them (e.g. nihilistic beliefs/passivity experiences)?

How distressed is she by them? Might there be evidence to support the impression that she has 'Belle Indifference' (a degree of distress that seems surprisingly low given the nature of the symptoms)?

Has she ever witnessed similar symptoms in other people (e.g. father)?

What is the impact of the symptoms? What can/can't she do – is there any secondary gain (e.g. can't go to school where she is being bullied)?

Have the symptoms been preceded by any clear life event/stressor (e.g. family break-up, exams, victimization etc.)? Does Sarah have any recognized physical health problems? Does she take any prescribed medicines?

Screen for the following:

Mood disorder

Anxiety disorder

Background school/home psychosocial history

Who is in the household?

Is there a history of physical/mental health problems?

Are there tensions in the home setting?

What is Sarah's academic and social functioning at school?

Risk

Are there any factors that increase the risk of Sarah having experienced recent abuse?

Is there any past history of self-harm?

Note: It is a good idea to make sure that you ask a few screening questions about risk in any station. A good initial question might be 'Do you have any concerns about Sarah's safety?' Sarah's symptoms could have been preceded by an adverse life experience, which may include experiences of abuse.

Address the father's question – 'Are you saying that she's faking it?'

Useful things to say in response to this question include:

- No, her experiences are clearly very real for her, and understandably worrying for her family. It is highly unlikely that she is faking it.
- However, so far physical investigations have not found a clear cause.

- Whilst one can never be 100 per cent sure that there is no physical contribution to her problems, all possibilities that are usually considered have been ruled out.
- The important thing to recognize is that she is still impaired due to problems with walking, so we need to think of ways of moving forward.
- In the absence of an obvious physical cause (and treatment that any such diagnosis might suggest), an alternative approach that can often be very useful is to think of how mental factors can influence the body.

Note: You may want to use somatic features of anxiety as an example. They are common experiences and provide a concrete instance of how our emotional state can affect our physical state.

- For some people, without them knowing it, troubles and stress can influence their body in such a way that things like altered sight, altered ability to move limbs and even fits can occur.

Ask if he has any questions.

Next steps

Thank the father for coming.

Let him know that you would like to discuss your meeting with your consultant and the rest of the multi-disciplinary Children's Liaison Mental Health team.

Tell the father that detailed plans will need to be based on joint working between Sarah, her family, and the clinicians on the paediatric ward (includes many professionals in addition to paediatricians e.g. physiotherapists, nursing staff).

Ongoing assessment will be required.

You will need to work closely with paediatricians.

PROBLEM SOLVING

Managing anger in others can be worked into many stations, so it is a good idea to develop skills in this area. These will of course also come in handy in the real world! The core is to be calm, measured, non-confrontational, and to demonstrate that you care about what the other person is saying, and have taken their concerns seriously. Additional strategies should come into play if the person becomes abusive, threatens assault or wants to lodge a complaint.

ADDITIONAL POINTS

It is particularly hard to screen for such 'internalizing' disorders in a reliable and valid manner via an informant. For exam purposes, in such a scenario it will be reasonable to ask the father 'Have you been worried about Sarah's mood recently? Do you feel she has been particularly low? Do you think she is troubled by anxiety?' For further examples of screening questions see the references below.

The differential diagnosis for medically unexplained symptoms includes:

- a physical cause that has not yet been diagnosed;
- a somatoform disorder;
- a dissociative [conversion] disorder;
- primary anxiety/depression with prominent physical symptoms interpreted as signs of a physical illness;
- a psychotic/delusional disorder;

- factitious disorder;
- malingering.

FURTHER READING

Eminson, D.M. (2007) Medically unexplained symptoms in children and adolescents. *Clinical Psychology Review*, *27* (7), 855–71.

STATION 7: Attention deficit hyperactivity disorder

KEY POINTS
Communication/empathy
ADHD history
Assessing comorbidities/differential diagnoses
Risk issues
Investigations
Explaining diagnosis

INTRODUCE YOURSELF

SET THE SCENE

Thank the mother for coming. Ask her what her understanding is of why you are meeting today.

Tell her that you have received a letter from Simon's GP mentioning that you wanted to meet with Child Mental Health Services about difficulties with Simon's behaviour.

Explain that you would like to ask her a few questions to try to understand things a bit better. What you discuss will be confidential. However, if your discussion raises concerns about safety, you may have to share these with other agencies in discussion with the family.

Acknowledge the absence of Simon:

Who is looking after him now?

Any idea why he is refusing to attend?

COMPLETING THE TASKS

ADHD history

It is a good idea in any initial outpatient assessment such as this to begin by getting a sense of the child's family and school context. Quickly establish:

Who else lives in the house?

Is Simon in mainstream/special school?

How is school going? Is there any evidence that Simon might have generalized learning difficulties/specific learning disabilities?

What is the nature of the difficulties as experienced by the mother? General questions include:

What are the informant's main concerns and how long have they been an issue?

Do problems occur across all settings (e.g. home, school)?

Are they associated with impairment (e.g. suspended from school, limiting what the family can do)?

What has been tried to address the problems so far (include parental disciplinary methods as well as formal support from within school or past CAMHS involvement)?

Has input received to date been of any benefit? If so – how? If not – any ideas why not?

How does the family deal with Simon's behavioural difficulties? Is physical chastisement ever used? To what extent might his behaviours be reinforced by the response of others (e.g. are outbursts reinforced by Simon eventually being given what he wants)?

Move on to a more targeted ADHD history, focusing on:

Hyperkinesis

High levels of physical activity

Fidgeting

Inattentiveness

How long can he stay on task?

Does he flit from one activity to another?

How easily is he distracted from a task?

If distracted, does he re-engage voluntarily or is prompting required?

Impulsivity

Does he think before acting (e.g. running across the road if interested in something)?

Can he wait his turn (e.g. queues)?

Does he blurt out answers or interrupt others when they are talking?

Establish that these began prior to age 7

Do they occur across settings (i.e. home and school)?

Are they impairing (e.g. suspended from school)?

Family history/care network

If not asked earlier – establish who is in the family and household.

Any problems with 'stress', slow development, substance use, ongoing contact with CAMHS in family members?

Has the family ever been known to Social Services?

Developmental history

Antenatal: Smoking, drugs, maternal health

Perinatal: Birth complications and need for special/intensive care

Early milestones

First words other than 'Mama, Papa'

First walking unaided

Previous school history

Is there any evidence that Simon might have generalized learning difficulties/specific learning disabilities?

Has he ever been granted a Statement of Educational Need (SEN)?

Assess comorbidities and differential diagnoses

Many comorbidities are also differential diagnoses for ADHD.

Consider and screen for the following (refer to diagnostic criteria for details of what to ask about):

Oppositional defiant disorder/conduct disorder

Generalized learning disability

Specific developmental disorder

Substance misuse

Depression

Risk issues

You will by this stage have some clues already (i.e. how parents deal with difficult behaviour, if Social Services have been involved).

Ask more directly e.g.:

Gently enquire about broken leg.

'I can imagine things can get very stressful trying to control Simon's behaviour. Do things ever get physical?'

'Does Simon ever get so angry that he hits out? Has anyone ever needed medical attention as a result?'

Is Simon at risk of harm due to his impulsivity (e.g. Does he have good road safety)?

Discussing the investigations you would like to perform

Biological

You would want to arrange a meeting with the child so that you can carry out a physical examination yourself.

Physical investigations might follow (baseline height/weight in case stimulant meds to be started, genetic investigations if dysmorphic, etc.).

Psychological

History and Mental state examination with Simon himself.

Connor's rating scale for teacher and parent.

Mention that you might want to do direct school observations yourself at a later stage.

If there is any suggestion that Simon may have a degree of unquantified Learning Disability, cognitive testing would be indicated, as inattention, hyperactivity and impulsivity required for ADHD diagnosis must be elevated relative to developmental stage of child (i.e. mental rather than chronological age).

If there is evidence that Simon has more specific learning problems (e.g. language delay), psychometric testing would be indicated.

Social

You could mention to the mother that after further assessment has been carried out, there may be helpful ways in which Social Services could get involved.

Explaining your likely diagnosis

You may want to say that whilst further information will have to be gathered, it seems likely that Simon's difficulties fall within what would be termed 'Attention Deficit Hyperactivity Disorder or ADHD'. Ask if she has heard of this condition.

Explain that:

- Attention deficit hyperactivity disorder is a term used in American diagnostic systems to describe a group of children who have early onset problems with hyperactivity, focusing their attention and being able to plan carefully before acting.
- If there are problems in all three of these areas, and they occur across different settings, then the term 'severe combined subtype ADHD' is used. This is equivalent to the UK term 'hyperkinetic disorder'.
- The condition affects boys more than girls.
- Both genetic and environmental factors play a role.
- Frontal brain systems that use a chemical called dopamine seem to be involved in ADHD.
- It is associated with worse outcomes in later life (mental health and psychosocial functioning).
- 40 to 60 per cent may carry on into adulthood.

Ask the mother if she has any questions.

PROBLEM SOLVING

Time management is key in a station like this with several components. Make sure you address each of the questions asked of you. This is especially hard in stations such as this that are essentially based around an 'initial assessment' scenario. In real life such an interview would take place over an hour or so.

Rather than trying to ask everything, ask questions in a structured way that will allow the examiner to see that you know the core information areas to be covered. So, rather than spending 3 minutes asking several questions about distractibility, make sure you have two or three questions for each of: inattentiveness, hyperactivity and impulsivity. Then quickly establish age of onset and impact before moving on.

ADDITIONAL POINTS

You should thank the mother for talking with you. Also explain that in order to be more certain of the nature of Simon's difficulties and how to best support him and his family, you will need to see him.

FURTHER READING

Taylor, D., Paton, C. & Kerwin, R. (2007) *The Maudsley Prescribing Guidelines*, 9th edn. London: Informa Healthcare, p. 281.

Taylor, E., Döpfner, M., Sergeant, J. et al. (2004) European clinical guidelines for hyperkinetic disorder – first upgrade. *European Child and Adolescent Psychiatry, 13* (Suppl. 1), i7–i30.

Chapter 5

Dr Justin Sauer

Learning disability psychiatry

◯ LINKED STATION 1

1a.

You are about to meet a member of staff from a local care home. They have brought a 37-year-old male resident, Mr Brian Harris, with Down's syndrome, to the A&E department following a change in his behaviour. They are concerned that he is withdrawn and no longer engaging in conversation. They think he has lost weight as he no longer eats well.

The triage nurse has asked for a psychiatric assessment as the patient has not allowed any investigations and has been pushing the nurses away when they try to examine him.

Prior to assessing the patient, gather collateral information that will inform your diagnosis.

1b.

This is Mr Harris. He has Down's syndrome and is much more withdrawn than usual.

Take a targeted history from this gentleman that will assist you in further management.

SINGLE STATIONS

2.

This is Michael Stern. He is 18 years old, has a learning disability and lives at home with his parents. His mother is his main carer. He also attends a special school.

Over the last few weeks he has become significantly more aggressive. This is mainly focused towards himself. He will bang his head repeatedly against the wall at home and he has been picking at his arms so that he has multiple skin lesions.

Assess this man and consider the important aetiological factors.

3.

Mr Roberts and his wife have come to see you. They had noticed that their son, now 4, had been slow to speak compared to his peers. He seemed to be clumsy and slower to learn in new situations.

He was seen by the paediatricians and diagnosed with fragile X syndrome following genetic testing.

The parents have been referred to your unit for advice because of his recent change in behaviour. They also want to know the risks of further children being born with this condition.

STATION 1

1a: Down's syndrome

KEY POINTS
History of presenting complaint
Behavioural history
Past psychiatric history
Social circumstances
Aetiological factors
Risk issues

INTRODUCE YOURSELF

'Hello, my name is Dr_____, one of the psychiatrists. Can I ask your name?'

SET THE SCENE

'Can I ask your role at the care home?'

'Could you tell me what's been happening for you to bring him to hospital today?'

COMPLETING THE TASKS

An accurate account of his change in behaviour is crucial:

How long has he been like this? When did it start?

Have the staff seen accounts/records of his previous behaviour?

Who knows him the longest? Would it be useful to speak to the GP/family?

Has anything changed e.g. how long has he been living in the current accommodation? (It transpires he's only recently moved in.)

Why did he move? What were the circumstances? Who was his previous primary carer?

Has he found it difficult to settle in? Has he made any friendships?

Have any close relationships changed (family/friend/staff/teacher)?

Have there been any bereavements?

Has there been a change in his routine?

Find out what the staff feel about him. Do they find him difficult to care for? If so, which aspects? Is this anything your team could help advise on?

In the aetiology, it is important to consider:

The environment (not happy with his accommodation or relations with staff).

Psychiatric illness (e.g. adjustment reaction/depression). He has some biological features of depression. Enquire about his sleep. Ask about his mood and irritability.

Organic causes (infection/hypothyroidism). Although only 37 years old, ask about any cognitive decline (risk of Alzheimer's disease (AD) with trisomy 21 – occurs 2 decades earlier).

Physical problems (e.g. pain/sensory impairment). Have the staff noticed he is avoiding urinating or is constipated?

Iatrogenic: Has he been started on medication recently or had any changes to dosages?

RISK

Enquire about any risky behaviour such as self-harm or voicing such thoughts. Have there been any previous attempts and what were the triggers? Has there been any aggression towards others? Does she think that anyone is taking advantage of him or behaving inappropriately with him?

PROBLEM SOLVING

There are a number of medical conditions associated with Down's syndrome. Has the GP been to see him and carried out any investigations? Explain that the following could be contributing to his presentation and ask about associated features of:

- hypothyroidism;
- obstructive sleep apnoea;
- epilepsy;
- visual or auditory impairments;
- gastrointestinal problems;
- cardiovascular conditions (mitral valve prolapse in adulthood);
- memory complaint (Alzheimer's disease).

ADDITIONAL POINTS

The life expectancy for this condition has improved considerably from the 20s to the 60s over the past 40 years. Bearing in mind the significant associated medical issues, it is recommended that they have regular health screening for thyroid function, cholesterol, blood pressure (BP), cardiovascular (including echo) and electroencephalogram (EEG) if required.

FURTHER READING

Baum, R.A., Nash, P.L., Foster, J.E., Spader, M., Ratliff-Schaub, K. & Coury, D.L. (2008) Primary care of children and adolescents with Down syndrome: an update. *Current Problems in Pediatric and Adolescent Health Care*, *38* (8), 241–61.

1b: Down's syndrome

KEY POINTS
Empathy and rapport
History of presenting complaint
Adequate reassurance
History of events
Aetiology – influences on behaviour
Risk issues

INTRODUCE YOURSELF

'Hello, my name is Dr____, it's nice to meet you.'

'Do you like to be called Mr Harris or Brian?'

SET THE SCENE

'How are you?'

'You seem to be sad. What's happened?'

'Is that why you don't want to talk?'

COMPLETING THE TASKS

This station follows on naturally from the first part of the link. You will hopefully have gained enough information to allow a more targeted interview.

You will need to be patient with Mr Harris and treat him with respect. Allow him enough time to answer questions. Keep your questioning simple and avoid complex ideas.

It seems to you that he is likely to be depressed and you follow that vein. If time allows you could expand your mental state examination.

Assessment of mood

Ask about his behaviour and why he is more withdrawn.

Has anything upsetting happened?

Ask if he becomes upset sometimes.

Does he ever become angry?

Does he ever cry/hurt himself/others?

Does he make it difficult for people to help him? Why?

Ask about previously pleasurable activities.

Ask what he thinks will happen to him. (The future)

What would he like to happen to him?

Does he want to get better?

Does he think he's been bad in some way? (Guilt)

Does he enjoy doing anything? (Anhedonia)

Ask about biological features of depression.

Assess for psychotic features (delusions/hallucinations).

Does he get muddled sometimes? (Cognition – explore further as required)

What does he think is wrong? (Insight)

Biological

Screening questions for hypothyroidism (e.g. do you prefer keeping warm?).

Ask about pain/physical discomfort.

You could ask about urinary or chest symptoms.

Ask about eyesight and hearing and whether they have worsened.

Social

Enquire about:

The move to the new home. Why had he moved? How has he settled in?

How does he get on with staff and residents?

Does he miss anyone?

Do they do things differently here? How? (Enquiries about routine)

Risk

Ask about suicidality. Ask if he felt threatened by anyone. Had anyone hurt him or upset him? If so, how? Had he felt like hurting anyone?

PROBLEM SOLVING

The main challenges are dealing with your own enthusiasm to get as much information as quickly as possible but at the same time interacting with someone who might be slow at answering and possibly difficult to interpret or engage. This is why you will need to demonstrate a rationale to your approach – a structure that makes sense to the examiner. It will be important to reassure the patient throughout and encourage him.

If the scenario were to progress and he asks about treatment, you should touch on both 'talking treatments' and 'medicine' for the treatment of depression.

ADDITIONAL POINTS

It is not uncommon for behavioural change to be attributed to the learning disability itself. Subsequently mental comorbidity such as depression or anxiety can often go untreated.

It is important to adopt a biopsychosocial model in your history taking and assessment so that all possibilities are considered. It is always useful to see the patient on their own, for part of the interview, so that they can answer for themselves and any pressure or coercion they feel will be lessened.

FURTHER READING

McGuire, D. & Chicoine, B. (2006) *Mental wellness in adults with Down syndrome: a guide to emotional and behavioural strengths and challenges*. USA: Woodbine House Inc. (8 Nov.).

STATION 2: Behavioural disturbance

> **KEY POINTS**
> Establish rapport
> Adequate reassurance
> Maximize communication
> History of events
> Aetiology – influences on behaviour
> Appropriate risk assessment

INTRODUCE YOURSELF

Do this normally – do not treat the patient like a child. Do not appear patronizing or over-familiar with him. Treat him with respect and if communication is difficult, adjust your style accordingly.

SET THE SCENE

'Your mum is worried about you – do you know why?'

'How have things been recently?'

'What happened to your arms?'

'Why have you done this?'

COMPLETING THE TASKS

Consider the aetiology using a biopsychosocial approach and enquire about the following in a way the patient can understand.

Related to the disability itself:	Specific conditions are known to have an association with behavioural disturbance e.g. Lesch–Nyhan syndrome, phenylketonuria, Cornelia de Lange syndrome, etc.
Psychiatric comorbidity:	e.g. depression, bipolar disorder, psychosis.
An organic disorder:	e.g. epilepsy, hypothyroidism, urinary tract infection (UTI).
Physical conditions:	e.g. constipation, oesophagitis/gastritis, dental caries (± pain), worsening sensory impairment (hearing/vision).
Iatrogenic:	medication: adverse effects (paradoxical agitation).
Substance misuse:	alcohol, amphetamines, solvents and withdrawal states.

Psychological

Look for evidence of emotional stress. Ask about familial relationships and recent stressors. Are there arguments at home or school? Consider any behavioural component to the self-harm and any positive gain. This should not be assumed to be 'attention-seeking behaviour' but rather a way of communicating distress or unpleasant feelings. More appropriate ways of communicating is something that a psychologist could assist with.

Social

Enquire about close relationships. Has anyone close to the family or friend/staff member from school moved away? Has the daily routine changed? Have they recently moved home or something changed at home?

PROBLEM SOLVING

This is a challenging station as you are attempting to take a history in a short period of time from someone who might not be forthcoming or who will be disturbed.

The actor will be instructed to give slow or delayed answers to your questions, so patience is key despite time pressures.

To help with communication you should:

- use simply phrased questions and concepts;
- use clear and direct language;
- keep reassuring the patient throughout;
- do not appear hurried or intimidating;
- allow time for answers – don't worry about silence;
- avoid jargon;
- use age-appropriate style and terminology;
- use body language/gesturing alongside speech if necessary;
- repeat questions if necessary.

ADDITIONAL POINTS

Risk assessment: always consider the possibility of physical, emotional or sexual abuse in vulnerable individuals. Ask about the self-harm and head-banging. Although such behaviours are most likely related to frustration or distress, you need to enquire about suicidality and homicidal thoughts.

Psychiatric illness is four times as common in learning disorders (LD) compared to the general population.

FURTHER READING

http://www.challengingbehaviour.org.uk. The Challenging Behaviour Foundation provides information and support to parents and carers of individuals with severe learning disabilities.

Emerson, E. (2001) *Challenging behaviour: analysis and intervention in people with severe intellectual disabilities*, 2nd edn. Cambridge: Cambridge University Press.

STATION 3: Fragile X syndrome

KEY POINTS
Empathy and rapport
Explanation of the condition
Exploring behavioural disturbance
Management advice
Genetic risk

INTRODUCE YOURSELF

'Hello, my name is Dr___, I'm one of the psychiatrists.'

SET THE SCENE

'Thank you for coming to see me today about your son. Can I ask his name?'

'I understand that you've seen the paediatric doctors recently. Is that correct?' 'Did they talk to you about his diagnosis?'

'It must be a worrying time for you since you found out about the diagnosis.'

'Can I ask what you already know about Fragile X Syndrome (FXS)?'

COMPLETING THE TASKS

Remember to talk in lay terms.

You could briefly demonstrate to the examiner your understanding of the condition by asking when the parents first became concerned. Had they noticed any unusual physical characteristics?

In FXS there is a problem with connective tissue development. Those with FXS can have double jointedness or lax joints. The skin may be soft, with a velvety texture. Testicular enlargement in men after puberty can be striking.

'Sometimes parents are concerned that their children's ears seem bigger than expected or with their child's face being large or longer. Are these things that you've noticed?'

Explain that these physical changes occur with FXS, particularly in boys (up to 80 per cent).

Intelligence may be impaired and 80 per cent of boys will have an IQ <70.

Behaviour

Ask about his current behaviour. Take a history of what is happening, frequency, triggers, how long it lasts and what seems to settle him, if anything.

Behaviour is often the presenting feature prior to formal diagnosis. Enquire about the following:

- speech disturbance (FXS speech has been described as jocular or cluttered);
- attentional deficit;
- mannerisms (commonly involving hands, flapping);

- autistic-like behaviour (accounts for perhaps 2 to 3 per cent of autism);
- sensory defensiveness (avoids loud noises, bright lighting, touch, strong smells);
- emotional instability;
- anxiety.

Management advice

A multi-disciplinary approach is advised and engagement with LD services is recommended.

Speech and language therapy

Can help with language development, impaired pronunciation and rate of speech. If speech is delayed they can help teach non-verbal ways of communicating.

Occupational therapy

Can help to adjust tasks and conditions to match his needs and abilities. It can also help with sensory defensiveness by using appropriate stimulatory or calming activities to alter his responses to sensations.

Physiotherapy

Can help to improve motor control, posture and balance. At school it can help a child who is easily over-stimulated or who avoids body contact to take part in sports.

Psychology

Can assist by teaching parents or teachers to identify why a child acts in certain ways and how to prevent distressing situations and to teach the child to cope with the distress.

Family support

Education: for child and family. It is also important that the school understand that he may have problems with auditory processing, concentration and abstract concepts.

Medication

Is used for behaviour where other interventions have been ineffective. Medication is not without risk of side effects and should be used cautiously. A proportion of children will need anticonvulsants for epilepsy and these drugs can also help with behavioural and mood instability. Sometimes different doses or combinations of medications are needed for maximum benefit. Stimulants such as methylphenidate can be of benefit where attention deficit or hyperactivity is pronounced. Similarly, aggression can be treated with mood stabilizers or antidepressants.

Risk to further child

FXS is the most common form of inherited intellectual disability. Although called FXS, the affected area isn't fragile at all. It's an area where there is an abnormal expansion of DNA material on the long arm of the X chromosome. Men have one X chromosome and women have two X chromosomes. Consequently this condition can affect both boys and girls.

As their son has the condition, he will have inherited it from his mother as she has passed on her X chromosome. As the mother has the premutation she will have a 50 per cent chance of passing it on to future sons and daughters.

You might suggest that formal genetic counselling is advisable if they are seriously considering more children. This service would be better able to advise on the chances of passing on the premutation or full mutation. Without the results of the parental genetic tests you would be unable to predict this accurately.

Should their son have children in the future, he will pass on the mutation to all his daughters, but to none of his sons.

PROBLEM SOLVING

It is important to consider the timescale of behavioural change. Enquire about other causes for this, for example an underlying physical illness (urinary tract infection (UTI)/pain), organic disorder (e.g. epilepsy) or concurrent mental illness.

Testing eyesight and hearing is essential. FXS is associated with short and long sightedness, squints and glue ear. These can aggravate speech and language problems and cause frustration.

ADDITIONAL POINTS

Follow-up and engagement with services is important to help the child as they develop. Epilepsy (20 per cent), challenging behaviour and mood disorders occur more frequently after puberty.

FXS usually occurs with an expansion of the FMR1 gene on the X chromosome, through CGG trinucleotide repeats. In the full mutation there are more than 200 repeats (normal <54).

Fragile X Society: http://www.fragilex.org.uk. UK registered charity providing support, information and friendship to families whose children and relatives have fragile X syndrome.

FURTHER READING

Hagerman, R.J. & Hagerman, P.J. (eds) (2002) *Fragile X syndrome – diagnosis, treatment and research*, 3rd edn. Baltimore, MD: John Hopkins University Press.

Chapter 6
Liaison psychiatry Dr Jayati Das-Munshi

O LINKED STATION 1

1a.

You are a liaison psychiatrist. The rheumatologist has asked you to see a lady who has been diagnosed with systemic lupus erythematosus (SLE) and antiphospholipid syndrome. Recent investigations, including magnetic resonance imaging (MRI), have indicated secondary small vessel disease.

She has been referred to you as she has become increasingly forgetful and reports that she frequently forgets where she was meant to be going when out driving her car.

Assess this lady's difficulties, carrying out any relevant brief cognitive testing.

1b.

The rheumatologist is interested to know your thoughts following your assessment.

Discuss this case with the referring practitioner and discuss how you think this lady should be managed from a psychiatric point of view.

O LINKED STATION 2

2a.

You are asked as a matter of urgency to see a young man who has stabbed himself and is refusing surgical treatment. The wound has been bandaged; however, the surgeons wish to take him to theatre and perform life-saving surgery, without which they feel he might die.

His mother reports that over the last year he has become more reclusive and withdrawn. In A&E he is mute and does not answer any of your questions.

You may wish to take notes as you will be asked to discuss his likely differential diagnosis and management with his mother, at the next station.

Take a history from this gentleman's mother and assess his capacity regarding consent to medical treatment. Assume that the gentleman is happy for you to communicate with his mother. You should not assess his capacity to consent to psychiatric treatment.

Feed back your findings to his mother.

2b.

The gentleman has been admitted to a surgical ward for treatment.

His mother would like to talk to you about her son's likely psychiatric diagnosis and treatment. She is fairly worried about the risk to himself if he were to go home from the surgical ward.

O LINKED STATION 3

3a.

You are asked to provide an opinion on a young lady referred by the Neurologists as she has become wheelchair bound and is no longer able to walk, over the last six months. All neurological investigations, including detailed neuro-imaging, have been reported as normal. She was the passenger in a tragic car accident six months previously, where her mother who was the driver was killed.

Take a history from this lady.

Conduct a mental status examination of this lady, eliciting any abnormal psychopathology.

Briefly summarize your findings to her father; assume that she has given consent for you to speak to her father.

You may wish to take notes as you will be asked to discuss this case in the next station.

3b.

The Neurology F2 doctor would like to discuss your findings and possible treatment and future prognosis with you.

Discuss your findings with the F2 doctor and outline the investigations, treatments and prognosis for this lady.

O LINKED STATION 4

4a.

You are a liaison psychiatrist. The surgical team ask you to see an elderly gentleman who was admitted two days ago for an elective surgical procedure. Post-operatively he has presented as 'confused' and uncooperative. His wife is by his bedside and is fairly concerned; she reports that he has a significant history of alcohol use. He has not yet been commenced on any treatment as the surgical team were not aware of his alcohol use.

Take a history from the gentleman's wife. You may want to take notes as in the next station you will be asked to discuss your findings and management.

You will not be asked to directly assess the gentleman in this station.

4b.

Discuss your findings with the surgical registrar. You should discuss the likely differential diagnosis, and advise them of further management.

SINGLE STATIONS

5

You are a liaison psychiatrist. The medical team call you to review an elderly man on a medical ward, who is being managed for an infective exacerbation of chronic obstructive airways disease. The medical F1 doctor reports that he has become 'acutely paranoid' and confused, frequently not knowing where he is. He believes that staff are trying to poison him and he refuses to eat or drink.

Assess this gentleman. There is also an F1 doctor present to whom you can speak to regarding this gentleman's recent medical management and any other collateral history you would like to enquire about.

Do not perform a full mini mental state exam or physical examination; however, you may wish to ask the patient a few relevant questions around cognition.

Spend the last minute summarizing your findings and the likely differential diagnosis to the F1 doctor, so that he may liaise with the rest of his team. You do not need to discuss management.

6

You are asked to see a young man in his 30s who has become increasingly anxious and depressed. He recently discovered that his partner is HIV positive.

The man is accompanied by his sister; assume that he has consented to your discussing his health with her.

Assess the gentleman and finish by explaining to him and his sister what you think the problem is and how you might go about managing it.

STATION 1

1a: Psychiatric lupus

KEY POINTS

Communication and empathy

Issues related to driving and cognitive impairment

Relevant history taking

Associated problems

Cognitive assessment

Feedback to patient

INTRODUCE YOURSELF

SET THE SCENE

Begin the station by introducing yourself to the patient. Explain that you have been asked by colleagues to have a brief discussion with her about her difficulties, and to provide a second opinion. Begin by asking her why she thinks she has been referred to you.

The candidate should make it clear that they are a psychiatrist and that the rheumatologists have asked for a second opinion. The candidate can begin the interview by informing the patient that they would like to ask her a few questions around her difficulties, including a few questions specifically testing her memory.

COMPLETING THE TASKS

1. Take a brief history
- Onset of difficulties, nature of difficulties, progression, in the context of SLE. Other exacerbating factors – adjusting to diagnosis, stressful life events, financial concerns e.g. secondary to loss of job.
- How memory problems have impacted on her functioning, including driving; e.g. does she need extra help for any activities of daily living, has she stopped work as a result?
- Screen for mood and anxiety disorders, psychotic symptoms, drug and alcohol use, other previous psychiatric history. Current medications – is she taking an antidepressant?

2. Brief risk assessment – including risk to self, driving. Communicate concerns around driving to patient.

3. Brief cognitive testing
- Mini mental state examination (MMSE) + frontal lobe tests.
- (If time permits, tailor to history): Additional simple questions e.g. knowledge of recent news events/current affairs, draw a clock face, parietal lobe tests, etc.

4. Thank the patient and conclude the station.

ADDITIONAL POINTS

This station should be handled in the same way as assessing memory problems in any other context (e.g. old-age psychiatry). It is important to ensure that a functional psychiatric illness, such as depression, is not masquerading as memory disturbance. Underlying vascular disease in the brain may also predispose to secondary mood and psychotic disorders.

The Driver and Vehicle Licensing Agency (DVLA) has issued fairly clear guidelines on driving for a number of conditions (see *For medical practitioners: at a glance guide to the current medical standards of fitness to drive*. DVLA: Swansea (2007). Available: http://www.dvla.gov.uk/media/pdf/medical/aagv1.pdf).

1b: Psychiatric lupus

KEY POINTS
Communication with a colleague
Differential diagnosis
History discussion
Psychiatric management
Further investigations
Driving and the DVLA

INTRODUCE YOURSELF

SET THE SCENE

Begin this station by introducing yourself to the examiner (referring practitioner). Thank him/her for the referral.

COMPLETING THE TASKS

Discuss your main findings and likely differential diagnosis.

Discuss management and further investigations.

Discuss the issue of driving and the DVLA.

ADDITIONAL POINTS

Likely differential diagnosis: Untreated depression, vascular dementia.

Further investigations:

(Biological investigations) urine drug screen; (if not already carried out by referrer): dementia screen – B12/folate/TFTs (thyroid function tests), other vascular risk factors, relevant neuroimaging.

⇧ (Psychological investigations) Formal neuropsychological assessment/testing. Objective rating scales for mood, e.g. Beck's Depressive Inventory both pre and post treatment with an antidepressant.

(Social investigations) Collateral history from a family member or friend would be extremely important to obtain. Occupational therapy assessment. Objective rating scales e.g. Global Assessment of Functioning might also be used.

Management:

The history and examination suggest that this lady may be suffering from co-morbid depression. Treat depression, and suggest to the referring practitioner that she should have her memory and mood reassessed at a suitable time point (e.g. 2–3 months). Offer to follow this patient up frequently in the initial stages of treatment. Suitable treatment might include a selective serotonin reuptake inhibitor (SSRI) (although note contraindications with increased risk of GI bleed if prescribed aspirin for pro-thrombotic tendencies (Taylor et al., 2007)), or other antidepressants such as mirtazapine or venlafaxine. Other possibilities might include psychological interventions (cognitive behavioural therapy (CBT)), although underlying cognitive impairment may limit how far the patient is able to take part in this therapy. She may benefit from supportive counselling if she is finding it difficult to adjust to the diagnosis. Simple aids could be suggested to help with her memory problems, e.g. dosette box for medications, a diary and wall clock with date for appointments, calendars, alarms.

- As this is a liaison psychiatry station, how the candidate discusses these possibilities with the referrer will be assessed.
- Suggest to the practitioner that you are concerned about this lady continuing to drive at this point in time, as she appears to have greatly impaired recent memory, and this could impact on her judgement. Indicate to the practitioner that you would suggest that she stops driving for now, and that she could be referred for further neuropsychological testing which may inform medical recommendations to the DVLA. She should also inform her insurers. The issue of driving could be revisited after her depressive illness has been adequately treated and her memory problems have been reassessed. If she can demonstrate that her skills are sufficiently retained and that the progression of the underlying brain impairment is slow, she may be able to drive subject to annual review/a formal driving assessment (DVLA, 2007).

FURTHER READING

DVLA (2007) *For medical practitioners: at a glance guide to the current medical standards of fitness to drive.* Swansea: DVLA. http://www.dvla.gov.uk/media/pdf/medical/aagv1.pdf

Taylor, D., Paton, C. & Kerwin, R. (2007) *The Maudsley Prescribing Guidelines*, 9th edn. London: Informa Health Care.

STATION 2

2a: Risk and consent to treatment

KEY POINTS

Empathy, rapport and communication skills

Attempts to communicate with the patient, who is mute

Check with patient if he is able/willing to communicate using other means (e.g. written instructions)

Relevant history taking from mother as patient is not communicative

Feed back findings to mother

INTRODUCE YOURSELF

SET THE SCENE

This is a difficult situation, and you can say so, as part of your opening introduction. Make attempts to establish rapport with the patient and their mother. Despite the gravity of the situation, you should assume that the patient has capacity unless you are able to prove otherwise.[1]

COMPLETING THE TASKS

1. Take a brief history. As the patient is not communicating at this stage, this should be done through the family member.
- Clarify age of patient.
- Circumstances leading to the current presentation; how was the patient found, what events preceded him stabbing himself?
- Onset and nature of any mental health difficulties, preceding the attempt by the patient to stab himself. Was there a clear change in mental state noted by his mother over preceding days/months?
- Is there a preceding history of potential prodromal features to a psychotic episode, e.g. social withdrawal, decline in functioning, apathy/loss of drive, odd behaviour?
- Or is there a possible preceding history of a mood disorder: stressful life events, history of affective symptoms/biological features of depression, noted by mother?
- History of previous bizarre behaviour or bizarre beliefs expressed to/noted by mother; is there a possible prior history of auditory hallucinations?
- Is there a previous psychiatric history, including previous attempts to harm self? Concerns by family member as to his self-harm/suicide risk?
- Is there a family history of psychosis, suicide, depression?
- Is there a history of illicit substance misuse/dependency (cannabis, cocaine, etc.), alcohol misuse or dependency?
- Is there any forensic history of note?

2. Assess the patient's mental state and capacity to accept or decline treatment.
- Mental state examination in this station will be merely an observation as you will not be able to communicate with the patient. It may be worth noting if he appears to be responding to internal stimuli (e.g. auditory or visual hallucinations), and you may wish to examine him, if appropriate, for associated catatonic features.

- In this station the patient is mute and will not be able to communicate with you either verbally or otherwise; however, you must show that you have made attempts to communicate adequately with the patient, and you may wish to check this with his relative.
- You may wish to check with his mother if her son has any pre-existing religious or cultural beliefs which might have affected his decision (e.g. Jehovah's witness, blood products, etc.).

3. Turn to the patient's mother and summarize your findings and likely diagnosis.
- Given the history and the patient's presentation (which represents a clear change in mental state indicative of an underlying mental disorder – which you will elaborate upon in the next station), it is likely that on balance of probabilities, this patient lacks capacity to consent to treatment for his injury.
- You should explain to his mother that given the urgency of the situation (life threatening) the medical team should be advised to act in his best interests; however, his capacity will need to be reassessed once his medical condition has been adequately managed.

ADDITIONAL POINTS

Candidate should explain that as this is a life-threatening situation, measures should be taken to act in the patient's best interests; however, his capacity for any further interventions should be reassessed when he has had treatment for the injury.

The history and clinical presentation noted in this station should allow you to summarize the likely differential diagnosis and likely management to the examiner in the next station. The marks awarded in this station are mostly for history taking, brief risk assessment, difficult communication, and brief case discussion (with the patient's mother).

The general principles around assessment of capacity still apply.[1] Based on the history it seems likely that the gentleman has an impairment or disturbance of the mind which at present makes him unable to make a decision regarding surgical treatment, and may be affecting his ability to weigh up and use information as part of the decision-making process. However, he is unable to communicate directly with you, and so you have been unable to **directly** assess whether he has fulfilled the basic functional tests of capacity, i.e. 1) Does he understand all relevant information; 2) Can he retain that information; 3) Can he use or weigh up that information as part of the decision-making process[1]? Based on a balance of probabilities you may argue that this gentleman at present lacks capacity regarding potential surgical treatment, and that a decision will need to be taken in his best interests.

---

1. Booklets on all aspects of the Mental Capacity Act can be downloaded from: http://www.dca.gov.uk/legal-policy/mental-capacity/publications.htm#mental.

2b: Risk and consent to treatment

KEY POINTS

Empathy and sensitivity towards the patient's mother

Clear discussion of likely diagnosis and differential diagnosis

Risk assessment

Discussion of other potential investigations which may be needed

Clear discussion of management in the short, medium and long term

Management and investigations should include a discussion of psychological and
   social as well as biological interventions

SET THE SCENE

Introduce yourself again to the patient's mother. The actress playing the role of the mother may initiate the discussion by explaining her concerns. You may therefore wish to start this station with a fairly open statement.

COMPLETING THE TASKS

1. Discuss the likely differential diagnosis: e.g. first-episode psychosis/paranoid schizophrenia, depression, drug-induced psychosis

2. Risk – Obtain further history from mother under relevant risk areas, elicit whether she has any other concerns around his risk and why she is concerned about him, if he were to go home.

- Risk to self (self-harm) – previous self-harm or suicide attempts, did he express his wish to harm himself to anyone beforehand, or was he secretive/attempted to avoid being found, after he stabbed himself?

- Risk to self (self-neglect) – Had he been eating and drinking adequately/any concerns about oral intake and weight loss? Any concerns over his personal care?

- Risk from others – Had his mother been concerned about his vulnerability to exploitation by others?

- Risk to others – Any associated forensic history, has he ever attempted to harm anyone else? Has he ever expressed a wish to harm others? Does he have children? Children on child protection register?

3. Further investigations might include:

- Biological – Urine drug screen (note recent National Institute for Health and Clinical Excellence (NICE) recommendations (2008) which have concluded that neuroimaging should not be a routine investigation in psychosis unless other organic causes are suspected), basic bloods including thyroid function tests, assessment of alcohol withdrawal if appropriate.

- Psychological – objective rating scales e.g. Brief Psychiatric Rating Scale (BPRS)/Beck Depression Inventory (BDI) if communicative.

- Social – further collateral history from other relatives/partner/other agencies e.g. if has children. Risk assessment can be enhanced through collateral history.

4. Management:

- You should explain that once he is medically stable you will want to reassess his mental state and consent to psychiatric treatment. You may have to consider an assessment under the Mental Health Act, with a view to an admission for a period of assessment. However, you would need to check with her son if he is willing to accept treatment informally first.

- Management: You may wish to consider (in short term): Medication e.g. commencing an atypical neuroleptic at the doses recommended by NICE guidelines (2002); 1:1 Registered Mental Nurse (RMN) input on surgical ward, given ongoing concerns around possible harm to himself; possibly suggest assessment under Section 5(2) of the Mental Health Act to surgical team if he attempts to leave and they are concerned about his risk to himself or his safety.
- Management (in longer term) (NICE, 2002): Referral to first onset psychosis team or community mental health team; consider Care Programme Approach. Monitor response to medication/side effects and titrate dose accordingly, provide support/referral to services for any substance misuse issues if appropriate, family therapy (if family agreeable), CBT or other psychological approaches if it was felt he would be able to work with this model of therapy, consider longer-term support for social skills, assistance with employment/further education goals/housing and benefits etc.

ADDITIONAL POINTS

The vignette indicates that risk assessment is an important part of this station and will influence your subsequent management plan.

Biological, psychological and social approaches should be considered when thinking about investigation and management of this patient.

FURTHER READING

NICE (February 2008) *Structural neuro-imaging in first episode psychosis.* http://www.nice.nhs.uk/nicemedia/pdf/TA136Guidance.pdf

NICE (December 2002) *Schizophrenia: core interventions in the treatment and management of schizophrenia in primary and secondary care.* Clinical guideline 1: http://www.nice.nhs.uk/nicemedia/pdf/CG1NICEguideline.pdf

STATION 3

3a: Dissociative (conversion) disorder

KEY POINTS

Communication, empathy

History taking: Exploration of circumstances surrounding the accident and her own beliefs around this (guilt, blame, views about the future)

Mental state examination and brief risk assessment

Patient's own beliefs of potential causation/aetiology

Patient's own views around accepting psychiatric treatment, including psychological treatments

Summarizing findings to lay relative

INTRODUCE YOURSELF

SET THE SCENE

Begin the station by explaining that you have been asked by your Neurology colleagues to provide an opinion on this lady's difficulties. Start off by asking her what her difficulties are and why she believes she has been referred to see you.

The candidate should make it clear that they are a psychiatrist and that the neurologists have asked for a second opinion. The candidate can begin the interview by informing the patient that they would like to ask her a few questions around her difficulties.

COMPLETING THE TASKS

1. Take a brief history.
- Demonstrate an empathic and sensitive approach to the patient, especially when exploring aspects of the accident with her. Elicit from the patient and her father whether they were in agreement with the referral or whether they feel that there is an underlying undiagnosed physical cause.
- Nature of difficulties, onset and chronology with respect to the accident.
- Other aspects of history: previous psychiatric or medical history, drug and alcohol use, prior premorbid functioning, previous childhood abuse, previous medical illnesses in childhood/time off school, illnesses in parents, long periods of sickness (Bass and May, 2002), current familial/social support, pending litigation, potential secondary gain from disability/the consequences of recovery versus ongoing disability (WHO, 1992), current input (e.g. physiotherapy) for her difficulties.
- Her view of the difficulties. What does she think is causing her mobility problems? What is her view on treatment; specifically, what is her view on psychological therapies? What is her view for the future? Does she think she can ever get better or does she view herself as permanently disabled?
- What has she been told by other medical practitioners? Has she had all results of investigations explained to her? Does she feel reassurance that neuroimaging and other investigations have been reported as normal?
- Mental state exam: Ensure that no abnormal or psychotic beliefs are apparent. Exclude depressive and anxiety symptomatology. Ensure that no symptoms indicative of an atypical grief reaction are present.

2. Thank the lady and conclude the discussion by briefly summarizing your findings to her and her father. Address any concerns which she or her father may have.

ADDITIONAL POINTS

Dissociative motor disorders are classically associated 'with traumatic events, insoluble and intolerable problems, or disturbed relationships', and have a psychogenic origin (WHO, 1992). Patients may show a 'striking denial' of obvious problems or difficulties, despite these being fairly apparent to observers, and may attribute distress to the resulting disability instead (WHO, 1992). Calm acceptance of disability ('belle indifference') may also be apparent (WHO, 1992), although this is not necessary for diagnosis and may be present in only 6–41 per cent of patients (Brown, 2006). For a diagnosis of a dissociative motor disorder, it should be possible to make a clear psychological formulation of why the patient is presenting in this way at this time (WHO, 1992).

⇧ Dissociative disorders frequently present with other comorbid psychiatric conditions, with comorbid mood and anxiety disorders reported in up to 80 per cent, and comorbid personality disorders also frequently reported (Ovsiew, 2006). Candidates should ensure that they have screened for other functional comorbidities, as presence of these will influence management decisions, discussed in the next station.

Explaining your thoughts to the patient and her father may on the surface appear difficult. However, a collaborative and flexible approach (suggested by Bass and May, 2002) when assessing patients with multiple functional somatic symptoms may also be relevant here. For example, interview cues such as 'I wonder if you've thought of it like this?', or making tentative 'reframing' links between the trauma and the onset/temporal sequence of the symptoms, may be helpful to the patient.

In an ideal situation you would have at least an hour (and possibly further interviews!) to see a patient like this, so you may also wish to conclude the interview by indicating that you would like to see them again, with more time in hand to explore some of the difficult issues touched upon in this very brief review.

FURTHER READING

Bass, C. & May S. (2002) Clinical review: ABC of psychological medicine. Chronic multiple functional somatic symptoms. *British Medical Journal, 325,* 323–6.

Brown, R.J. (2006) Chapter 16: Dissociation & conversion in psychogenic illness; in M. Hallett, S. Fahn, J. Jankovic, A.E. Lang, C.R. Cloninger & S.C. Yudofsky (eds) *Psychogenic Movement Disorders: Neurology & Neuropsychiatry.* Philadelphia: AAN Press.

Ovsiew, F. (2006) Chapter 14: An overview of the psychiatric approach to conversions disorder; in M. Hallett, S. Fahn, J. Jankovic, A.E. Lang, C.R. Cloninger & S.C. Yudofsky (eds) *Psychogenic Movement Disorders: Neurology & Neuropsychiatry.* Philadelphia: AAN Press.

WHO (1992) *The ICD-10 classification of mental and behavioural disorders: Clinical descriptions and diagnostic guidelines.* Geneva: WHO.

3b: Dissociative (conversion) disorder

> **KEY POINTS**
> Communication with a colleague
> Differential diagnosis
> Brief summary of relevant/salient findings
> Psychiatric management, in the medium and long term
> Likely prognosis

INTRODUCE YOURSELF

SET THE SCENE

Begin this station by introducing yourself to the referring practitioner (F2 doctor). Thank him/her for the referral.

COMPLETING THE TASKS

1. Discuss your main findings and likely differential diagnosis.
- The history and examination suggest that this lady is suffering from a fairly clear dissociative motor disorder.
- You should highlight to the referrer whether or not you thought there was any other psychiatric comorbidity present, such as major depression, anxiety, or substance misuse.
- You may wish to highlight to the referrer aspects of the history in support of this diagnosis.

2. Discuss further investigations and management.
- You may want to highlight to the referrer that this is a complicated presentation and you would usually want more time to conduct the assessment, and that part of your plan might be to review this lady and her father again, in order to gain further information.
- You should discuss management with the referrer in the same way as for other stations, i.e.:

Biological:	**Investigations:** Obtain confirmation that there is no comorbid history of illicit substance misuse, possibly by obtaining a urine drug screen, check bloods and ensure that these are normal. You may want to specify thyroid function tests to exclude underlying endocrine abnormalities. **Management:** Treat a depressive/anxiety disorder if there is evidence of this on mental status examination; suggest an SSRI as appropriate. She may need a referral to physiotherapy if there is evidence of atrophy of leg muscles, and input from the physiotherapist may also include a programme of graded exercise (Gill and bass, 1997).
Psychological:	**Investigations:** Psychological rating scales such as the Beck Depression Inventory (BDI) (Beck et al., 1961) or the Hospital Anxiety and Depression Rating scale (Zigmond and Smaith, 1983) are useful for objective measures of depression or anxiety. If she is clinically depressed, the BDI can also be used to monitor response to treatment. **Management:** Cognitive behavioural therapy may be appropriate if she can demonstrate the ability to fruitfully use this approach, and is keen to consider this. Bereavement counselling may be appropriate if there are unresolved grief issues related to the accident. You may also want to suggest suitable literature or self-help books, and suggest patient/user groups for added support (Gill and Bass, 1997). It may be important to involve the patient's father/social network in any programme of psychological therapy, especially if secondary gain has become prominent, for example in supporting the family to allow the patient to become independent over maintaining a passive/dependent role (Gill and Bass, 1997).
Social:	**Investigations:** Suggest that you would like to obtain further collateral medical and social history from this lady's GP. You may want to explore this lady's social network, and pre-morbid role/social functioning in further detail at the next review (this may provide clues to other unconscious motives). **Management:** This should be tailored to her social circumstances. If at all possible, a return to work/education may play an important part in longer-term rehabilitation, although in some cases work may be another form of stress to the patient, and could impede rehabilitation (Gill and Bass, 1997).

3. Give an indication of longer-term follow-up and prognosis.

These cases can be difficult to manage, although positive factors relating to her prognosis include clear onset following a psychological stressor, good pre-morbid functioning and family/social support networks, and a recent onset with short associated history (Gill and Bass, 1997).

ADDITIONAL POINTS

As this section focuses on management it may be fruitful to divide up aetiology into 'predisposing', 'precipitating' and 'maintaining' factors, and suggest strategies to deal with each, using a bio-psychosocial framework.

FURTHER READING

Bass, C. & May, S. (2002) Clinical review: ABC of psychological medicine. Chronic multiple functional somatic symptoms. *British Medical Journal*, *325*, 323–6.

Beck, A.T., Ward, C.H., Mendelson, M., Mock, J. & Erbaugh, J. (1961) An inventory for measuring depression. *Archives of General Psychiatry*, *4*, 53–63.

Gill, D. & Bass, C. (1997) Somatoform & dissociative disorders: assessment & treatment. *Advances in Psychiatric Treatment*, *3*, 9–16.

Zigmond, A.S. & Snaith, R.P. (1983) The Hospital Anxiety & Depression Rating Scale. *Acta Psychiatrica Scandinavica*, *67*, 361–70.

STATION 4

4a: Alcohol problems on a surgical ward

KEY POINTS
Communication skills, professionalism
History taking from an informant (patient's wife)
Alcohol history taking, focus on reaching a differential diagnosis

INTRODUCE YOURSELF

SET THE SCENE

Introduce yourself to the patient's wife. Begin by explaining that you have been asked by the surgical team to provide an opinion on her husband's confusion. Aside from focusing on alcohol use, you should also enquire after other possible causes contributing to her husband's confusional state. Clues to the diagnosis will be apparent by getting a clear picture of his pre-morbid functioning, as well as onset of the current presentation and reported psychopathology. The vignette suggests that alcohol use is an important part of the presentation, so you should ensure that you leave enough time to take an adequate alcohol history.

COMPLETING THE TASKS

1. Take a corroborative history from the gentleman's wife.
- When did she first notice that he was more confused? Was his confusional state fairly sudden/acute in onset (onset pre or post operative procedure?)
- Clarify from his wife in what way he is 'confused' (e.g. disorientated, paranoid, not recognizing her, memory difficulties and confabulation). Is there evidence of night-time confusion? Evidence of agitation? Is there evidence of clouding of consciousness/sensorium? Are there tactile disturbances (Kosten and O'Connor, 2003)?
- Has he been hallucinating? (Visual e.g. Lilliputian, insects] or auditory hallucinations?) Have there been any concerns around his behaviour, e.g. agitation, anxiety? Is there a tremor? Is he sweating (Kosten and O'Connor, 2003)?
- Is there a previous history of medical or psychiatric comorbidity? Is he prescribed any medication? Is there a previous history of admission for alcohol detoxification/input from alcohol detoxification services? Is there a history of psychiatric service involvement? Is there a previous history of delirium tremens or severe alcohol withdrawal/alcohol-withdrawal-related seizures? Is there a history of (other) illicit substance misuse?
- Pre-morbid functioning: Is there a pre-existing history of memory problems/cognitive impairment? What was his level of functioning prior to admission – was this affected by his alcohol use and/or memory problems? Was there a pre-morbid history of apathy, increased dependency on wife for activities of daily living etc., prior to admission?

2. Take a detailed alcohol history from his wife:
- When was his last drink (NB: signs of alcohol withdrawal peak within 24–48 hours (Taylor et al., 2007))?
- Current (pre-admission) alcohol use (drinks every day or days off from alcohol use?); what is his current pattern of use, what time does he usually have his first drink, and how much is his average daily intake (units)? Has there been evidence of narrowing of drinking repertoire (WHO, 1992)?
- Does she think he has problems controlling onset, levels, and termination of use? Does he crave alcohol? Does he ever drink to blackout? At home, is he secretive with respect to his alcohol use? Does he drink to the detriment of other interests/activities? Have there been any medical, psychological or social consequences to him from alcohol use? Does he continue to drink despite this? Is there evidence of tolerance? Has his wife ever noted features of alcohol withdrawal?
- Does she know how old he was when he first started to drink and when his alcohol use first started to escalate? Has he had any periods of abstinence or input from Alcoholics Anonymous?

ADDITIONAL POINTS

The primary diagnosis should be severe alcohol withdrawal or alcohol-withdrawal-associated confusional state ('delirium tremens') on a background of alcohol dependence (Taylor et al., 2007). This is a life-threatening condition associated with convulsions (Kosten and O'Connor, 2003). Delirium tremens is characterized by clouding of sensorium or acute confusional state, tactile disturbances, auditory and visual hallucinations, agitation and severe tremor (Kosten and O'Connor, 2003). Be also vigilant to a possible diagnosis of Wernicke's encephalopathy, characterized by a classic triad of confusion, ataxia and ophthalmoplegia (Thompson et al., 2002). It is more common than usually thought, and frequently missed or under-treated (Thompson et al., 2002). All patients presenting with

⇧ severe alcohol withdrawal should always be treated with parenteral thiamine (Taylor et al., 2007; Kosten and O'Connor, 2003).

For a diagnosis of alcohol dependence (F10.2) according to ICD-10, there should be evidence of the presence of a 'cluster of behavioural, cognitive, and physiological phenomena that develop after repeated substance use and that typically include a strong desire to take the drug, difficulties in controlling its use, persisting in its use despite harmful consequences, a higher priority given to drug use than to other activities and obligations, increased tolerance, and sometimes a physical withdrawal state' (Taylor et al., 2007).

FURTHER READING

Kosten, T.R. & O'Connor, P.G. (2003) Management of drug and alcohol withdrawal. *New England Journal of Medicine*, 348, 1786–95.

Taylor, D., Paton, C. & Kerwin, R. (2007) *The Maudsley Prescribing Guidelines*, 9th edn. London: Informa Healthcare, p. 465.

Thomson, A.D., Cook, C.H.C., Touquet, R. & Henry, J.A. (2002) Invited special article: The Royal College of Physicians Report on Alcohol: Guidelines for managing Wernicke's encephalopathy in the Accident and Emergency Department. *Alcohol & Alcoholism*, 37 (6), 513–21.

WHO (1992) *The ICD-10 classification of mental and behavioural disorders: Clinical descriptions and diagnostic guidelines*. Geneva: WHO.

4b: Management of alcohol problems on a surgical ward

KEY POINTS

Communication skills, professionalism

Concise summary of findings with salient features

Discussion of further information or details of any investigations/examinations that the candidate would like to perform/obtain. This may include suggesting further input from the medical team.

Likely differential diagnosis

Discussion of management (immediate/ acute management)

Discussion of management (longer term)

INTRODUCE YOURSELF

SET THE SCENE

Introduce yourself to the Surgical Registrar.

COMPLETING THE TASKS

1. Begin by summarizing your findings, focusing on salient points gleaned from the previous station.

2. Discuss the likely differential diagnosis (acute confusional state secondary to alcohol

withdrawal/delirium tremens, acute confusional state secondary to other causes, Wernicke's encephalopathy).

3. Explain that you would want further information prior to confirming diagnosis:
- This should include interview and examination of the patient (MMSE, other tests of cognition, clinical examination – signs of alcohol withdrawal (Taylor et al., 2007) and neurological examination. If there was a pre-morbid history of memory problems with acute-onset confusional state then also consider causes of acute-on-chronic confusional states (e.g. superimposed on a possible dementia).
- Further investigations – Basic bloods including full blood count (FBC), urea and electrolytes (U&Es), liver function tests (LFTs), septic screen, urine drug screen, breathalyser (for blood alcohol concentration). Computed tomography (CT)/MRI brain scan if neurological features evident, or a history of pre-morbid memory problems present.

4. Discuss the management (acute/immediate management)
- If severe withdrawal from alcohol is suspected, suggest intravenous (IV) diazepam. As seizures may be a feature of severe withdrawal/delirium tremens, the candidate may also be inclined to suggest an opinion from the medical team, particularly as electrolyte abnormalities may occur and parenteral fluid support may be needed (Taylor et al., 2007; Kosten and O'Connor, 2003).
- If less severe, commence on regime of chlordiazepoxide or diazepam. Consider oxazepam if there are concerns over the patient's liver function. (Good candidates may give an example of an appropriate treatment regime with example dosing (Taylor et al., 2007)).
- 'Stat' dose of benzodiazepine, depending on blood alcohol concentration and withdrawal features (Taylor et al., 2007).
- Titrate dose to alcohol withdrawal symptoms (candidate could suggest the use of objective rating scales for surgical nursing staff to use on the ward (e.g. Clinical Institute Withdrawal Assessment of Alcohol scale, revised (CIWA-Ar) (Sullivan et al., 1989)). In addition, pulse and blood pressure should be monitored. In severe withdrawal institute frequent (1–2 hourly) monitoring of observations (Kosten and O'Connor, 2003).
- Commence dose reduction of benzodiazepine after initial period of assessment (24 hours). This should be tailored to patient's withdrawal symptoms; general rule of thumb is to reduce by 20 per cent of baseline dose each day (Taylor et al., 2007). The candidate may also suggest prn Benzodiazepine for 'break-through' symptoms.
- All patients presenting with features of alcohol dependence should also be commenced on intramuscular (i.m.) thiamine, to prevent development of Wernicke's encephalopathy. Intravenous thiamine is preferred if a diagnosis of Wernicke–Korsakov is suspected. Give for five days, followed by oral thiamine supplementation (Taylor et al., 2007; Thomson et al., 2002).

5. Discuss the management (medium/longer term)
- The candidate should suggest that they will return to review the patient's mental state post-detoxification, for signs of cognitive impairment, or psychopathology.
- The candidate may suggest assessing the patient's motivation at this time to address his alcohol use.
- Post successful detoxification, the patient should be given details of self-referral to local alcohol services, or hospital liaison alcohol services (if available). Psychosocial measures will be needed to maintain long-term abstinence (individual/motivational input, group psychological input, etc.).
- If there is evidence of cognitive impairment, the candidate may suggest neuroimaging and referral to Older Adult services for follow-up (especially if there is evidence of impact on functioning and the possibility of underlying cognitive

impairment). Suggest occupational therapy (OT) assessment if there are related concerns over functioning at home.

- The candidate should recommend to the surgical team that the patient is discharged with thiamine supplements.

ADDITIONAL POINTS

As this is a diagnosis and management station a helpful structure would be:

- Present the likely differential diagnosis (suggest most likely diagnosis first). Support the differential diagnoses by salient findings gleaned from the history which you gathered in the first station.
- List any further investigations or assessments you may need to complete (as you have not seen the patient yet, a good starting point would be to run through examination of the patient, and the clinical features you would look for).
- Discuss the management: Acute management should be followed by medium- to longer-term management. Consider the 'bio-psychosocial' model for this section of the station.

The Clinical Institute Withdrawal Assessment of Alcohol scale (CIWA-Ar) is a 10-item scale measuring features of alcohol withdrawal over a variety of domains. Each section is scored from 0–7. For severe withdrawal, patients score >15. For moderate withdrawal, patients score 8–15. In mild withdrawal, patients score <8 (Taylor et al., 2007). High-scoring patients are at an increased risk of convulsions and delirium (Kosten and O'Connor, 2003).

Wernicke's encephalopathy is a frequently under-diagnosed condition, associated with high levels of morbidity and mortality. The classic clinical triad of confusion, ataxia and ophthalmoplegia is in fact seen in less than a third. Untreated, Wernicke's encephalopathy proceeds to Korsakoff's psychosis, with high personal and social costs. Malnutrition with chronic alcohol use are risk factors for the development of Wernicke's encephalopathy (Thomson et al., 2002). Current treatment recommendations suggest 'one pair IM/IV ampoules high potency B-complex vitamins daily over 3–5 days' (Taylor et al., 2007), as oral thiamine is poorly absorbed (Thomson et al., 2002). Glucose should not be given without thiamine as this may precipitate Wernicke's encephalopathy (Taylor et al., 2007; Thomson et al., 2002).

FURTHER READING

Kosten, T.R. & O'Connor, P.G. (2003) Management of drug and alcohol withdrawal. *New England Journal of Medicine*, 348, 1786–95.

Sullivan, J.T. et al. (1989) Assessment of alcohol withdrawal: the revised Clinical Institute Withdrawal Assessment for Alcohol scale (CIWA-Ar). *British Journal of Addiction*, 84, 1353–7.

Taylor, D., Paton, C. & Kerwin, R. (2007) *The Maudsley Prescribing Guidelines*, 9th edn. London: Informa Healthcare, p. 465.

Thomson, A.D., Cook, C.H.C., Touquet, R. & Henry, J.A. (2002) Invited special article: The Royal College of Physicians Report on Alcohol: Guidelines for managing Wernicke's encephalopathy in the Accident and Emergency Department. *Alcohol & Alcoholism*, 37 (6), 513–21.

STATION 5: Acute confusional state

KEY POINTS

Communication skills, professionalism

History taking from patient

Mental state exam and very brief cognitive assessment of patient

Collateral history taking from attending FY1 doctor

Brief summary of correct diagnosis and likely differential diagnosis to F1 doctor

---

INTRODUCE YOURSELF

SET THE SCENE

Introduce yourself to the patient and to the medical F1 doctor. Begin by explaining to the patient that you have been asked by the medical team to provide an opinion regarding current difficulties. Given the vignette you should already be considering possible organic causes for the presentation, so you may wish to make apparent at this stage that you will want to ask the patient questions around his orientation, as well as review the history and recent medical management/medications with the F1 doctor.

COMPLETING THE TASKS

1. Take a brief history and mental state examination from the patient.
- Clarify with the patient why he has not been eating and drinking. Does he have any other abnormal or delusional beliefs?
- Is there a current or previous history of alcohol or substance misuse?
- Mental state exam and brief cognitive assessment: Is the patient orientated and lucid?

2. Brief history from the F1 doctor:
- How long has he been an in-patient, and when did the team first notice the problems? Did the change in mental state come on abruptly or gradually? Has there been an associated history of fluctuating lucidity/disorientation/changes to consciousness and attention? Is there an associated history of visual hallucinations? Any obvious changes to the patient's sleep–wake cycle, or emotional disturbances e.g. emotional lability?
- Is there a previous history of psychiatric problems or memory problems? Previous history of delirium? What is the state of his current physical health and are there any other medical problems of note? Has he been prescribed any new medications (e.g. steroids, antibiotics)? Had his family expressed any concerns around pre-morbid memory and functioning?
- What is the team's future medical plan? What have been the results of any relevant investigations?

3. Summarize findings and likely differential diagnosis to the F1 doctor.

ADDITIONAL POINTS

ICD-10 defines delirium as an 'etiologically non-specific syndrome characterised by concurrent disturbances of consciousness and attention, perception, thinking, memory, psychomotor behaviour, emotion and the sleep-wake cycle' (WHO, 1992). If there is no previous psychiatric history of note and the problems are of

⇧ relatively recent and rapid onset (usually less than six months) then delirium or acute confusional state should be considered. According to ICD-10 criteria, for a diagnosis of delirium, symptoms in each of the areas should be present: 1) impairment of consciousness and attention; 2) global disturbance of cognition, with perceptual disturbances (which usually tend to be visual hallucinations); 3) psychomotor disturbances; 4) emotional disturbances.

Other potential differential diagnoses might include a mood disorder, an acute psychotic episode, or (pre-existing) dementia/delirium superimposed on dementia.

Potential causes of an acute confusional state in this case might include: infection (chest infection, urinary tract infection), medications/polypharmacy (steroids, antibiotics).

Risk factors for delirium include: older age (Burns et al., 2004), medical and psychiatric comorbidity (Burns et al., 2004), underlying cognitive impairment (e.g. dementia) (Fick et al., 2002; Burns et al., 2004), psychoactive drug use (Taylor et al., 2007), polypharmacy (Taylor et al., 2007), and male sex (Burns et al., 2004). Risk factors for delirium can be characterized as predisposing versus precipitating (Burns et al., 2007).

FURTHER READING

Burns, A., Gallagley, A. & Byrne, J. (2004) Delirium. *Journal of Neurology Neurosurgery and Psychiatry*, 75, 362–67.

Fick, D.M., Agostini, J.V. & Inouye, S. (2002) Delirium superimposed on dementia: A systematic review. *Journal of the American Geriatrics Society, 50* (10), 1723–32.

Taylor, D., Paton, C. & Kerwin, R. (2007) *The Maudsley Prescribing Guidelines*, 9th edn. London: Informa Healthcare, p. 465.

WHO. (1992) *The ICD-10 classification of mental and behavioural disorders: Clinical descriptions and diagnostic guidelines.* Geneva: WHO.

STATION 6: Anxiety and HIV

KEY POINTS
Empathy, rapport
History taking from patient
Mental state exam
Assessment of psychopathology
Brief summary of likely diagnosis, with management plan

INTRODUCE YOURSELF

SET THE SCENE

Introduce yourself to the gentleman and his sister. Explain that you wanted to ask him a few questions around his health; it may be worth checking again if he is happy to discuss all matters in front of his sister, given the sensitive nature of the difficulties.

COMPLETING THE TASKS

1. Take a brief history from the gentleman; his sister will be able to provide a collateral history.
- Clarify onset of difficulties. Has there been a discernible change in mental state, if so when did this occur? When did his sister notice the changes? When did the changes to mental state come on, with respect to receiving the news about his partner's health?
- What is the situation with his current partner – is it a stable and long-term relationship or more recent? How did he find out about his partner's diagnosis? When did he find this out?
- Has he any concerns around his own health? Any plans for HIV testing himself and pre-/post-test counselling?
- Other relevant factors in history – previous psychiatric history of note, current medications, family history, drug and alcohol use.

2. Mental state examination:
- Assess for psychopathology, especially for mood and anxiety symptoms.
- Risk assessment – risk to himself (self-harm/suicide) or through neglect. Risk to others – ask about current sexual practices/other practices which could put others at risk of potential HIV infection (injecting drug use/needle sharing etc.).
- For the risk assessment his sister will provide helpful collateral history, especially around risk to himself.

3. Summarize the main points discussed during the interview and finish with a brief differential diagnosis and management plan, explained to the patient in simple jargon-free terms.
- Likely differential diagnosis could include: adjustment disorder, major depression, or an anxiety disorder (WHO, 1992).
- Advise HIV pre-test counselling, safer practices, informing sexual partners, etc.
- Suggest SSRI if he meets clinical criteria for depression or an anxiety disorder.
- Suggest psychological support – either CBT if depressed/anxiety or supportive counselling if there are outstanding issues around his health and his relationships.

ADDITIONAL POINTS

Note the difference between an Adjustment Disorder and an Acute Stress Reaction, as described in ICD-10 (WHO, 1992). To meet criteria for an Acute Stress Reaction (F43.0) there should be evidence of 'exposure to an exceptional mental or physical stressor' and symptoms should come on within one hour of the stressor. Conversely, to meet criteria for an Adjustment Disorder (F43.2), there should be evidence of 'an identifiable psycho-social stressor, not of an unusual or catastrophic type, within one month of onset of symptoms'. Symptoms may be similar to those noted within the 'neurotic, stress-related and somatoform disorders' or 'affective disorders', but should not be of a severity to indicate a separate diagnosis of these.

FURTHER READING

WHO (1992) *The ICD-10 classification of mental and behavioural disorders: Clinical descriptions and diagnostic guidelines.* Geneva: WHO.

Chapter 7

Forensic psychiatry

Dr Marc Lyall

○ LINKED STATION 1

1a.

As a psychiatry trainee you have been called to assess a young woman who is in police custody charged with shoplifting. She has a history of deliberate self-harm. While in the police station she has made superficial cuts to her forearm with a disposable razor that she had hidden.

Take a history of her self-harming behaviour and assess the risk of suicide and of further self-harm in the short term.

1b.

The woman has given her consent for you to explain her situation to the custody sergeant.

Explain to the police officer your risk assessment and advise him on how to manage the situation.

○ LINKED STATION 2

2a.

This woman became depressed after her husband left her. She was extremely distressed and presented herself to A&E where she was seen by the liaison nurse.

She agreed to an informal psychiatric admission to the ward and settled extremely quickly. It was recommended that she start lofepramine at night and she has cooperated with this.

She would now like to leave hospital and return home. There are no grounds currently to detain her under the Mental Health Act.

During her admission she disclosed to another patient detailed plans on how she intends to kill her husband.

She has a history of violence towards her husband.

Take a relevant history and mental state.

2b.

Following your interview in the previous station you have arranged to meet with her husband.

Discuss how you intend to manage his wife and any other issues you consider of relevance.

O LINKED STATION 3

3a.

You are a psychiatry trainee. You have been asked by the prison doctor to assess a 45-year-old man in prison. He is charged with attempted murder. He has assaulted other inmates while in prison. The man has spoken to a number of prison officers about hearing the 'voice of God' commanding him to attack others.

Assess the risk of the man acting violently to others in prison. Is the man fit to plead?

3b.

You have made your assessment of the man in the previous station.

Over the telephone, summarize your findings to your supervising consultant and discuss your proposed management plan.

SINGLE STATIONS

4.

You are a psychiatry trainee. You have been called to the Emergency Department of a local hospital to see a young man who is under arrest for an alleged offence of arson. He has suffered burns but is now physically well.

Take a forensic history with particular reference to fire-setting.

5.

This patient, who is in her 20s, has attended the emergency clinic complaining of low mood. She claims a longstanding history of 'feeling depressed' since adolescence.

You discover that she has had a row with a neighbour who complained that she was playing music loudly. This led to a physical fight.

You uncover a past history of previous violence to property and assaultative behaviour. She admits to having been extremely violent towards her ex-partner.

She wants to know what you can do to help her with her regular angry outbursts.

1. Take a relevant history to determine the diagnosis.
2. How do you intend to assist her?

6.

You have been asked to see this 30-year-old police officer in your clinic. She was referred by the general practitioner (GP) as she had attended A&E with minor injuries on at least 6 occasions over the last few months. These had included injuries to her hands from punching walls and a laceration to her face from an argument with someone at her partner's place of work.

The police have also been to her home address following calls from the neighbours concerned about domestic violence, which she found completely humiliating.

The letter from the GP includes details of a conversation with her brother setting out her belief that her husband is having an affair and the brother's opinion that this is absolutely not the case.

She has also apparently been misusing both her work time and police information to keep track of her husband's activities.

1. Elicit the main features of what you believe is the likely diagnosis.

2. Assess the risk to others and of self-harm/suicide.

7.

You are psychiatry trainee working in outpatients. You are asked to see a 63-year-old man with a history of bipolar affective disorder. The man lives in a housing association flat. His GP has been informed by his housing officer that whenever she has visited over the past 2 months he has answered the door with his trousers undone exposing his penis. He has corrected his attire when told this and has appeared embarrassed. The housing officer has noticed pornographic magazines spread openly around the man's living room.

Take a history of the man's behaviour, any other sexually abnormal behaviour and carry out a focused mental state examination.

STATION 1

1a: Risk assessment in a police station

> **KEY POINTS**
> Appropriate empathy
> Explains professional role and the boundaries of confidentiality
> Explores this episode of self-harm: precipitants, method of self-harm, desired
> outcome of self-harm
> Explores past episodes of self-harm
> Assesses current ideas and intent of suicide and self-harm
> Discusses future risk of self-harm, including factors that would increase and
> decrease this risk

INTRODUCE YOURSELF

'Hello. I'm Dr_____, I work at the (hospital) as a doctor. I'm not a police officer. I've been asked to see you today because of worries that you've hurt yourself.'

SET THE SCENE

Start with general open questions, perhaps about the patient's experience in police custody. The woman is likely to be angry, anxious and distressed – establishing trust and empathy will be necessary before an accurate assessment can be undertaken.

COMPLETING THE TASKS

The task is to complete a brief but comprehensive assessment of the risk of self-harm and suicide in a woman who is in police custody. Past episodes of self-harming should be explored: what were the circumstances, what was the method of self-harm (lacerating self, burning, 'head banging'), what was the intent of the self-harm, was there any planning, what was the patient's attitude afterwards? A history of the current episode should be taken; in particular, what was the aim and how does the woman feel now? Factors affecting the future risk of self-harm should be elicited.

Her access to the means to self-harm while in custody should be explored, bearing in mind that she will have been searched on reception into the custody suite but nonetheless has managed to secrete a razor blade.

Detailed psychiatric or substance misuse histories are not required but these areas should be concisely explored, and some attempt should be made to assess her current level of substance misuse.

A detailed forensic history or an account of the current criminal allegation is not needed.

PROBLEM SOLVING

Candidates should anticipate that the woman is likely to be distressed. She will require reassurance as to the candidate's role and intentions. The boundaries of confidentiality are important: these should be maintained unless she consents to the release of information or there appears to be a significant risk to her safety.

ADDITIONAL POINTS

Good candidates might suggest to the woman that they will gather background information from her GP and any mental health professionals who have been involved in her care to date.

Around a third of deaths in police custody are due to self-harm or suicide. The most common form of self-harm/suicide in custody is through the tying of ligatures.

Predictors of repetition of self-harm include: number of previous episodes; features of personality disorder; a history of violence; alcoholism; being unmarried and of low socioeconomic status.

Predictors of suicide after deliberate self-harm: evidence of serious intent; continuing wish to die; previous acts of self-harm; depressive disorder; substance misuse; dissocial personality disorder; social isolation; unemployment; older age group; male sex.

FURTHER READING

Kreitman, N. & Casey, P. (1988) Repetition of parasuicide: an epidemiological and clinical study. *British Journal of Psychiatry, 153*, 792.

Lohner, J. & Konrad, N. (2006) Deliberate self-harm and suicide attempts in custody: distinguishing features in male inmate's self injurious behaviour. *International Journal of Law and Psychiatry, 29* (5): 370–85.

Shaw, J. & Turnbull, P. (2006) Suicide in custody. *Psychiatry, 5* (8): 286–8.

1b: Risk assessment and advice on management

KEY POINTS
Communicates with a non-medically trained professional appropriately
Explains professional role and issues of confidentiality
Offers practical suggestions to manage the risk of self-harm
Describes current ideas and intent of suicide and self-harm
Explains findings in relation to the future risk of self-harm
Suggests avenues through which the police officer can access further help

INTRODUCE YOURSELF

'Hello. I'm Dr_____, I'm the on-call psychiatrist and I've just been to see Ms ... Can I speak to you somewhere privately where we won't be disturbed? Is this a good place?'

SET THE SCENE

Ask if the patient's injuries have been assessed by the police doctor (Forensic Medical Examiner). If not, you should request that this happens.

Taking a brief account of the events surrounding her arrest and self-harm from the police officer would be useful, not least to see if they concur with the patient's description.

COMPLETING THE TASKS

The difficulty in this station is to communicate the woman's future risk of self-harm and suicide in a way that is understandable to the police officer and avoids discussing unnecessary details of the woman's history. The police officer's understanding of mental health issues is likely to be limited. However, the officer will wish to avoid any danger of the woman harming herself again or attempting suicide.

A formulation of risk will form the basis of your discussion with the police officer. It will be based on the history and mental state but also factors likely to increase the risk of self-harm or dangerous behaviour. The following questions will need to have been considered.

How serious is the risk?

Is the risk specific or general?

How immediate is the risk?

How volatile is the risk?

What specific treatment, and which management plan, can best reduce the risk?

Giving practical advice, such as organizing a search of the woman's cell, ensuring that an adequate level of observation is maintained and detailing the factors that might increase the risk of self-harm in the short term, would be important.

The police are likely to want to know whether she has a mental illness. If in your opinion she does, detention under the Mental Health Act will need to be considered.

PROBLEM SOLVING

Giving the right amount of information, neither so little that the risk of self-harm/suicide cannot be managed nor so much that the woman's confidentiality is unnecessarily breached, can be made easier if the rules being followed by the candidate are discussed explicitly with the police officer at the beginning. The candidate might want to make it clear that they can only disclose information to manage the risk the woman poses to herself. If they are asked to comment on issues not relating to this, their response needs to be clear but polite.

ADDITIONAL POINTS

A good candidate would have some knowledge of a police custody suite and an understanding that prisoners are searched and that varying levels of observation can be used. They should be aware of the role of the Forensic Medical Examiner ('police surgeon'), Approved Social Worker, woman's legal representative and the potential use of the Mental Health Act 1983.

STATION 2

2a: Duty to warn

KEY POINTS
Communicates appropriately, displaying empathy
Takes a detailed account of threats
Assesses past forensic history
Assesses substance misuse
Performs a focused mental state examination
Assesses the risk of violence

INTRODUCE YOURSELF

'Hello I'm Dr____, I work here on the ward. I wanted to speak to you about your plans for when you leave hospital.'

SET THE SCENE

The course of the interview will be largely determined by the patient's attitude to being questioned. The discussion could initially be framed as a way of planning the care package for her discharge, before later moving on to the specifics of the risk that she poses to others.

COMPLETING THE TASKS

History taking

The history needs to focus on factors that are related to the risk that the woman poses to her husband.

Has there been previous violence towards others, including her husband? Any forensic history?

Will she disclose any plans to harm her husband? If so, what are the details of these plans: has she considered how to harm him, when to act against him, how to avoid detection, how to defend herself against (presumably) a stronger 'opponent'? Does the patient know where her husband is living? Does she have access to weapons e.g. guns or knives? Is there evidence of jealousy (delusional jealousy)? Does she identify any others that could potentially be victims?

More generally, is there evidence of rootlessness or 'social restlessness', for example few relationships, frequent changes of address or employment? Has she complied historically with treatment and psychiatric aftercare?

What is her use of alcohol and illicit drugs, especially stimulants such as cocaine and amphetamines? Has past intoxication been associated with violence?

Always ask about children.

Is her husband aware of the way she feels or plans she has?

Mental state examination

Look for evidence of any threat/control override symptoms: firmly held beliefs of persecution by others (persecutory delusions), or of mind or body being controlled or interfered with by external forces (delusions of passivity).

Assess the patient for the presence of emotions that are known to be related to violence, for example irritability, anger, hostility, suspiciousness.

What is her level of insight? Will she comply with treatment in the community, including with medication?

Has the patient got the capacity to consent to you speaking to her husband about risk issues? If yes, would the patient consent to disclosure of the threats that she has made?

PROBLEM SOLVING

The patient might well be guarded about her plans with regard to her husband. An open and empathetic style of interviewing will be important. If the patient refuses to talk about the threats she will need to be informed, tactfully and in a way that doesn't put others at risk, that she has been overheard describing what she might do to her husband. She will need to be challenged directly about these ideas.

2b: Duty to warn

KEY POINTS

Introduces self appropriately

Displays empathetic style

Explains issue of confidentiality

Describes risk to husband

Gives advice on managing the risk

Answers questions appropriately

INTRODUCE YOURSELF

'Hello. I'm Dr_____, I'm your wife's doctor.'

SET THE SCENE

The man is anxious and will be looking to you for support and assistance. He is likely to be shocked and upset by his wife's threats.

COMPLETING THE TASKS

The management of your patient depends on the level of risk, guided by the assessment carried out in the previous station.

If the patient does not want you to share the details of her clinical state with her husband, how much information needs to be shared with the husband in order to manage the risk that is posed? Only the minimum necessary to manage the risk: for example, the circumstances in which violence is likely and how this risk could be managed should be disclosed.

Explain to her husband that you will try to persuade his wife to remain in hospital, treat any underlying mental illness, arrange temporary accommodation away from him and offer close support and monitoring through the home treatment team. Inform him that there will be ongoing careful assessment for detention under the Mental Health Act 1983.

Other options could include advising her husband to seek a non-molestation order, which could be made by a court if it was felt that the husband was at significant risk and the couple have had a child together; otherwise legal action could be taken under the Protection from Harassment Act.

Offer out-of-hours 'crisis' numbers for mental health services and advise him to inform the police urgently if he feels under threat.

PROBLEM SOLVING

Explaining to the husband the legal limitations on your ability to share information will be helpful. What he is likely to want is practical advice. However, the resources available to mental health services to aid him are limited as the focus of care is on his wife. This needs to be explained.

ADDITIONAL POINTS

If the patient has capacity but refuses to consent to disclosure, the grounds for breaking confidentiality are a matter of judgement and involve weighing the risk of disclosing information against the risk of non-disclosure. If the matter is of overriding public interest, for example if there is a risk of violence, then there is a right to disclose (as described in the Royal College of Psychiatrists guidance, 'Good Psychiatric Practice: Confidentiality and Information Sharing'); arguably, if the risk is considered significant and is focused on a particular individual, there is a duty to disclose information which safeguards that individual. In essence, the question is what would be supported by the Bolam/Bolitho test i.e. by a reasonable body of medical practitioners based on logical evidence.

If in doubt, the clinician should discuss the matter with a senior colleague, their medical defence organization or their Trust's solicitors. Whatever decision is taken will need to be justified in writing in the clinical notes.

FURTHER READING

Adshead, G. (1999) Duties of psychiatrists: treat the patient or protect the public? *Advances in Psychiatric Treatment*, 5, 321–8.

Mackay, R.D. (1990) Dangerous patients, third party safety and psychiatrists' duties – walking the Tarasoff tightrope. *Medicine, Science and the Law*, 30 (1), 52–6.

Royal College of Psychiatrists (2006). *Good psychiatric practice: confidentiality and information sharing.* Council Report CR133

STATION 3

3a: Prison assessment

KEY POINTS
Communicates appropriately and with empathy
Explains professional role and boundaries of confidentiality
Explores past episodes of violence
Elicits current ideas of violence and intent
Performs focused mental state examination
Assesses fitness to plead

INTRODUCE YOURSELF

'Hello. I'm Dr_____, I work at the (hospital). I'm not a prison officer. I've been asked to see you today to see how you are.'

SET THE SCENE

'Could you tell me a little bit about what it's been like in prison?'

'I understand that there have been some fights with other inmates – can you tell me about them?'

It is important to be empathetic and non-judgemental.

COMPLETING THE TASKS

Assess ideas, intent and plan to act violently. Look to take a focused history and conduct a mental state examination targeted towards relevant areas.

Was the attempted murder the first incidence of violence? If not, who were the victims of previous violence, what were the circumstances, what was the man's mental state at the time?

Regarding the alleged attempted murder: who was the victim, what was the man's intention, did he have symptoms of mental illness at the time (for example, delusional beliefs/command hallucinations concerning the alleged victim), what was the degree of planning, how does he view what happened in hindsight? (Note: the man has not been convicted. He might not wish to discuss the allegation. If he does describe what happened, the candidate should give an assurance that the details of what he describes will be kept in confidence and not relayed to the police or the courts.)

In terms of the prison assaults: who were the victims and what was their link to the prisoner, was a weapon used, what was the man's motivation (for example, does he want to be transferred to hospital), how did the assaults end?

Has the man any ideas, intent or plans for future violence? If so, who are the likely victims, when might the assaults take place, are there any protective factors which, if present, might reduce the chances of assault, are there any factors that might trigger an assault?

A mental state examination should be conducted focusing on his level of irritability, hostility, the presence of delusional beliefs of control and persecution, beliefs about particular individuals, hallucinations, especially command-type auditory hallucinations, level of insight and in particular the man's attitude towards antipsychotic medication.

Fitness to plead

The criteria for establishing fitness were laid out in the case of R v Pritchard (1836) 7 C&P 303. An assessment should consist of a judgement of capacity to: understand the criminal charge the patient faces; understand what it means to enter a plea (i.e. guilty or not guilty); instruct a legal representative; understand the role of the judge and jury; challenge a juror; follow proceedings in court. What is important is the current mental state, not the mental state at the time of the alleged offence.

Some example questions:

Do you know what the police say you have done?

Do you know the difference between saying 'guilty' and 'not guilty?'

Can you tell your solicitor your side of things?

If you think a witness in court is not right in what they say, who would you tell?

Do you know what it means if they say you can object to some of the people on the jury in your case?

When assessing the patient's mental state a particular focus should be on aspects that might interfere with his ability to concentrate on proceedings and delusional ideas which could affect his willingness to cooperate with the legal process. The degree to which the patient is distracted by any hallucinations should be investigated. Delusional ideas of persecution or grandeur might be especially problematic if they concern people in court.

PROBLEM SOLVING

Confidentiality is an issue in this station. Candidates need to explain their role and be clear about their purpose in carrying out an assessment (i.e. to facilitate appropriate healthcare, not to provide information to the criminal justice system for use in any trial).

The patient is likely to be hostile and suspicious of seeing a doctor. Given his history of violence, the candidate needs to be aware of their own safety.

ADDITIONAL POINTS

Several large-scale epidemiological studies (for example, the MacArthur risk assessment study) have found an increased rate of violence in patients with psychosis. Specific symptoms such as ideas of 'threat and control override' increase the risk of violence, as do the presence of anger and distress associated with delusional beliefs. Substance misuse, psychopathy and demographic factors (for example age and sex) are also strongly associated with the rate of violence in mentally ill patients.

FURTHER READING

Buchanan, A. (1999) Risk and dangerousness. *Psychological Medicine*, 29, 465–73.

Maden, A. (2007) *Treating violence.* Oxford: Oxford University Press.

Mullen, P. (1997) Assessing the risk of interpersonal violence in the mentally ill'. *Advances in Psychiatric Treatment*, 3, 166–73.

3b: Prison assessment

> **KEY POINTS**
> Communicates using appropriate and accurate terminology
> Explains circumstances of the assessment
> Accurately summarizes history obtained
> Offers practical suggestions to manage the immediate risk
> Describes longer-term risk management plan
> Responds appropriately to questions

INTRODUCE YOURSELF

'Hello. I've visited the prison today to see Mr____. I wanted to talk to you about my assessment and what should happen next.'

SET THE SCENE

Explain to the consultant the circumstances of your visiting the prison: that you have assessed the patient only briefly but that you're worried about the risk that he might pose to other inmates.

COMPLETING THE TASKS

The consultant will need to know relevant background information about the prisoner. This will include brief details of the alleged attempted murder and information about the assaults in prison. The man's mental state should be described. Any ideas, intent or plan to be violent again also need to be conveyed.

Advice on immediate management should include a suggestion that the prisoner be placed on an enhanced observation level and that their access to potential weapons, for example razor blades, should be limited. If he has made threats to specific inmates, particular measures to protect them should be discussed.

An assessment of his mental health will inform future medical management. An admission to the prison healthcare wing is likely to be appropriate. He should be reviewed regularly by the prison psychiatric in-reach team. Antipsychotic medication should be offered, although treatment cannot be enforced.

Obtaining further history from past medical records is likely to be helpful. His solicitor might be able to provide further details of the current charge. If the man's mental state means that the court case is not going to be able to proceed then informing his solicitor, with the prisoner's consent, would be useful.

In the longer term he might need treatment in hospital, especially if he is refusing to accept medication. This could be brought about either through a court ordered transfer (in England and Wales under the provisions of Section 36 of the Mental Health Act 1983), or by the Ministry of Justice (in England and Wales) making an order to transfer him to prison (under Section 48 of the Mental Health Act). If this is needed, given the seriousness of the offence and his assaults in prison, management in a secure unit will be necessary.

PROBLEM SOLVING

The prison environment is an unusual one and for candidates who haven't visited a prison it might be hard to imagine. However, the basics of risk assessment are transferable to any environment. The management of the risk of violence, whether in prison or in hospital, has common features, notably enhanced observation and limitation of access to weapons and potential victims.

ADDITIONAL POINTS

Good candidates will have knowledge of the '2052SH' ('ACCT') document which is used by prison officers to monitor prisoners who are considered likely to pose a risk to themselves or others.

STATION 4: Fire-setting

KEY POINTS
Communicates appropriately and empathetically
Explains professional role and boundaries of confidentiality
Takes a history of this episode of fire-setting, including precipitants and desired
     outcome
Explores motivations for setting fire
Discusses past episodes of fire-setting
Takes a general forensic history

INTRODUCE YOURSELF

'Hello. I'm Dr_____, I work here at the hospital, not for the police. Are you happy to talk to me about the events that brought you to hospital today?'

SET THE SCENE

An important aspect of the task is to be empathetic and non-judgemental. The patient will need to be informed about the general confidentiality of the interview and reassured that information will not be disclosed to the police unless there appears to be a significant risk to a named individual.

COMPLETING THE TASKS

Take a history of the current incident. What happened? Was there any forethought? What degree of planning was there? Was an accelerant (e.g. petrol) used? What was the intention in setting the fire (e.g. to get help; financial; to harm others?). Was any consideration given as to how the fire would spread? Any attempt at concealment? Conversely, was the fire set with the aim that it would be easily discovered? Did the patient call the emergency services? Did they wait and watch the fire? Were they alone?

Assess the man's mental state at the time of setting the fire: use of substances including alcohol, suicidal ideas and intent, presence of depression, irritability, anxiety, anger, 'tension', delusional ideas, perceptual abnormalities.

Take a more general forensic history: evidence of childhood conduct disorder (truanting, bullying, expulsion from school, early age of first contact with the police), previous convictions, age at first conviction, first custodial sentence, previous offences of fire-setting, sexual offences, violent offences, any hospital order disposals.

Assess for any social skills deficits, including the ability to communicate distress, any suggestion of learning disability or pervasive developmental disorder (e.g. autism/Asperger's syndrome). To clarify this, ask about birth problems, developmental milestones, academic achievements and friends at school. Try to gauge the person's level of self-esteem: childhood bullying, peer rejection and social isolation are often seen in patients who set fires.

PROBLEM SOLVING

Time might run short in this station as the candidate needs to take a comprehensive history and the patient is likely to be a somewhat reluctant interviewee. Having a good structure in approaching the task is important: concentrate first on the present incident, and then consider past episodes. Discuss each episode systematically, establishing the motivations for the behaviour, any short-term triggers for fire-setting and the outcome.

ADDITIONAL POINTS

Most cases of arson are not related to mental illness. A good candidate will acknowledge this in their questioning by investigating whether the fire-setting is likely to lead to financial benefit, perhaps through an insurance payout. Pyromania, achieving sexual satisfaction through fire-setting, is a rare condition but some attempt to explore this would be helpful. If time allows, trying to establish a pattern of fire-setting would be impressive, for example discussing with the patient positive and negative reinforcers, such as the relief of tension and the communication of distress to others.

FURTHER READING

Jackson, H. (1994) Assessment of fire-setters. In M. McMurran & J. Hodge (eds) *The assessment of criminal behaviours in secure settings*. London: Jessica Kingsley, pp. 94–126.

Prins, H. (1999) The motivations of arsonists – reflections of research and practice. *The British Journal of Forensic Practice*, *1* (1), 6–11.

Puri, B.K., Baxter, R. & Cordess, C. (1995) Characteristics of fire-setters. A study and proposed multiaxial psychiatric classification. *British Journal of Psychiatry*, *166*, 393–6.

STATION 5: Dissocial personality disorder

KEY POINTS
Communicates empathetically
Builds rapport
Takes detailed personal history
Takes detailed forensic history
Assesses for the presence of comorbidity
Discusses treatment options

INTRODUCE YOURSELF
'Hello. I'm Dr____. How can I help you?'

SET THE SCENE
The patient has come seeking help, a major step, and is likely to need reassurance around issues of confidentiality and the types of assistance that mental health services can offer.

COMPLETING THE TASKS

History taking

A comprehensive history needs to be taken.

Family history: exposure to parental violence; parental substance misuse; parental criminality. What was her experience of parental support – was she fearful of her parents? Did she feel able to confide in an adult figure? Did she suffer any abusive experiences?

Personal history: birth trauma; prematurity; developmental milestones. Schooling: oppositional behaviour; relationships with teachers and peers; truancy; detention; suspension; exclusion. Academic progress: evidence of dyslexia or specific learning problems. Occupational history: has she been able to keep employment; attitude towards authority figures; any conflict with fellow workers.

Relationship history: pattern of past relationships; promiscuity; experience of cohabiting with others; past violence in relationships. Why have relationships ended? Presence of legal injunctions? Any children; if so, have social services been involved in the care of children?

Forensic history: previous offences; cautions; disposal – imprisonment? How has she responded to sanctions in the past e.g. did she comply with the conditions of any community (probation) order or did she re-offend after conviction? Who have been the past victims of her violence? Has she been aggressive to those who are especially vulnerable e.g. children, mental health patients, animals? What have been the circumstances of past violence? Does she display any remorse for past victims or empathy towards them? Eliciting any fantasies of violence or torture would be useful.

Substance misuse: both alcohol and illicit drugs; symptoms of dependence on substances. Has her substance misuse been associated with offending? If so, in what way

– has she offended when intoxicated, when in a state of, withdrawal, or to pay for substances?

Is there evidence of broader impulsivity, for example impulsive deliberate self-harm, gambling, risk taking?

An important aspect of her mental state that requires assessment is her mood state, for example is her irritability associated with depression, anxiety or hypomania/mania?

Treatment options

Treatment could be as an outpatient or inpatient, either as a voluntary patient or detained under the Mental Health Act, dependent on the ongoing risk that she poses to others.

Attempting to build a therapeutic alliance during this initial interview will be important. Validating the effort that she has made will be useful e.g. 'it's a very important first step that you're here today'. Explore her motivations for attendance.

Try to establish firm boundaries and begin to draw up a treatment contract with the patient, perhaps by suggesting: 'It's often useful if we establish right at the start how we can help you and what you need to do.'

Treat any mental illness or substance misuse.

If outpatient psychological therapy is to be offered the options include structured problem solving and group or individual anger management. There is limited evidence for the use of medication but possibilities would include flupenthixol, olanzapine, lithium and fluoxetine. Avoid prescribing benzodiazepines.

Remember to be aware of your own safety during the interview. Where are the alarms situated? Are colleagues aware that you are seeing the patient? Is the room set up adequately?

PROBLEM SOLVING

There is little time in the station to establish the diagnosis of a personality disorder. Useful information is likely to come from concentrating on the quality of the patient's relationships. Distinguishing an emotionally unstable from a dissocial personality disorder might also be difficult as both often share common historical features. In reality, comorbidity between 'cluster B' conditions is common; clinical psychopaths, on average, have three other personality disorders.

ADDITIONAL POINTS

The term dissocial personality disorder describes the tendency to be antisocial, commit criminal acts, show little remorse, blame others for your actions and not to learn from past mistakes; often it is first seen during childhood with difficulties at home and school.

In reality, taking a collateral history would be necessary in this case. Asking the patient's permission to speak to someone who knows her well would indicate to the examiner that the candidate is aware of this.

Other options for treatment might include attendance at a day hospital, or admission to a therapeutic community.

FURTHER READING

Fagin, L. (2004) Management of personality disorders in acute in-patient settings. Part 2: Less common personality disorders. *Advances in Psychiatric Treatment, 10*, 100–6.

McMurran, M. (2004) *NHS national programme on forensic mental health research and development. Expert paper: personality disorders.* London: Department of Health. http://www.dh.gov.uk/en/Researchanddevelopment/A-Z/Forensicmentalhealth/DH_4069012.

Tyrer, P. & Bateman, A. (2004) Drug treatment of personality disorder. *Advances in Psychiatric Treatment, 10*, 289–98.

STATION 6: Delusional jealousy

KEY POINTS
Introduces self appropriately
Establishes rapport
Take a history of the presenting complaint
Identifies and elucidates delusional ideas
Assesses risk to others
Assesses risk to self

INTRODUCE YOURSELF
'Hello. I'm Dr____. Thank you for coming today. How can I help you?'

SET THE SCENE
Establishing how the patient views her attendance at the appointment will be important early on in the interview. In her mind, her husband is to blame for her difficulties and she is likely to be resistant to the idea that mental health treatment could assist her.

COMPLETING THE TASKS
Main features of diagnosis
The patient is suffering from delusional jealousy and the core symptom is that she believes, on false grounds, that her partner has been sexually unfaithful.

The strength of the patient's belief in her partner's infidelity needs to be established.

The 'evidence' for this belief is important to elicit. How has this been obtained? Often patients will examine their partner's underwear for signs of sexual contact, check mobile phones and phone records, follow the person, employ a private detective, repeatedly interrogate their partners.

Taking a psychosexual history is important. What has been the quality of the patient's past intimate relationships? Have there been past episodes of similar behaviour? If so, what happened? Were the courts involved?

What is the patient's affect: anger, misery, irritability, apprehension?

Are there any links between the patient's behaviour and the use of alcohol, cocaine or amphetamines? Is there any evidence of an organic cause, such as temporal lobe epilepsy?

Is the delusional belief encapsulated or is it part of another mental disorder, for example depression, schizophrenia or a personality disorder (paranoid, antisocial)?

Risk assessment

First, consider the risk to the patient's partner and to those whom she perceives to be having an affair with her husband.

We know that she has been violent. Who has she considered attacking? What was the cause of the injuries with which she has attended hospital? If there has been violence, what happened, was there a trigger, why did it stop?

What has been the patient's husband's response? Has this made the situation worse?

The patient in this case is a police officer, which might increase the risk she poses to others. Does she have access to weapons or otherwise confidential information about others, especially her husband's alleged partners?

The risk to self also needs to be discussed. The patient is evidently very distressed by her husband's supposed behaviour. Whether she has experienced suicidal ideas and has any intent or plan to harm herself needs to be elicited, as do potential triggers to acting against herself and protective factors against this.

PROBLEM SOLVING

One of the key problems with this station will be engaging the patient in the assessment; the patient is upset and firmly believes that her husband is committing adultery. The candidate will need to show good communication skills and attempt to show the patient that her own behaviour is causing her distress. Empathy will be important, without colluding or unfairly supporting the patient's belief about her husband.

ADDITIONAL POINTS

The risk to others in cases of a delusional disorder can be significant. A good candidate, as well as assessing risk, will make some attempt to consider risk management. Options include detention under the Mental Health Act or arranging an informal admission to hospital. Treatment with antipsychotic medication, at the same doses as in schizophrenia, either as an outpatient or inpatient will need to be considered. Psychological treatment, in the form of cognitive behavioural therapy, if the patient will allow this, might be useful; as might working to ensure that the patient's partner does not provoke further conflict with their reaction to the allegations. If the risk to the partner's husband is great, geographically separating the patient from her husband might be necessary.

FURTHER READING

Kingham, M. & Gordon, H. (2004) Aspects of morbid jealousy. *Advances in Psychiatric Treatment*, 10, 207–15.

Michael, A. et al. (1995) Morbid jealousy in alcoholism. *British Journal of Psychiatry*, 167(5), 668–72.

STATION 7: Abnormal sexual behaviour

> **KEY POINTS**
> Demonstrates appropriate communication skills
> Elicits a description of current behaviour
> Takes an account of past behaviour
> Takes a psychosexual history
> Assesses mood state
> Performs a brief cognitive examination

INTRODUCE YOURSELF

'Hello. I'm Dr____. Thank you very much for coming today. I'm one of the junior doctors and I thought it was important for us to meet to see how you are getting on.'

SET THE SCENE

The patient might well be embarrassed and distressed at coming to the appointment. This should be quickly acknowledged and the overall structure of the assessment should be explained, as should the duty of confidentiality.

COMPLETING THE TASKS

Whether this is a case of exhibitionism, sheer forgetfulness, or the likely prelude to more serious sexual offending needs to be established.

Take an account of the sexually inappropriate behaviour:

What did the patient do? What effect did he believe his actions would have, and what was the effect that he wanted to have, for example to make the housing officer fearful, to be caught or as the start of a sexual encounter? Was the housing officer the intended victim and if so, why?

Was exposing himself sexually arousing? Was his penis erect or flaccid? Did he masturbate afterwards?

How much planning was involved? Was the patient intoxicated at the time? What was his mental state: any evidence of mania/hypomania such as an elevated mood, increased energy, quick thoughts, insomnia, lack of fatigue, elevated self-regard, loss of concentration, grandiose ideation, etc? Was the man anxious and did exposing himself make him feel less so?

Is there any evidence that the man was confused? Was he taking any disinhibiting medications at time, for example benzodiazepines? Does he suffer from any physical illnesses, such as diabetes, or a recent head injury that have might have affected his psychological state?

What is his current attitude to what he did? Embarrassment? Entitlement? Pleasure? Does he want treatment?

In view of his age, particularly if this is new behaviour, screen for any cognitive decline. Have there been any episodes of forgetfulness? Has he suffered any form of functional decline: how well does he manage to live independently and complete tasks such as shopping, self-care, travelling around? Has anyone remarked to him about a decline in his memory?

The type of pornography in the flat needs to be established. How often does he purchase pornography – is it always of the same type? Does he access internet pornography?

Taking a psychosexual history will be key. Consider whether he has previously been married or had cohabiting partners.

Is there any evidence of paraphilia as shown by fantasy beliefs, past behaviour or sexual ideas about children? Is the man hypersexual? Discuss the level of his sexual preoccupation as judged by the frequency of masturbation, number of sexual partners and description of 'uncontrollable' urges.

A more wide-ranging forensic history, with a view to establishing any general antisocial attitudes, will be important. Has he offended in the past? Any sexual offences – past exhibitionism or contact sexual offences (e.g. indecent assault, rape)? Has he undertaken a sex offender treatment programme before?

Consider also his use of alcohol and illicit drugs.

Does he have any regular or predictable access to children? If so, does he present a sexual risk to them?

A mental state examination needs to be focused on the man's current affective state, symptoms of psychosis and his cognitive functioning, in particular his orientation and his long- and short-term memory.

PROBLEM SOLVING

This is potentially an embarrassing situation for the patient. Fantasy beliefs, particularly if they concern paraphilic activities, might be difficult to elicit: normalizing the issue of sex and being clear with the patient that everyone has sexual ideas could assist. Notwithstanding the difficulty, the situation is potentially serious and a clear assessment of risk needs to be undertaken.

ADDITIONAL POINTS

Most cases of exhibitionism involve young, emotionally immature young men who are not sexually excited by the behaviour. A smaller group of perpetrators have a more dissocial personality structure. They tend to experience a sense of sadistic pleasure by exposing themselves and typically masturbate during or after the exposure.

If exhibitionism starts for the first time in this age group, psychosis and organic brain damage need to be excluded as a cause.

FURTHER READING

Gordon, H. & Grubin, D. (2004) Psychiatric aspects of the assessment and treatment of sex offenders. *Advances in Psychiatric Treatment*, 10, 73–80.

Series, H. & Degano, P. (2005) Hypersexuality in dementia. *Advances in Psychiatric Treatment*, 11, 424–31.

Chapter 8

Psychotherapy

Dr Dinesh Sinha

○ LINKED STATION 1

1a.

You have been asked to take a call from a patient you have seen once since joining the Community Mental health team (CMHT). She has a diagnosis of anxiety and depression, but is known as a 'difficult patient' by the team. She has had several care co-coordinators. It is Friday at 4.45 pm and she is insisting on being seen immediately by you and threatening self-harm if you are not available.

Using techniques learnt in psychotherapy, talk to her and see how you are able to help.

1b.

The patient you have just spoken to is discussed in the team meeting. She is very needy and rapidly engages with care workers. There can often be situations where people are left feeling very anxious for her. A lot of intervention is provided but the patient will often use the intervention, be grateful for it, but then not make any lasting change to her presentation. Her heavy use of alcohol is assumed to account at least in part for this.

The team manager has referred her to psychology for cognitive behavioural therapy (CBT). She only attended some of those sessions, but was appreciative of the help offered. The manager believes a deeper approach may help her.

Discuss a referral for psychodynamic psychotherapy with your team manager.

○ LINKED STATION 2

2a.

You are meeting a patient for the first of 12 sessions of CBT.

Work out with the patient what will happen in the therapy and attempt to answer any queries the patient may have.

2b.

You have now seen your patient for three sessions of CBT and he has explained in some detail his difficulties in social situations. He can find it hard to function socially and spends much of his free time at home. He feels his career is also affected. He has often felt a failure when describing past episodes of being in social situations.

Discuss a behavioural experiment with him.

⊙ LINKED STATION 3

3a.

A patient has presented to A&E having taken an overdose. She has an unclear diagnosis, with several mentioned in the records. She initially wanted help but is now refusing treatment. A&E staff are concerned about her physical state, but she will not allow them to examine her.

Assess this patient. In the next station you will be asked to consider the case psychodynamically.

3b.

The patient you have just seen has been admitted to your ward. Her case notes clarify her diagnosis as chronic depression with significant borderline traits. The patient now appears paranoid and talks about hearing voices. Nursing staff are unimpressed and feel her bed could be better used. They feel angry towards her (and you for admitting her) and are suspicious of her motives.

Discuss a psychodynamic formulation and case management with the newly appointed consultant. He does not know the patient and wonders if she could be discharged.

SINGLE STATIONS

4.

This patient has a diagnosis of post-traumatic stress disorder (PTSD) and wants help.

Discuss possible psychotherapeutic options available.

5.

You are seeing a patient for the first time. He has been on the waiting list for psychotherapy for a year. He has a history of having been in multiple foster placements. He seems hesitant and gives practical reasons for not being able to commence therapy.

Conduct the business meeting to discuss starting psychotherapy.

6.

You are seeing a patient with bipolar affective disorder who has been known to the team for several years. She is very angry with the consultant who admitted her to the ward earlier that year under section (previously she had been informal) and is refusing to see him. She is seeing you in the clinic for the first time as she is threatening to stop all her medication and to terminate contact with the team.

Speak to this patient and attempt engagement and discussion regarding the future.

7.

This patient is a senior executive in an advertising firm. In the records you note that she has once-weekly private therapy. She tells you things have been well despite a hectic life. She has a diagnosis of depression with a history of self-harm attempts a long time ago. She was brought up by her father after her mother left when she was 6. She has not had a community psychiatric nurse (CPN) for the last few months and the GP believes she is now less well.

Speak to this patient and use your experience of psychodynamic psychotherapy to interpret her presentation.

STATION 1

1a: Psychotherapeutic techniques in patient management

KEY POINTS

Interview technique – open questions

Ability to put patient at ease

Engage patient in dialogue

Building a therapeutic alliance – moving her away from a confrontation

Communication skills – engaging her in issues which are of importance to her

Understanding of transference and knowledge of counter-transference

Talking calmly with an angry/anxious patient

INTRODUCE YOURSELF

SET THE SCENE

You will need to find out why the patient has called you. If the patient is very angry/abusive you may have to do some boundary setting, suggesting that she needs to calm down and call you back when she is able to talk. Addressing the patient formally helps by reminding the patient of the setting. If she is anxious and wants to talk, your being able to set the boundary and an enquiry with open questions will help her start talking to you as it will indicate your availability to take in her projections. The object (you) needs to demonstrate both robustness and openness.

COMPLETING THE TASKS

You will need to hear her complaints and anxieties without feeling pushed to solve them instantaneously. What may help is if you are able to keep in mind that a patient who has only recently begun to see you and then finds it hard to let go (at the end of the week) has issues around separation. This may then get presented in a manner with a number of grievances, which will leave you feeling you are doing something very wrong by leaving her at the start of the weekend. The temptation can be to become collusive and agree to meet her or to be dismissive (which is how she fears you will be, that the separation means that you are dismissing her). You need to talk to her about what is worrying her, point out that you will be meeting again and engage with her more adult aspects. Remaining calm when the patient is clearly in a state of panic/anger will be important. You will have to take her self-harm threats seriously while also coaxing out why she is presenting like that. The attempt to connect emotionally with her experience of loss will help more than simply providing her with a practical solution.

Patients are often thought about based on their existing diagnosis. The diagnosis may undergo revision over time but long-term patients who present in a needy way, such as this patient, can be thought of as having prominent attachment difficulties that manifest with separation issues. The interplay of functional symptoms overlying deeper personality issues needs to be kept in mind for such patients.

PROBLEM SOLVING

The emphasis could remain on the patient managing until you meet next time. However, this may well depend on the history of the patient and the level of risk that she presents with. There is only so much you can offer in the time available. You must attempt to have a discussion with her, which includes issues of risk. If she is not able to offer you an assurance of her capacity to keep herself safe then you must suggest to her other ways in which she can seek help. This can usually include speaking to the crisis team or making contact with her GP/A&E.

ADDITIONAL POINTS

Keeping the conversation going without being pushed to terminate the phone call or agreeing to see the patient after hours (when it is time for you to go home) is primary.

Completing a risk assessment on the patient with regard to the threat to self-harm and giving additional follow-up advice.

Boundary setting.

Comment on anxiety.

Remind patient of your ongoing involvement.

FURTHER READING

Diamond, D., Stovall-McClough, C., Clarkin, J.F. & Levy, K.N. (2003) Patient–therapist attachment in the treatment of borderline personality disorder. *Bulletin of the Menninger Clinic*, 67 (3), 227–59.

Rosenfeld, H. (1987) *Impasse and interpretation*. London: Tavistock.

1b: Assessment for psychodynamic psychotherapy

KEY POINTS

Discussion with a colleague
Communication skills
Discussing a clinical scenario
Thinking of alternatives
Knowledge of psychological interventions
Consideration of team working
Risk evaluation

INTRODUCE YOURSELF

SET THE SCENE

The discussion will be with the manager, who may have some knowledge of psychotherapy but perhaps not of its details in terms of making a referral. You should start by asking her for her views about the patient. The information that is conveyed would guide the discussion and decision.

COMPLETING THE TASKS

The manager describes the young woman as being someone who also has drug and alcohol difficulties. There is a sense of chaos from the description of the patient. Although seemingly engaged with services, it is also very much on her terms and you could point out her inability to make use of what has been offered so far. She can make use of the support but psychotherapy is not an intervention to provide support per se. Such information should alert you to the possibility that this may not be the best time for the patient to be engaging in a psychotherapy intervention. Motivation is a key ingredient in the process of any psychological intervention.

Further questioning of the manager would reveal ongoing and prolific use of substances, including alcohol. The manager admits that the patient at times continues to use crack cocaine along with the methadone which she gets from drug services. Patients who are addicted to substances do poorly in therapy and the difficulty is that the relationship is with the substance rather than with the therapist. Also, as painful issues will come up in the process of therapy the patient's capacity to manage without drugs will be put increasingly under strain, if it is not yet proven that she can manage without them for a sustained period before commencing therapy.

As part of the discussion it comes to light that she has been resistant to discharge even when things seem to be going well for her. You could discuss the sense of an underlying narcissism in the patient's more easily apparent neediness. There is a feeling that somehow everyone needs to be available to her and the engagement is often on her terms only. She does not easily tolerate boundaries and the anxiety felt and responded to by professionals is evidence of the rampant projective identification at work. At times she has been to see the team psychologist but then has disengaged when the material begins to move towards more sensitive areas. Her difficulty with being able to think of her emotional state bodes ill for any deeper explorative work. Patients need to have some ego strength and curiosity about themselves to engage in long-term work. This patient does appear to be able to engage, though this does tend to be as a helpless recipient.

PROBLEM SOLVING

Your colleague may be feeling pressure from the patient and the discussion of the referral could be the need for a third person to intervene in a stuck relationship. A formulation could be the need for a firm paternal presence in thinking of this patient and to help set the boundaries. In this way, thinking about the need and motivation of the patient would be helpful for the manager to separate herself from the projections of the patient. Further risk evaluation (the patient is not currently self-harming or suicidal) would help guide consideration of the alternatives. She may currently only be able to use supportive psychological interventions that help her reduce her addiction and promote psychological thinking.

ADDITIONAL POINTS

Patients with an active dependence on substances are not good candidates for explorative psychological interventions.

Patients need to be sufficiently motivated and curious about themselves.

Options of supportive versus explorative therapies can be considered.

Discussion of difficult clinical scenarios can be a helpful way of promoting enquiry about a patient.

Ego strength and engagement are important considerations for long-term psychodynamic psychotherapy.

FURTHER READING

Holmes, J. (1991) *Textbook of psychotherapy and psychiatric practice.* Edinburgh: Churchill Livingston.

Storr, A. (1990) *The art of psychotherapy.* London: Routledge.

STATION 2

2a: CBT first session

KEY POINTS
Knowledge of CBT
Answering questions from a patient
Empathy
Ability to put patient at ease
Engage patient in dialogue
Building a therapeutic alliance

INTRODUCE YOURSELF

SET THE SCENE

The patient will be meeting you for the first time. You will need to introduce yourself, explaining who you are and what your role is. The aim of CBT – of enabling the patient to acquire skills with which they can function better – can be pursued from the beginning of the meeting when you could explain to them that you will not be someone who will be simply instructing them on what to do to get better. You will be working alongside them in discovering more about themselves and learning skills that they could then use both in and out of the sessions.

COMPLETING THE TASKS

At the beginning you could both agree on items in the agenda for the session. You need to discuss the frame of sessions, including the length, place, progress since last seen (bridge), current difficulties, aims from therapy, knowledge of CBT, homework/work outside sessions and summary. They might have further questions which could be around the anxiety of starting therapy. An acknowledgement of anxious feelings along with an enquiring and encouraging stance will help the patient feel more at ease with you.

You will need to ask them how they have been since they went on the waiting list. This can be followed up by a discussion of what their current knowledge of CBT is and how CBT may help them in understanding their difficulties. You should introduce the central role of thoughts to mood/feelings and also to behaviour. The trick will be to allow the patient lots of room to ask questions while allowing new information about the duration/structure and possible content of sessions to be introduced in the first session. Drawing a simple diagram linking all of these together with a reinforcement loop can help.

PROBLEM SOLVING

Some patients could ask if there is any evidence that this therapy works. You could cite NICE guidelines which are based on systematic reviews of current relevant evidence and make specific recommendations about the use of CBT. Avoid the use of technical jargon and try to present the information to the patient in simple terms. Allowing the patient to express their doubts and reservations as the session progresses will help in setting up a therapeutic alliance. You could explain that homework is about the work done in therapy continuing outside the sessions and that behavioural experiments are opportunities to allow the skills which are being learnt to be tested in the real world.

ADDITIONAL POINTS

It is a here-and-now therapy.

There are typically 8–20 sessions over a few months.

The therapy is collaborative with the therapist.

Problem solving, diary keeping, homework.

Has been shown to be useful in depression and anxiety.

Weekly sessions involve problem solving and reviewing diary-keeping and homework set from the last session.

FURTHER READING

Beck, A.T. (1987) Cognitive models of depression. *Journal of Cognitive Psychotherapy*, *1* (1), 5–37.

Greenberger, D. & Padesky, C. (1996) *Mind over mood*. New York: The Guilford Press.

2b: CBT follow-up session

KEY POINTS
Collaborative work with the patient
Explaining the theory
Exploring anxieties
Engage patient in a dialogue
Building a therapeutic alliance
Ability to put patient at ease
Imparting knowledge of CBT

INTRODUCE YOURSELF

SET THE SCENE

The behavioural task is a useful tool in CBT and one of the important ways in which the patient carries on the work outside the sessions. It enables the patient to translate the theory into practice and provides the therapy with an *in vivo* experiment to discuss and base further work on. It can give the patient a very real sense of picking up the skills being discussed and a sense of mastery over the problems for which they have sought therapy.

COMPLETING THE TASKS

The rationale for the behavioural task needs to be explained to the patient. If this is the first such task in the therapy the patient will be understandably anxious. Allow enough space for questions from the patient. The task for a patient with social anxiety has to be carefully graded to be a step up from what they may be currently able to achieve and yet not too much. You could, for example, discuss a small setting with just a few people like at work, which may be an opportunity to experiment, with a patient who finds it very hard to talk in social situations. He may be able initially to talk over coffee with a colleague before the task becomes more challenging and complex. Too much too soon can leave a patient feeling more of a failure and stymies attempts at change. Thus, graded exposure to increasingly difficult tasks provides a sense of mastery over the problem. Later there may be more challenging tasks which could be set up, which could include different settings and levels of tasks to be achieved. The setting of the task, the people involved, the patient's anxieties and fears and the actual task (talk for 5 minutes over coffee) need to be considered and agreed upon. Making clear notes and encouraging the patient to keep a record of the task also helps, as does imagining and discussing a situation (cognitive rehearsal).

The patient could have catastrophic outcomes in mind and going through this, following the model of thoughts, behaviour and consequences in the setting, will help him gain a more realistic perspective. It will also lead you and him to consider strategies to help in the task. This may include using distraction techniques preceding the task to reduce anxiety or the use of cue cards to help carry through the actual task. Role-play (modelling) also helps by providing a taste of the experience in a contained setting where the task can be rehearsed and misgivings addressed.

PROBLEM SOLVING

Adequate contingency planning to anticipate known reasons for avoidance and failure to complete a task is important. After the task there may be an opportunity to use a feedback survey to evaluate task completion properly. This behavioural feedback can help provide a more balanced report, which can be used to question the black-and-white thinking. Further work on automatic thoughts and clarification of rules, assumptions and beliefs will help the patient understand his difficulties.

ADDITIONAL POINTS

Address the patient's anxieties.

Agree on the details of the experiment.

Explore the sequence of events needed to complete the experiment.

Decide how to evaluate completion.

STATION 3

3a: Overdose in A&E

KEY POINTS
Interview technique – open questions
Empathy and communication skills
Managing anxiety in a challenging situation
Understanding of transference
Knowledge of counter-transference
Risk evaluation

INTRODUCE YOURSELF

SET THE SCENE

Perhaps start by asking the patient, 'What has brought you here today?' The emphasis at the beginning needs to be on finding out what's happened using open questions but without creating an atmosphere of confrontation, which could be persecuting for the patient. Her responses will then guide you into the body of the task.

COMPLETING THE TASKS

In talking to the patient you have to try to find out what has happened, including the reason for the overdose, to understand why she has presented (her motivation to seek help) and what is the problem in accepting treatment. This could include eliciting any odd beliefs and her orientation. Questions about her mood and difficulties might elicit a lifetime of feeling low and repeated self-harm. Comment on the shift in her from initially seeking help to then finally refusing help. Now, when help is available, does she feel anxious or unsafe? After this you could present her with options that are available, along with the risks and benefits (in a concise way) of each.

The actor might have instructions to engage with you fleetingly and then ask what you think would help. If you mention the need for an inpatient assessment or community follow-up she will refuse and try to leave. Having sought help she is then in the midst of such intense anxiety that the object very quickly shifts from being good to bad and she is easily frustrated. These are features of a patient in a paranoid schizoid position, which is an ongoing feature in borderline personality disorder, though it can also affect other individuals in situations of stress. You could ask about her feelings of rejection when she does not get exactly what she needs. This makes use of your counter-transference, such as feelings of anxiety about how to deal with the situation, followed by a sense of being unsure of what goes wrong in your conversation with the patient, even feeling you have done something to provoke the patient to try to leave and being left with feelings of rejection.

PROBLEM SOLVING

This could include having to deal with your own frustration when talking to such a patient, as you need to be calm when the patient is agitated and anxious, without appearing to be detached. While talking to the patient, you would also need to avoid being authoritarian, and instead try to give her a sense of having options. Comments on her having sought help and the importance of that not getting missed would be helpful here. Parts of her are acting in opposition. Appealing to the more adult part of her is one way to engage with her limited awareness of needing help.

ADDITIONAL POINTS

The patient will ask questions which you will need to answer. As the interview progresses, you will also need to ask questions regarding risk relating to suicidal ideation, planning and intent as far as possible. Further, there could be a discussion with the examiner in the next station about the heightened risk associated if she were to have a diagnosis such as personality disorder. An investigation of psychosocial precipitants and their link to a signature in her presentations should be attempted.

FURTHER READING

Gabbard, G. (2000) *Psychodynamic psychiatry in clinical practice.* Washington, DC: American Psychiatric Press Inc., Section III: Dynamic Approaches to Axis II Disorders.

Seiner, J. (1987) The interplay between pathological organizations and the paranoid-schizoid and depressive positions. *International Journal of Psycho-Analysis, 68,* 69–80.

3b: Borderline personality disorder

KEY POINTS
Knowledge of defensive manoeuvres
Linking the psychiatric presentation with psychodynamic formulation
Understanding of transference
Knowledge of counter-transference
Risk evaluation

INTRODUCE YOURSELF

SET THE SCENE

The consultant wants information about the patient and your opinion of what you think may be going on. You need to start the discussion keeping in mind that there are already strong opinions about her. You should summarize the circumstances surrounding her admission and mention the need for more collateral information. You could comment on the brief time you have had to assess the patient so far and the fact that you have no previous knowledge of her prior to this admission.

COMPLETING THE TASKS

Keep an open mind about the patient. Patients with borderline presentations can arouse deep splits and conflict amongst staff involved in their treatment. Indeed, they can often present with affective and psychotic disturbances, which can coexist, causing additional difficulties. Along with this there may already be comorbid alcohol and drugs misuse. Think about splitting fairly early on in your discussion where the patient is trying to manage opposing feelings by lodging them in different members of staff. The patient is unable to consider good and bad qualities as being in the same person and the extreme reactions in the ward staff appear to mirror this problem. This can be linked in your discussion with the response to such feelings about the patient in the staff (which includes you), which can be understood by the defence of projective identification employed unconsciously by the patient. The emphasis of your understanding must be on the responses of the various staff members being all part of the presentation of the patient. Try to hold these opposing feelings together to deal with the patient in the most helpful way, which would include evaluation and boundary setting. Discussing the use the patient makes of relationships with objects can add some depth to this discussion. The good and bad split refers to the inability to hold a whole object and the predominance of part objects in the internal world.

You may then be asked about her possible discharge from the ward and whether you agree with one or other staff members who have strong feelings about the patient being on the ward. Being able to link your own feelings about these differing opinions with the patient's confusion about being on the ward will emphasize the need for joined-up thinking between the various professionals. It is known that long periods of inpatient treatment are not helpful for such patients.

PROBLEM SOLVING

You should emphasize the need for risk assessment in managing the patient in the ward and also the importance of the continuity of care into the community setting. If her mental state is stable, discharge should be considered early, along with a clear plan on how to manage crises in the community, preferably with the involvement of a limited and small group of caseworkers. Discussion with care workers in the community helps manage splits and provides the patient with some sense of being thought about, though any sense of being discharged is likely to provoke persecutory responses.

ADDITIONAL POINTS

Avoid splitting.

Emphasize the need for joined-up thinking.

Consistent boundary setting.

Assessment of the presentation including risk evaluation.

Short-term respite admissions better than long-term admissions.

Community management is best done through a clear-cut contract with fixed members of staff.

FURTHER READING

Bateman, A. & Holmes, J. (2003) *Introduction to psychoanalysis. Contemporary theory and practice.* London: Routledge.

Hinshelwood, R.D. (1999) The difficult patient. *British Journal of Psychiatry, 174*, 187–90.

STATION 4: PTSD – treatment options

> **KEY POINTS**
> Collaborative decision taken with the patient
> Explaining the theory and choices
> Explaining best practice
> Exploring anxieties and answering questions
> Engaging patient in a dialogue
> Empathy

INTRODUCE YOURSELF

SET THE SCENE

The patient could present in quite a helpless and anxious manner. On the other hand, you may be confronted by a patient who has researched the internet and wants a particular type of therapy. You have to be mindful of the need to discuss options and try to help the patient arrive at a decision without pushing a decision onto the patient.

COMPLETING THE TASKS

Guidelines need to be considered, but not necessarily adhered to rigidly. The patient should be informed about the various alternatives on offer for the treatment of PTSD (knowledge of NICE guidelines is important). The options include pharmacological and psychological interventions. The level and timing of intervention will depend on the period since the trauma. In the first 4 weeks 'watchful waiting' is all that is indicated, with a follow-up appointment. If the symptoms have lasted for over 3 months then trauma-focused psychological treatment should be carried out (CBT) or eye movement desensitization and reprocessing (EMDR). The treatment centres on psychoeducation, exposure and cognitive restructuring. Exposure can be imaginal, *in vivo* and real-life situational. The model for CBT therapy is somewhat along the lines of any anxiety disorder, incorporating the feedback loop, anticipatory anxiety, avoidance behaviours and misperception/misunderstanding of (physical and emotional) cues. When the trauma is discussed in therapy, a much longer period of treatment may be required than the usual 8–12 sessions. This is particularly important as CBT sessions will have to be focused through the course of the longer term in order not to lose sight of the treatment aims. The restructuring aims to target unhelpful thinking and uses thought records to identify automatic thoughts. The patient may insist on the use of pharmacological therapy which is not first-line treatment. The use of specific antidepressants (like paroxetine and mirtazapine) is advocated and can also be used as an adjunct to the psychological intervention. Presenting all the options available and encouraging discussion will also help soothe a confrontational patient.

PROBLEM SOLVING

Being able to think of the alternatives and weighing up the options can help the patient's engagement with the eventual treatment, and the decision a patient may then reach should be respected. You could speak of the evidence base (quality of evidence) used for the recommendations (e.g. for CBT) whilst making it clear that there are options to choose from.

ADDITIONAL POINTS

CBT attempts to modify cognitions, assumptions, beliefs and behaviours and aims to influence disturbed emotions. Through the identification of irrational thoughts and beliefs leading to negative emotions and maladaptive behaviours, the aim is to replace them with more realistic and positive alternatives.

EMDR is a method of psychotherapy designed to treat trauma and anxiety-related disorders. It combines well-established therapeutic methods, including imaginable exposure, cognitive restructuring and self-control techniques, into specific structured protocols, which are modified to meet the unique needs of each person.

FURTHER READING

Bisson, J. & Andrew, M. (2005) Psychological treatment of post-traumatic stress disorder (PTSD). *Cochrane Database of Systematic Reviews*, (2):CD003388.[abstract].

NICE CG026; *Post-traumatic Stress Disorder; Anxiety: Management of post-traumatic stress disorder in adults in primary, secondary and community care.* March 2005.

STATION 5: Psychodynamic psychotherapy

> **KEY POINTS**
> Interview technique – open questions
> Eliciting feelings of anxiety
> Communication skills
> Understanding of transference and counter-transference
> Helping the patient with ambivalence without being persecutory or dismissive
> Helping the patient with a difficult decision

INTRODUCE YOURSELF

Introduce yourself and acknowledge that the patient has been on the waiting list for some time.

SET THE SCENE

You should explain that the meeting is not a therapy session but to agree to start therapy with you as the therapist i.e. a business meeting. This will be particularly important for such a patient who has a history of being recurrently moved on and thus with possible difficulties around attachment and separation.

COMPLETING THE TASKS

The business meeting gives the therapist the opportunity to learn about the person, to understand his troubles and to formulate ideas about treatment. During the initial session, factors such as the frequency and length of sessions should be discussed. The therapeutic dyad is important in psychodynamic psychotherapy. It is within this context that positive changes in the patient's outlook and behaviours are able to unfold. The therapist maintains a consistently neutral and accepting stance and is trained to listen objectively without criticism.

The patient is likely to have had a prolonged assessment (usually 2–3 sessions) with another therapist when he was entered onto the waiting list and there could be feelings of resentment about having been moved again to yet another person to actually commence therapy. He may insist that he does not need therapy any longer. He could also say that he is now working or hoping to begin work and so can only do therapy if it is offered to him in the evenings. You could ask what his expectation was, as therapy in NHS settings is usually only in working hours and he should have been aware of this when he went onto the waiting list. The aim throughout is to encourage a dialogue and acknowledge feelings of anxiety or anger. All of this needs to be done with the emphasis on not converting the business meeting into a therapy session. The discussion needs to consider the balance of claustrophobic anxiety (the patient feels trapped when therapy is available) and agoraphobic anxiety (he does not want to be left out, hence remains on the waiting list).

The patient may then tell you that he is afraid of what he will find out about himself in the therapy. He may have feelings of anxiety about being picked up and then left by you. You should introduce the structure of the sessions, which would be once weekly at a fixed time and day. You will need to be explicit about the length of the therapy which is being offered, which is usually from 12 to 18 months. As you continue to talk the patient may then seem to become less dismissive. Acknowledging the patient's anxieties while at the same time pointing out that he has been waiting for a long time for therapy and opening up further dialogue about this will help him to make a decision. Be mindful that while you can help him to think about what may be difficult, the decision on whether to start or not, in the end, is his.

ADDITIONAL POINTS

This is not an easy station. The patient and you have to struggle with feelings of anxiety and rejection. The manner in which you handle this situation, where the patient may be uncontained or very dismissive in the way he talks to you, will be crucial. Such a patient could bring up powerful feelings of wanting to get him into therapy or, if he persistently refuses, to get rid of him and go along with his stated wish not to commence therapy. Awareness of the counter-transference is thus very important to convey to the examiner that you are emotionally involved with the patient's dilemma while at the same time not caught up in an enactment.

Psychodynamic psychotherapy aims to help find relief from emotional pain and is based on the theories of psychoanalysis. It is similar to psychoanalysis in attributing emotional difficulties to unconscious motives and conflicts. It differs from classical psychoanalysis in not necessarily accepting that these unconscious motives and conflicts are ultimately sexual in nature. Psychodynamic psychotherapy is employed for a variety of problems, including prolonged sadness, anxiety, sexual difficulties, and persistent feelings of isolation and loneliness. Sessions can be one to three days per week, with greater frequency allowing for more in-depth treatment, and usually last for 45–50 minutes. It is not usually possible at the outset of treatment to determine precisely the number of sessions that will be necessary.

FURTHER READING

Bateman, A. & Fonagy, P. (2004) *Psychotherapy for borderline personality disorder.* Oxford: Oxford University Press.

Hughes, P. (1999) *Dynamic psychotherapy explained.* Oxford: Radcliffe Medical Press.

STATION 6: Managing anger

KEY POINTS
Empathy and rapport
Not reacting to provocation
Ability to manage hostile projections
Thinking about the counter-transference

INTRODUCE YOURSELF

SET THE SCENE

The patient is very angry and ready to have a fight with you regarding her medication. This could become a point of disagreement, with her insistence that she comes off it and your anxiety that this does not happen with a history of relapse on stopping treatment. It is important that you start with an open statement such as acknowledging she has a lot to talk about with you and allowing her to have her say without seeming to be ready to disagree.

COMPLETING THE TASKS

She may launch into a provocative account of how she feels she was 'put' into hospital by the consultant who did not know her well (in spite of having seen her for years). The actor would then tell you that she is planning to start a family, how she feels completely well and all your team has done is to leave her in more difficulty. She intends to stop her medications and withdraw from the team. She will not be coming to any more of these 'useless' clinic appointments and now you seem just like the consultant too. Initially you need to acknowledge that she is feeling angry, as this may serve to diffuse her anger. For a patient like this, a 'mentalization' manoeuvre of working out her state of mind can help shift her into a more explorative state.

A lot of this is an evacuation of her resentment, which you simply need to be able to bear and make some sense of. There is a lot, though, in the content and process of what is being said which could be helpful in this consultation. The anger could also mask anxiety about what might happen with you. For someone who has had a long period of contact with the service this meeting may be both a chance to air her grievance and also a reparative attempt. Good listening is key. Don't dismiss her thoughts about wanting to start a family. This should be explored. Of course, this idea could refer to fantasy of a successful union with you (unlike that with the consultant recently) and the birth of a shared understanding. Also, this discussion would feel more hopeful, away from the point of contention (the argument about the medication). This may help her begin to talk about plans and think about her needs. Clearly there is an aspect of the patient which does want to be thought about (she has turned up for the appointment after all) and that is the aspect you need to try to engage. When the patient begins to talk to you, you could begin to think of the disruption which falling ill causes to her life and the need to be mindful of this given her plans for the future.

PROBLEM SOLVING

Depending on your handling of the initial stages of the station, you may see a calmer period in the conversation where her ambivalence about accepting her illness and the effects of this upon her can be talked about. On the other hand, she could well turn back onto the grievance and thus demonstrate her ambivalence in her interaction. The further you can progress into the conversation and address the future while acknowledging her grievance and also her wish for care, the better are the chances to engage her with her more concerned part.

The mother and feeding baby dyad could be one way of thinking about this interaction. The baby needs a feed and at the same time has to express her fury at not having the breast. The rageful destructive fantasies are expressed in the initial biting of the breast until the persistent and containing mother can soothe the infant to feed.

ADDITIONAL POINTS

Has she stopped the medication because she wants to have a baby?

Is she in a relationship?

Do not get caught up with the provocation.

Consider your counter-transference – the rage from the patient and your feeling trapped with her could be her difficulty with her emotional states where she has to process a lot by herself, like a hungry infant which is expected to manage its hunger by itself until the breast returns.

Focus on the future so that the hopeful aspects of the patient's interaction can begin to be thought about, even if some of the plans may seem unrealistic.

FURTHER READING

Cavell, T.A. & Malcolm, K.T. (2006) *Anger, aggression and interventions for interpersonal violence.* London: Routledge.

STATION 7: Psychodynamic interpretation

KEY POINTS
Establishing rapport
Responding thoughtfully to dismissal
Dealing with narcissism
Exploring risk
Empathy for a defended patient and consideration of the need for the defence

INTRODUCE YOURSELF

SET THE SCENE

You might start by asking the patient how she has been. She is likely to respond by giving you a lot of detail about her busy life. She has been flying all over the world presenting to senior businessmen. She goes on to mention that she has been puzzled about why she is not able to get out of bed on some days. You need to highlight the discrepancy and ask her more about this, otherwise she might continue to dazzle you with her 'functioning' aspects which may present a false picture.

COMPLETING THE TASKS

It is important to make an emotional link with this patient who herself seems to function in a cut-off way, making a manic flight away from her more depressive feelings. When you question her about the days when she is not able to get out of bed, she says she has no idea but also gives you some sense of everything not being well within her. She says this has only happened now for the past 2–3 months. You might mention the impact of the loss of her care coordinator around the same time. She might accept that this could be a factor and that she does not feel that good. She mentions an incident 2 weeks ago where she had gone into the shop to buy some medication for a cold and instead bought several packets of paracetamol. She had never thought much about this and had certainly not wanted, or planned, to overdose. You might now feel anxious, a shift away from the slightly cut-off and even irritated feeling at the beginning while she discussed her work. Despite the task set, you will need to consider a risk screen.

Ask about what's coming up in therapy for her and if she has been going. It transpires that she has been so busy in the past few months that she has missed several sessions. This is another example of the scotomization of her needs by moving away from the space where her experience of loss could be considered. The patient is struggling to process her loss, seeming to be stuck in a stage of denial about it. This is acting out of her background where she achieved a lot early on while seemingly managing the loss of her mother. The problem with this is that her feelings of rage and hurt are ignored and instead turned inwards, as captured in the faltering motivation to work and purchase of tablets.

You could now have a discussion about her blocking out and point out that there is a process going on where the frame that is available to help her think of her emotional state is being left. Perhaps in leaving her therapist waiting she is acting out how left and messed about she feels, though this is only a fleeting triumph.

PROBLEM SOLVING

The patient might ask for more medication, as this is what has helped her in the past. She thinks this is what will help her and lapses back into telling you about all the meetings which are coming up ahead and the plans for travel which are part of this.

You could feel very controlled by this patient and when you try to point her to her therapy she seems to have shifted the discussion to something intellectual. She bristles when you suggest her feelings of loss and her controlling you in the consultation is another example of her method of seeking to ensure distance from the object that makes her feel needy. You may try pointing out the shift in your discussion and must attempt to avoid giving in to her pressure to prescribe, and eventually she may come round again when you remind her of her therapy which is, after all, available to her. You could also point out that you are now available too in the outpatient appointments to monitor her.

ADDITIONAL POINTS

The task captures the difficulty with mourning.

Move away from the patient's cut-off state of denial.

The patient's response to making emotional contact is to seek to control the emotion/object. You must take this up with the patient.

Scotomization is a defensive process by which the person fails (consciously) to perceive circumscribed areas of his environmental situation or of himself (as in a visual scotoma – a blank area in the visual field).

FURTHER READING

Rosenfeld, H. (1971) A clinical approach to the psychoanalytic theory of the life and death instincts: an investigation into the aggressive aspects of narcissism. *International Journal of Psycho-Analysis*, 52, 169–78.

Chapter 9
Personality

Dr Justin Sauer

O LINKED STATION 1

1a.

You receive a referral asking that you review a medical patient who is now physically fit.

This woman initially presented to A&E having taken an overdose of ibuprofen and paracetamol.

The charge nurse has informed you that she is 'a right nuisance', taking up an acute bed when it should have been used more appropriately. You are told of several presentations to the same unit over the last 6 months.

You are also told that she has been known to mental health for a number of years since moving to this area. In that time she has had a number of different care coordinators and believes her team to be 'useless'.

Gather relevant information that will help you in considering a diagnosis.

She has been told in the past that she has a personality disorder and wants to know what this means.

1b.

You decide following your assessment that you would like to admit this patient to a psychiatric ward. You consider that the risk of repeated overdose is currently high and she agrees to an informal admission. The consultant on call agrees with your plan, but the staff on the psychiatric ward are not happy with the decision. The ward manager gets involved and asks to meet with you.

Discuss your management plan with the ward manager.

SINGLE STATIONS

2.

You have been asked to assess this patient who has attended clinic. He has a diagnosis of paranoid personality disorder (PPD). He did not turn up for his previous two appointments. As part of your consultation:

Elicit the main features of PPD.

Discuss management options with him.

3.

You are seeing this gentleman in your clinic. The general practitioner (GP) has written to you as he believes he has an unusual personality.

He gives you little useful information as he is really not sure what to do. There is no significant past psychiatric or medical history and no regular medication.

He hopes you are able to shed some light on what is going on.

Assess this patient's personality.

For dissocial personality see Chapter 7.

STATION 1

1a: Borderline personality disorder (BPD)

KEY POINTS
Empathy
Dealing with hostility
Diagnostic evaluation
Features of emotionally unstable personality disorder
Explaining personality disorder – lay terms
Risk issues

INTRODUCE YOURSELF

'Hello, my name is Dr____, I'm one of the psychiatrists.'

SET THE SCENE

'I've been asked by the medical team to come and see you. Would it be OK if we spoke about how you were just before you came into hospital?'

'Could you tell me what happened?'

COMPLETING THE TASKS

We have been conveniently told that she has been diagnosed with a personality disorder in the past. No doubt from the history you will be thinking of an emotionally unstable personality disorder and you should focus your interview to consider this. However, be seen to make your own mind up and screen for other major psychopathology.

Gather relevant information that will help you in considering a diagnosis

An empathic response is needed, as are firm boundaries. Explore the events leading up to the overdose and her intentions.

Enquire about the previous attendances at A&E and the context of these presentations.

Ask when she first came in to contact with mental health services, what diagnosis she was given, treatments she received and whether they helped her. What happened in the relationships with her care coordinators and why did they break down?

Screen for affective disorder, psychotic illness and other personality disorders (question 3 – this chapter).

You must attempt to elicit the following features for an emotionally unstable diagnosis (although all are not necessary).

Emotionally unstable PD (impulsive type)

Unstable mood:	'Do you find your mood varies from day to day or from week to week?'
Desultory:	'Do you have goals in life which tend to change depending on how you are feeling, for instance?'

Explosivity:	'We all get upset from time to time. Do certain people upset you from time to time? What usually happens when you become upset?'
Quarrelsome:	'We all have arguments and often this is important in relationships. Do you have many arguments in your everyday life?'
Unpredictability:	'Do you find yourself losing control in certain situations and perhaps becoming upset, even aggressive?' – Outbursts of violence or threatening behaviour are common, especially when subject to criticism.

Emotionally unstable PD (borderline type)

Relationship difficulties/ crises:	'Have you had any relationship difficulties recently?' They are often involved in intense and unstable relationships with frequent emotional crises and fear of abandonment. There is subsequently often self-harm, suicide threats or attempts in a bid to get help.
Self-harm:	'Sometimes people's unwanted thoughts and feelings become so much that they feel like harming themselves. Has anything like that happened to you?' 'Have you harmed yourself in the past?'
Feelings of emptiness:	'Do you feel low and particularly empty from time to time?' Such feelings tend to be chronic.
Poor self-image:	'How do you feel about yourself most of the time?' Their self-image, aims, sexual preferences are often unclear or disturbed.

Both subtypes show impulsive behaviour and a lack of self-control.

She has been told in the past that she has a personality disorder and wants to know what this means

'By the time we are young adults we usually have developed our individual personalities so that we behave, think and react in our own ways. Most people's personality remains fairly constant throughout their lives, allowing them to get on fairly well with people, most of the time. This is not the case for everyone, mind you. It is not uncommon for some of us to develop personalities that are less comfortable with ourselves and sometimes others. Often these differences in personality have been present for a long time, usually from childhood. We're not exactly sure why this happens. Some of it may be due to our genetic make-up and some of it can be due to our childhood development and experiences. It does mean that some people have difficulties with personal relationships and friendships, dealing with feelings or emotions and difficulty controlling their temper.'

RISK

Self-harm and suicidal threats might lead to admission and often this process can be counter-therapeutic for such people. However, a diagnosis of BPD should not compromise a thorough risk assessment and each presentation should be considered in its own right. A drug overdose as described could have been a serious suicide attempt and admission an appropriate approach. Although in this station you have not been asked to make such decisions, you should always consider risk, and a few screening questions, including asking about illicit substance misuse and alcohol, will let the examiner know you are a sensible psychiatrist.

PROBLEM SOLVING

Bear in mind that the patient is likely to be angry and discontented with the help they have received so far. While you might be the focus of their distress, it is important to remain calm and in control.

ADDITIONAL POINTS

People with BPD find it difficult to be alone, which often leads to a desperate search for a partner. This invariably leads to ill-suited partnerships, promiscuity and turbulent interpersonal relationships. Such individuals also show mood swings and will often appear to be in a crisis. Apparent psychosis can be a feature, such as hallucinations, but they are usually transitory and doubtful.

BPD prevalence in the community is 2 per cent and in psychiatric inpatients approximately 15 per cent. The development of BPD may have a genetic influence, but early childhood sexual abuse, and dysfunctional environments where children fail to identify their own emotional states and don't experience validation of their own experiences and emotions, are thought to be important. Later they show poor tolerance for distress, oversimplified problem-solving skills, unrealistic goals, shame, self-hate and impulsivity.

It has been suggested that the outcome is now better than previously thought, with some improvement in most people over a 5-year period.

FURTHER READING

Royal College of Psychiatrists health information leaflets for patients: http://www.rcpsych.ac.uk/mentalhealthinfo.aspx

World Health Organization (1992) *The ICD-10 classification of mental and behavioural disorders; clinical descriptions and diagnostic guidelines.* Geneva: WHO.

1b: BPD management

KEY POINTS
Dealing with a colleague
Acknowledging staff tension
Working as a team
Providing support to the team
Treatment plan
Risk assessment

INTRODUCE YOURSELF

'Hello, my name is Dr_____, nice to meet you.'

SET THE SCENE

Recognizing that you understand that some of the staff might disagree with the admission is important and could help diffuse any resentment. You could also acknowledge that the patient might induce strong feelings (counter-transference experiences) in some of the staff as we know she has fallen out with carers and believes them to be useless. It would be useful to explain to the manager the circumstances of her presentation and overdose and why you believe she needed an admission on this occasion. You could then set about discussing how together you should manage the admission. It is important to explain that the ward, as a place of safety, will provide her with some temporary stability, at a time when everything else in her life is extremely chaotic.

COMPLETING THE TASKS

Discuss your management plan with the ward manager.

Explain that you will complete a full history and physical examination of the patient as well as obtaining the results of investigations she has had at the general hospital. You will be looking to obtain as much information as possible from collateral sources, including the GP, community mental health team (CMHT) and family members/partner (with her consent).

Gabbard's (2000) principles in managing patients with BPD would be a sensible approach for the inpatient team:

Maintain flexibility:	Take into account the patient's ego strength, psychological mindedness, intellect and emotional state when considering supportive or interpretive psychological treatment.
Establish conditions that keep the patient safe:	Set boundaries regarding repeated hospitalization, suicidal behaviour, use of drugs and alcohol and inappropriate crossing of professional boundaries.
Tolerate anger, aggression and hate:	Defensive countermeasures, trying to prove staff are in fact good, angry responses and rejections are likely to lead to disengagement.
Promote reflection:	'What do you think are the consequences of the overdose?' 'How do you think I felt when you said that to me?'
Set necessary limits:	Particularly where behaviour threatens staff or the therapeutic relationship.
Establish and maintain the therapeutic alliance:	Regularly revisit the aims and goals of the therapeutic contract.
Avoid splitting between psychotherapy and medication:	Responses to prescribed medication must form part of the therapeutic interactions and be openly discussed if medication is resisted, sabotaged or abused. They may need reminding that medication benefits are modest.
Avoid or understand splitting between members of staff:	Recognize that they may show opposing attitudes within short periods, which can be confusing for staff.
Monitor counter-transference feelings:	Allow staff to share embarrassing or difficult feelings induced by the patient.

Psychotherapy

There are a variety of psychological treatment options for BPD, both individual therapy and group therapy. Approaches include cognitive analytical therapy (CAT) and dialectical behaviour therapy (DBT). Both are individual, time limited, structured and focused therapies.

DBT integrates individual psychotherapy (looking at the therapist–client relationship) with concurrent skills training (mindfulness, tolerance of distress, focus on acceptance, access to skills generalization) and team consultation for therapists. The focus is on addressing chronic para-suicidal behaviour. Treatment lasts 3 to 6 months. Direct and telephone contact is involved. Aims are to increase mindfulness, interpersonal effectiveness and emotion regulation.

CAT is a collaborative approach using letters, reformulations and diagrams, and links target problems with life experiences.

Other options would be attendance at, or admission to, a therapeutic community or psychodynamic psychotherapy.

Medication

Evidence for using medications is limited but they can confer some benefits, particularly for crises:

Antidepressants:	SSRIs for aggression, impulsivity and affective dysregulation symptoms or SNRIs if they are ineffective.
Mood stabilizers:	lithium, carbamazepine and valproate semisodium can sometimes help with anger and impulsivity. Some reports also suggest that a significant proportion of BPD patients have bipolar spectrum disorder.
Antipsychotics:	atypicals for psychotic features.
Benzodiazepines:	whilst best avoided, have been used for significant anxiety (clonazepam).

General

Good communication with all parties involved is essential.

Identification and treatment of any comorbidities, e.g. depression, anxiety, hypomania.

Collaboratively set goals – 'What do you want from treatment? What would be a good outcome for you?'

Draw up a treatment contract.

There are no 'quick fixes', but treatment can influence small positive changes.

RISK

The suicide rate in BPD is similar to that in affective disorders and schizophrenia. An ongoing risk assessment is needed, the result of which is shared with other clinicians who are involved in the patient's care.

PROBLEM SOLVING

You should offer to discuss concerns that the staff have and consider ways you might deal with these. Suggesting a session with staff where you could discuss the case and personality disorders in more detail would be useful. If a ward psychologist is available, their involvement can also help when teams are divided over issues. It is important to have a consistent approach to the patient.

ADDITIONAL POINTS

Reasons to admit (personality disorders) (Fagin 2004):
- crisis intervention – reduce suicide risk or harm to others;
- comorbid psychiatric illness;
- chaotic behaviour – endangering patient and therapeutic engagement;
- to stabilize medication regimes;
- review of diagnosis and treatment plan;
- risk assessment.

FURTHER READING

Fagin, L. (2004) Management of personality disorders in acute in-patient settings. Part 1: Borderline personality disorders. *Advances in Psychiatric Treatment*, *10*, 93–9.

Gabbard, G.O. (2000) *Psychodynamic psychiatry in clinical practice*. Washington, DC: American Psychiatric Press.

STATION 2: Paranoid personality

KEY POINTS
Empathy
Clear communication
Dealing with hostility and suspiciousness
Eliciting personality features
Management options
Risk issues

INTRODUCE YOURSELF

'Hello, my name is Dr_____, I'm one of the psychiatrists.'

SET THE SCENE

Thank him for coming to see you in clinic today. Explain that you've not met before and that you want to find out how he has been.

You could also mention that he had missed several appointments: 'I notice that we haven't seen you for a while. Sometimes when people have a lot going on in their lives or they're stressed, they don't want to attend appointments. Has anything like that been happening to you?'

COMPLETING THE TASKS

Elicit the main features of PPD

According to the ICD-10 diagnostic guidelines, PPD is characterized by:

- excessive sensitiveness to setbacks and rebuffs;
- bearing persistent grudges;
- suspiciousness, misconstruing neutral or friendly actions of others as hostile or contemptuous;
- combative and tenacious sense of personal rights;
- recurrent suspicions, without justification, regarding sexual fidelity of partner;
- excessive self-importance;
- preoccupation with unsubstantiated 'conspiratorial' explanations of events, personal and in the world at large.

Often others become frustrated with their persistent suspiciousness and accusations. They tend to distort reality, but their thoughts are not actually delusional. They continuously look to seek confirmation of their suspicions and conspiratorial explanations of events.

Discuss management options with him

You would want to take a full history and mental state examination. A collateral history would also be informative.

Psychotherapy
Psychological approaches are difficult, as building a trusting and intimate relationship with a therapist is often unworkable, but they are the treatment of choice as long as the patient demonstrates insight and is prepared to engage. Dynamic psychotherapy may be too demanding, but if successfully initiated the therapist should be aware that ambitious interpretations may be met with resistance and breaking-off of treatment. Group psychotherapy can help reduce suspiciousness and improve socialization, but frequently such sessions are not tolerated.

Medication
The evidence base for effective pharmacotherapy is weak. Antipsychotics can help with agitation and hyper-vigilance. Antidepressants can help with affective and anxiety symptoms. Short periods of benzodiazepines have also been used for marked anxiety and agitation, although there is the risk of dependence and they are generally out of favour.

RISK

Occasionally their thoughts can lead to violence against those they suspect. If, during the course of the interview, they express anger towards others, explore this further.

You can limit the likelihood of aggression towards yourself by not invading their space (i.e. not getting too close), not embarrassing them or using an accusatory interview style.

PROBLEM SOLVING

You need to be aware of his likely sensitivity and suspiciousness. The use of normalization can be helpful here. Typically these individuals do not do well with authority figures, such as doctors. This is often an obstacle to engaging with services. Such individuals feel that others are trying to get the better of them, to deceive or fool them. It is likely that during the interview you will be subject to accusations and insults and you need to remain polite but not defensive. It is possible that any suggestions you make are rejected or criticized.

ADDITIONAL POINTS

Pervasive personality disorder (PDD) patients are hypersensitive to potential slights, are suspicious and have a hyper-vigilant view of the world. They persistently scan for signs of potential danger and rarely relax their suspicion. These features make it difficult to form enjoyable relationships and others often drift away. Acquaintances will view them as secretive, prickly and devious. Unlike paranoid syndromes, in PPD ideas or themes are not of a delusional nature and there are no hallucinatory experiences.

FURTHER READING

Bateman, A.W. & Tyrer, P. (2004) Psychological treatment for personality disorder. *Advances in Psychiatric Treatment*, *10*, 378–88.

World Health Organization (1992) *The ICD-10 classification of mental and behavioural disorders; clinical descriptions and diagnostic guidelines.* Geneva: WHO.

STATION 3: Personality assessment

KEY POINTS
Communication
Rapport
Components of personality
Traits elicited
Risk issues

INTRODUCE YOURSELF

'Hello, my name is Dr____, I'm one of the psychiatrists.'

SETTING THE SCENE

Explain that you have received a letter from his doctor and ask if he knows why the GP has referred him. If he is unsure then you could describe how his doctor felt that things didn't seem to be going so well for him in his personal life and relationships, which is why he had asked that you see him. Did this seem correct to him? Ask if you could talk to him, to find out how things have been recently.

COMPLETING THE TASKS

Assess this patient's personality.

In an attempt to avoid this scenario ending up as a list of questions (examiners do not like lists), useful information can be gleaned from identifying how the individual has behaved in certain situations.

You should have questions in mind from each personality disorder that will allow you to tease out which is most likely (some examples are given below). Try to get an overall impression and scan for personality traits.

Ask about:
 Character 'Can you tell me what kind of person you are?'
 'How would you describe your own personality?'
 'If you were with other people, say at a party or at work, how do you behave?'
  Reserved/timid (anankastic)
  Shy/self-conscious/anxious (avoidant)
  Fussy/difficult/meticulous/punctual (anankastic)
  Selfish/self-centred (paranoid)
  Centre of attention (histrionic)
  Sensitive/suspicious (paranoid)
  Resentful/jealous (paranoid)
 Attitudes of others – 'How would people that know you describe your personality?'
 Attitudes to others – 'What do you think of other people, for example your friends or people at work?'
 Habits Risk-taking behaviour (± criminal behaviour) (dissocial)
 Food, smoking, alcohol, drugs
 Reactions to stress 'How would you cope in an extremely stressful situation, for example you lose your job or somebody is rude to you?'
 Temperament 'What are you like if you get angry?'
  'Has your temper ever got you into trouble?'(dissocial)
  'Do you ever think you are irresponsible?' (dissocial)
  'Do you get into lots of arguments?' (impulsive)
  'How do you respond to criticism?' (anxious/paranoid)
  'Are you ever very emotional?' (histrionic/borderline)
 Friendships and relationships 'How do you get on with other people?' (paranoid)
  'Do you have many friends?' (schizoid)
  'Do you feel close to your friends?' (schizoid/dissocial)
  'Do your friendships last?' (dissocial)
  'Do you trust other people?' (impulsive/paranoid)
  'Have you ever had serious arguments with a partner? How did you handle this?' (borderline)
  'Do you think you depend on other people to get by?'(dependent)
 Fantasy thinking 'What do you dream of or wish for?'
  'Do you ever daydream about things? Tell me more about this' (schizoid)
 Prevailing mood 'What is your mood like for most of the time. Predominantly cheery/gloomy?'
 It is important to exclude an affective disorder by screening for depressive/manic psychopathology. If confirmed, establish time course.
 Leisure Asking about their free time and what they enjoy can provide information on whether they prefer social or more solitary activities, sedate or energetic activities.

RISK

When asking about mood and dissocial traits it is an opportunity to screen for suicidal and homicidal ideation.

PROBLEM SOLVING

It can be a tense moment in a scenario if the actor turns to you and asks 'Do I have a personality disorder?' It would be prudent to say that it is difficult to make this diagnosis after one meeting and without the benefit of more collateral information. However, do mention if they have traits of a particular personality disorder (ICD-10).

It is challenging to form an accurate opinion on personality in such a short time and also based entirely on the individual's opinion of himself. However, such is the nature of the exam that one at least needs to attempt this.

It could be quite depressing to focus on entirely negative personality traits and the person might feel somewhat persecuted. Enquire also about their positive qualities.

ADDITIONAL POINTS

A useful mnemonic for personality assessment is 'CHART FAME'.

Character

HAbits

Reaction to stress

Temperament

FAntasy thinking

Mood (prevailing)

Enduring relationships

FURTHER READING

Leff, J.P. (1992) *Psychiatric Examination in Clinical Practice*, rev. edn. Oxford: Wiley-Blackwell.

World Health Organization (1992) *The ICD-10 classification of mental and behavioural disorders; clinical descriptions and diagnostic guidelines*. Geneva: WHO.

Chapter 10

Perinatal psychiatry
Dr Justin Sauer

O LINKED STATION 1

1a.

A general practitioner has referred this patient to you. She gave birth to a baby boy 2 months ago and over the last 5 weeks has been tearful and feeling 'low'. Her partner works in a very busy city job and comes back late in the evenings. She has no other children and no siblings herself. Her parents live in Spain and she sees them perhaps once a year. Several of her close friends do have children and live in the area, but she has preferred not to socialize with them for several weeks now.

Elicit a psychiatric history from this woman.

1b.

You meet with her partner who has taken time off work to see you. He explains that he is trying to be as supportive as he can, but that his job is extremely demanding.

He wants to know what is wrong with his girlfriend and what he should do to help.

O LINKED STATION 2

2a.

This is Mrs Leighton. She is reported by her sister to have been behaving quite strangely. Rather than attend your outpatient clinic you have been asked to visit her at home as she has a 2-week-old baby.

Try to elicit the relevant features from the mental state and assess the risks.

2b.

You return to the community team base where you meet the team manager. She has been concerned about Mrs Leighton following the referral and asks what the plan should be following your assessment.

SINGLE STATIONS

3.

This woman has a history of bipolar illness. Her illness has been well controlled over the last 8 years with lithium.

Today she informs you that she has had a positive pregnancy test and thinks she must be 6–8 weeks pregnant. She has been in a stable relationship with her boyfriend for 4 years and has decided to keep the baby.

As you look through her records you note that she also takes regular diazepam.

Her medications are:

Lithium (Priadel) 600mg nocte

Diazepam 20mg regular (up to 40mg/day)

Manage this situation.

4.

This is Mrs Gray. She is a patient of yours and you have been seeing her in clinic for anxiety related mainly to concerns about death and ill health. She has been physically well.

You started her on fluoxetine a year ago, which had a modest effect. She had since informed you that she was keen to start a family and had stopped the antidepressant. Her anxiety worsened and you referred her for a course of cognitive behavioural therapy (CBT). She had responded well, although she required more sessions than anticipated and needed several top-up sessions.

She was able to conceive and handled the physical manifestations of pregnancy well.

She had a healthy baby boy 5 days ago and has asked to see you urgently. Your secretary has squeezed her into your already overbooked clinic.

Review Mrs Gray in your clinic.

STATION 1

1a: Postnatal depression

> **KEY POINTS**
> Empathy and rapport
> History of presenting complaint
> Past psychiatric history
> Social circumstances
> Risk issues
> Brief mental state to elicit psychopathology

INTRODUCE YOURSELF

'Hello my name is Dr_____, thanks for coming to see me today.'

SET THE SCENE

'I have a letter from your GP who is concerned about you.'

Ask an open question about how she has been feeling recently.

Supportive statements will demonstrate your understanding of her situation and encourage good rapport, e.g.

'The weeks after delivery are often extremely stressful.'

'It's very common to feel this way after the baby is born.'

Then hone in by using more closed questions where appropriate

COMPLETING THE TASKS

You need to take a psychiatric history and show the examiner you have considered the likely differential diagnoses, namely:

- postnatal blues;
- postnatal depression;
- puerperal psychosis.

The timescale and history in this case makes postnatal depression (PND) more likely:

- usually within 3 months of delivery;
- 10–15 per cent of women;
- likely to be similar to non-puerperal depressive episode.

Enquire about low mood, reduced interests, energy, low self-esteem, tearfulness, anxiety, concerns about the baby and its health, coping with the new routine, are they breastfeeding and if so has this been problematic.

Ask about sleep disturbance (not associated with the baby), guilt, feelings of inadequacy as a mother.

Ask about previous psychiatric history of depression and family history of mental illness.

RISK

Who is looking after the baby?

Is the patient already known to mental health services?

Is she taking any medication?

Ask about suicidal ideation, fear or wish to harm the baby (and others).

Ask about other children or minors she has contact with.

How does her partner think she is doing and how is their relationship?

If there are concerns about the safety of the child or the mother you will need to discuss the case with her partner and Social Services.

Although not specifically requested, it would look professional if in the last few moments of the station you explained to the patient what you believed was happening and reassured her that there would be help for her during this difficult time.

Important areas in the history (risk factors for PND)

History of:

- depression;
- pre-menstrual mood symptoms;
- sexual abuse in earlier life;
- loss e.g. miscarriage, abortion, baby or family member;
- poor relationship with their partner;
- poor relationship with their mother;
- very young or much older mothers;
- lack of adequate community support;
- presence of anti-thyroid antibodies during pregnancy;
- feelings of ambivalence about their baby or parenthood.

PROBLEM SOLVING

As well as the community mental health team offering support, there are a number of organizations that can help:

Association for Postnatal Illness:	Provides support to mothers suffering from postnatal illness.
CRY-SIS:	Provides self-help and support for families with excessively crying and sleepless babies, 365 days a year.
Meet-A-Mum-Association (MAMA):	Self-help groups for mothers with small children and specific help and support to women suffering from postnatal depression.
National Childbirth Trust:	Advice, support and counselling on all aspects of childbirth and early parenthood.
The Samaritans:	Provides confidential emotional support to any person who is suicidal or despairing.

ADDITIONAL POINTS

Midwives, health visitors or doctors often use the Edinburgh Postnatal Depression Scale – a 10-item questionnaire – as a screening tool.

10–15 per cent incidence of PND in the first 6 weeks following childbirth.

The onset of depression is now increasingly recognized before giving birth (antenatal depression).

FURTHER READING

Kumar, R. & Robson, K. (1984) 5–10 per cent women attending obstetric clinics have psychiatric disturbance. *British Journal of Psychiatry*, *144*, 35–47.

Wheatley, S. (2005) *Coping with postnatal depression*. London: Sheldon Press.

1b: Discussion with partner

KEY POINTS
Developing rapport
Explanation of PND in lay terms
Exploring risk
Management of PND
Support available

INTRODUCE YOURSELF

'Hello my name is Dr_____, nice to meet you. I've just met your partner.'

SET THE SCENE

If the link station did not warn you that you are about to discuss her case with someone else you might not have asked about confidentiality and sharing information – you should none the less raise the issue.

COMPLETING THE TASKS

What is wrong with my girlfriend?

Explain that you believe she has postnatal depression. Ask if he has heard of this. Depression is different from just 'feeling sad'. When you are depressed your mood is low most of the day and on most days. Most cases of PND start within a month of giving birth, but it can start up to 6 months later. Around 1 in every 10 women has PND after having a baby and it needs to be treated or it can last for months.

Has he recognized any of the following in his partner?

Depression:	Feeling low, unhappy and miserable for much or all of the time.
Irritability:	Irritable with other children, occasionally with your baby, but most often with you.
Tired:	Beyond what would be expected with a new baby.
Sleepless:	Despite feeling tired, difficulty sleeping. Early morning wakening.
Appetite:	Loss of appetite (occasionally comfort eating associated with guilt).
Enjoyment:	Have you noticed that she doesn't enjoy anything?
Sex:	Reduced interest in sex that goes beyond complications associated with childbirth. Does he feel rejected by this?
Guilty:	Has he noticed she feels guilty about things, that she is responsible for how she feels or for things that she is finding difficult?
Relationship with baby:	Has he spoken with her about how she feels about the baby? Some mothers describe feeling detached from the newborn.

Confirm with him that these clinical features are consistent with the diagnosis.

What can he do to help?

Don't be surprised or saddened if your partner confesses that she has felt dreadful since the birth of the baby. It is important to take time to listen to your partner and make sure that she gets the support and encouragement she needs. PND is common and can be helped effectively. She is not to blame in any way as PND is an illness. Get advice on how to help, but also make sure that you have some support yourself. Helping with the practical/domestic tasks e.g. shopping, housework can make a significant difference. You might also help with the child care e.g. feeding or changing the baby. Sympathetic listening, patience, warmth and remaining positive are the rule.

If this is a first baby, it is easy to feel sidelined both by the baby and by your partner's needs. Try not to feel resentful.

PND can be helped by support from family and friends and also the GP and health visitor. More severe PND will need input from mental health professionals.

RISK

Revisit the risk factors from the previous station.

Has she ever described things being so dark that she wished she was dead, or that both she and her baby would be better off dead?

Does he have concerns about her ability to care for the baby?

Could she get the support from a member of the family – e.g. a grandparent? Could her parents come from Spain?

Can he take time off work?

What is his opinion about a psychiatric admission and social service involvement?

Has he ever felt at the end of his tether? Is he able, for example, to manage a crying baby and disturbed nights?

PROBLEM SOLVING

A discussion about management options might ensue:

Counselling, self-help groups: Many general practices have a counsellor and health visitors can help treat PND. Maximize family and community support, and organize assistance with childcare if necessary.

Psychotherapy: CBT can help. This can be arranged through her GP, a community psychiatric nurse (CPN), psychologist or a psychiatrist. There are still long waiting lists in some areas.

Antidepressants: tricyclic antidepressants (TCAs) – but seek advice, especially if breast feeding.

Antidepressants can take 2–4 weeks before there is any noticeable benefit.

Admission: if severely depressed or risk factors outweigh community treatment (Mother and Baby Unit if bed available). Electroconvulsive therapy (ECT) is not contraindicated, but is considered only if other options have failed or the mother is extremely unwell.

ADDITIONAL POINTS

ICD-10 does not classify puerperal disorders separately unless they do not meet the criteria for disorders classified elsewhere. Section F53, mental and behavioural disorders associated with the puerperium, not elsewhere classified, can be used in such circumstances.

There is not always a clear precipitant for PND. It can occur without any obvious stressors. Similarly, having some or all of the associated risk factors does not mean that someone will definitely develop PND.

FURTHER READING

Cox, J.L., Holden, J.M. & Sagovsky, R. (1987) Edinburgh Postnatal Depression Scale (EPDS). *British Journal of Psychiatry*, *150*, 782–6.

Eberhard-Gran, M. et al. (2002) Depression in postpartum and non-postpartum women: prevalence and risk factors. *Acta Psychiatrica Scandinavica*, *106*, 426–33.

Hoffbrand, S., Howard, L. & Crawley, H. (2001) Antidepressant treatment for post-natal depression. *Cochrane Database of Systematic Reviews*, 2.

STATION 2

2a: Puerperal psychosis

KEY POINTS
Sensitive communication
Empathy and rapport
Eliciting psychopathology from the mental state
Evaluating the risk following assessment

INTRODUCE YOURSELF

'Hello Mrs Leighton, my name is Dr_____, I'm one of the psychiatrists. Would it be OK if we had a talk?'

SET THE SCENE

'How have you been since you had the baby?'

'I would like to ask you if anything has been troubling you. What have been the main difficulties?'

'Have you ever seen a psychiatrist before? What was this for?'

COMPLETING THE TASKS

Relevant mental state

Not knowing what will be relevant, ensure that her mental state is fully assessed. You can then focus in on areas of psychopathology. Pay attention to affective or schizophrenic features (manic features, delusions involving the baby, which may or may not be mood congruent, labile affect).

Mental state examination

Appearance and behaviour: Dishevelled/unkempt, movement disorder (catatonia), restlessness (extrapyramidal side effects (EPSE)), rapport, eye contact
Speech: Rate, rhythm, volume
Mood: Subjective and objective affect (? flat, anhedonic)
Somatic features
Self-esteem, guilt

Suicide, ideation and intent

Thoughts — Form (e.g. derailment – loosening of associations, flight of ideas/incoherence – world salad, knight's-move thinking, neologisms)
Content, what they are actually thinking (delusions, overvalued ideas, passivity, etc.)
Perceptions — Auditory, visual, olfactory, gustatory, tactile hallucinations
Mood congruence?
Cognitive state — Mini mental state examination (MMSE) (abbreviated if little time or not relevant)
Insight — Her concept of what is happening
Is it due to mental illness?
Do/could medicines help you?
Would you take medication to help? (Adherence)

Suggested approach (generic) on assessing thoughts, beliefs and perceptions.

Formal thought disorder is an abnormality in the mechanism of thinking, expressed as abnormal speech.

1 Formal thought disorder

***** Any actor would find this difficult to mimic – be prepared none the less*****

Formal thought disorder (FTD) would soon become apparent during the consultation.

Can you think clearly or is there any interference with your thoughts (passivity/concentration)?

You should be able to recognize:

- derailment (loosening of associations, flight of ideas);
- incoherence (world salad, knights move thinking);
- neologisms;
- tangentialty.

2 Thought possession

I would like to ask you some routine questions that we ask of everybody we see (normalizing). Would that be OK?

*****Open questions to start*******

> Are you able to think clearly or is anything interfering with your thoughts?

> Are thoughts put into your head which are not your own? (thought insertion)

> Do you hear your own thoughts spoken aloud so that people standing near to you could hear them too? (thought broadcast)

> Can you ever hear your own thoughts echoed or repeated? (thought echo/running commentary)

> Are your own thoughts ever removed from your head as though someone or something was taking them out? (thought withdrawal)

> Do your thoughts ever stop suddenly and unexpectedly, when your thinking was fine moments before? (thought stopping)

Explore any psychopathology involving her child.

3 Thought content, delusions

*****Open questions to start*******

Sometimes I see people who have had unusual things happening to them; has anything like this happened to you? (normalizing)

Patient says 'what do you mean?'

> For example, some people feel they are under the control of some force or power other than themselves; has this been happening to you? (delusions of control)

> Do people drop hints about you or say things with a double meaning? (delusions of reference)

> Do things seem to be specially arranged? (delusional misinterpretation/misidentification)

> Is anyone or anything trying to hurt or harm you in any way? (delusions of persecution)

> Has anything happened recently which has been very meaningful or of great significance to you? (delusional perception, e.g. 'traffic light changed to red and I knew I had been chosen to lead my people')

4 Perceptions

*****Open questions to start*****

> Does your mind ever seem to play tricks on you? or

Have you been having experiences that you have found difficult to explain?

Do you ever seem to hear **voices** or noises when there is no one else about, with nothing else to explain it?

What do the voices say?
Do you hear one voice or more?
Do they talk to each other?
Do they talk specifically about you?
Are the voices/noises in your mind or can you hear them through your ears?

Ask about command hallucinations.

Do you ever **see** things (? gas), like visions that other people could not see?

Do you ever **smell** things (? gas) that other people don't notice?

Do you ever **taste** things and find they are unusual, unlike other people's experiences?

Do you ever **feel** things, like someone touching you, but find there is no one there?

Risk assessment (also refer to risk issues in the PND scenario)

Ask about thoughts of self-harm.

Ask about intention to self-harm.

Ask about death wish.

Assess the seriousness of the death wish.

Ask about thoughts of wanting to harm others.

Does she have thoughts about wanting to harm her baby?

Also cover:

use of alcohol and drugs;

unemployment;

single/widowed/divorced;

any supportive relationships;

any professional support (health visitor, care manager, support worker);

other children or vulnerable people (elderly/disabled);

history of self-harm and/or violence towards others (including children);

previous psychiatric history and relationship with services;

adherence to previous treatments.

PROBLEM SOLVING

Try to explain to the patient what is happening. If the patient asks about her diagnosis, be sensitive but honest and explain in lay terms what has happened to her. Explain that you would want to do a few more tests to exclude a physical cause, but that you believe she has what doctors call a 'puerperal psychosis'. 'Puerperal' means the 6 weeks after having a baby and 'psychosis' a serious mental illness. So 'puerperal psychosis' is a serious mental illness, affecting women shortly after they have given birth. You could explain further if she is well enough to attend to the conversation.

ADDITIONAL POINTS

0.2 per cent live births

Increased risk especially during the first 2 weeks after delivery

Usually abrupt onset

Ask about mood, hallucinations and delusions

Fluctuation in mental state, with perplexity, restlessness, anxiety

Enquire about manic features **affective psychosis most common**, including severe insomnia in the absence of baby crying.

FURTHER READING

NICE Clinical Guideline 45 (2007) *Antenatal and postnatal mental health: clinical management and service guidance.* London: National Institute for Clinical Excellence.

2b: Management plan

KEY POINTS
Interacting with a team member
Relaying your findings from the previous station
Key points in the mental state
Risk assessment and areas of concern
Management plan

INTRODUCE YOURSELF

Remember this is a colleague you are supposed to know.

SET THE SCENE

'Hi, how are you? I've just been to see Mrs Leighton. Is now a good time to discuss this lady's mental state and think about what we should do?'

COMPLETING THE TASKS

Feed back your assessment

Spend a few moments giving a case summary. Present the main findings in terms of psychopathology and risk issues. You will not have time or want to present in full as this is primarily a management station.

It is a good idea to take notes in the first half of a link station, especially if you are going to have to present in the second. Ensure, however, that any writing does not interfere with the patient–doctor relationship. Do not spend all the time looking at your papers.

Discuss management plan with team manager

Suggest that the first thing is to exclude an organic aetiology and that you need to request urgent investigations. Suggest speaking to the obstetrics team for advice. If her physical health is a concern she will need to be assessed by the on-call medical team or by A&E staff.

You need to speak to her sister or any other contacts to get a better sense of her current presentation and how it has evolved and over what timescale. You also need to ask about any past mental health and family history.

Depending on her presentation, admission is often necessary in the interests of safety. A mother and baby unit would be best to minimize interference with the mother–baby bond. If the risk is such that the baby needs to be removed, it is important to plan reintroducing the baby as soon as it is safe to do so. Home treatment might be possible but will depend on how the patient presents and other support available.

Investigations

Rule out an organic aetiology e.g. infection (retained products or other), thromboembolic event, medication adverse effects, delirium. Bloods will need to be taken, including full blood count (FBC), urea and electrolytes (U&Es), thyroid function tests (TFTs), liver function tests (LFTs). She will need her blood pressure, pulse and oxygen saturations taken as well as full physical examination.

Management

Biological

Antipsychotic treatment. Discuss with specialist unit and drug information. There is limited data to form a strong evidence base.

Any medication prescribed needs to be carefully considered if the mother is breastfeeding.

If not breastfeeding, anticonvulsants and lithium may have a role where manic features predominate.

ECT can be effective and is reserved for severe cases.

Psychological

Supportive counselling

Psychotherapy once receptive

Psychoeducation

Social

Practical support for the mother e.g. feeding, washing, nappy changing and playing.

Increased support from family and partner.

Support for the partner where necessary, especially if there are other children.

Education and information for the family.

Involvement of Social Services who will want to assess mother and family and are likely to be involved with supervised care and home visits once mentally well enough.

Engagement with local community mental health team (CMHT) whilst an inpatient.

Help enrolling with a support group – continue on discharge – like the Association for Post Natal Illness, whose members are women who have survived puerperal psychosis or postnatal depression, and who are ready to befriend and support other sufferers.

RISK

Always consider the risk to the mother and the baby.

PROBLEM SOLVING

The risk of further puerperal psychosis is at least 1 in 5 – probably greater still in the case of manic-depression. Careful supervision is needed if a woman who has had such an illness has another baby, especially in the early days after the birth. Treatment can then be given at once if there is any sign of the illness returning. However, half the women who suffer a puerperal psychosis never become mentally ill again.

ADDITIONAL POINTS

Predisposing factors are a personal or family history of psychosis.

It affects around 1 in 500 women and starts within days or weeks of childbirth.

Most women make a full recovery, but an episode of puerperal psychosis is a risk factor for future psychosis after a subsequent birth.

FURTHER READING

Terp, I.M. et al. (1998) Post partum psychoses. Clinical diagnosis and relative risk of admission after parturition. *British Journal of Psychiatry*, *172*, 521–6.

STATION 3: Bipolar disorder and pregnancy

KEY POINTS
Empathy and rapport
History of her bipolar illness
Risk of continuing treatment
Risks of discontinuing treatment
Advice on benzodiazepine usage
Management plan

INTRODUCE YOURSELF

'Hello, my name is Dr_____, I'm one of the psychiatrists.'

SET THE SCENE

'I understand you're pregnant, is that something you're pleased about?'

'Well, congratulations. It's important that we have this time to talk because we need to try to make sure that your baby stays healthy and at the same time try to keep your mental health stable.'

'Do you know anything about lithium and pregnancy?'

COMPLETING THE TASKS

Managing this situation will involve: building up a shared understanding – 'what do you understand about bipolar illness and pregnancy?' Has she had any other pregnancies? 'Have you had any ideas about your medication?' Enquire about the history of her illness and whether relapses have involved mostly hypomanic/manic or depressive episodes. How many relapses has she had? What were the triggers? What medication has worked best for her?

1. Advising her on the risks/benefits of lithium

Lithium – max risk is 2–6 weeks after conception. Relative risk 10–20 times control but absolute risk 1:1000 of cardiac malformation (Ebstein's anomaly). Other adverse effects include neonatal goitre and reversible adverse effects, including hypotonia, lethargy, cardiac arrhythmias and respiratory difficulties. Ordinarily, slow withdrawal from lithium is advisable. However, danger period is already past – therefore detailed ultrasound and echocardiography at 6 and 18 weeks. Watch for persistent vomiting, fluid retention – need 4-weekly lithium levels then weekly after 36 weeks; also regular electrolytes.

Try to advise that she is maintained on the lowest possible dose and that she and baby are monitored frequently rather than stopping altogether as she had been well for so long.

2. Informing her of alternatives

If she decides to stop lithium, suggest alternative medications and the need for more support from the team. There is limited evidence for most drugs in pregnancy but an antipsychotic, for example olanzapine, could be suggested. Other mood stabilizers are used but not without risk.

3. Advising her on the risk of relapse

The patient should be informed of the potential risks involved should she stop her medication, in terms of relapsing illness and subsequent inability to care for the baby, but also the potential risks to the foetus if she continues her medication.

Very high (8-fold) risk of relapse in post-partum period. If she stops medication during pregnancy there is a risk to herself through relapse, possible self-harm and suicide, and potential risk to the child through neglect and/or violence.

Therefore, treatment of bipolar illness is advisable because of the risk of relapse. Should she decide to stop the medication her mental health team and GP/midwife should provide regular support and monitoring of her mental state throughout the pregnancy. Should she continue with medication then the foetus should undergo regular monitoring.

4. Advising her on the risks of benzodiazepine (BZD) usage

Attempt to clarify exactly how much diazepam she takes on a daily basis. There is some evidence that high dose and use in the first trimester increase risk of oral clefts. They are best avoided, but should be withdrawn slowly to avoid seizures. She will be particularly vulnerable if the lithium and diazepam are both withdrawn. If she is keen to stop medication it is strongly advised that she withdraw one drug first, gradually, and then she could reassess how she was feeling before stopping the second. A formal detoxification or admission to hospital for BZD withdrawal would be safer. She also needs to be informed about the withdrawal state from benzodiazepines in newborns – 'floppy baby syndrome', characterized by lethargy, irritability, reduced muscle tone and respiratory depression.

5. Discussing a possible management plan

It would be important to involve the partner. Offer education – leaflets, internet sites. Consider drawing up an advance directive for treatment. Share knowledge with obstetric professionals, GP, midwife.

Advise delivery in hospital. Consider making plans if she relapses to admit to a specialist psychiatric unit. Involve the perinatal psychiatry team. Watch for cardiac arrhythmia with lithium. Lithium levels within 24 hours.

Psychological therapies (individual supportive psychotherapy, anxiety management) can also be offered alongside or in place of medication if she insists on drug withdrawal.

PROBLEM SOLVING

It is important that the patient is fully informed of the risks to the foetus of taking lithium and BZDs in pregnancy and the risk of relapse without treatment so that she can make an informed choice. Considering the significant risks, failure to inform in such cases can lead to litigation.

The current consensus is that all decisions carry risk, but that mental health complications outweigh the risk of medication.

ADDITIONAL POINTS

Women with a history of bipolar affective disorder have up to a 25 per cent chance of an affective psychosis following childbirth.

The aim is to limit exposure to illness and/or treatment.

Mood stabilizers in pregnancy

Lithium should be avoided where possible due to risk of malformation.

Sodium valproate and carbamazepine are also linked to foetal malformations (spina bifida) and should be avoided.

Folate supplementation should be recommended even if the above are not prescribed.

No mood stabilizers are though to be entirely safe.

Breastfeeding

Little/no evidence base exists.

Mood stabilizers

Lithium has been reported to cause infant toxicity and should be avoided.

Small amounts of carbamazepine, valproate and lamotrigine are thought to pass into breast milk. The general advice would be not to breastfeed but in those patients who do, baby must be monitored for evidence of drug effects and toxicity.

Benzodiazepines, especially diazepam, excreted – can cause sedation, lethargy, weight loss.

Expressing and discarding milk from peak plasma times can help limit infant exposure to drugs.

Use the lowest therapeutic doses if continuing with medication.

Try to avoid drugs with long half-lives.

Try to take drugs once daily before the baby's longest sleep (usually nocte), to avoid peak plasma levels.

ECT has been used with good effect in pregnancy.

FURTHER READING

Kohen, D. (2004) Psychotropic medication in pregnancy. *Advances in Psychiatric Treatment*, 10, 59–66.

Taylor, D., Paton, C. & Kerwin, R. (2007) *The Maudsley Prescribing Guidelines*, 9th edn. London: Informa Health Care.

STATION 4: Baby blues

KEY POINTS
Empathy and rapport
Considering the differential diagnosis
Exploring anxiety symptoms
Advice and management plan

INTRODUCE YOURSELF

You are supposed to know this patient – so it would seem odd to introduce yourself as if this was your first meeting.

SET THE SCENE

Start by saying it's good to see her again and congratulating her on her baby. You could ask what she has decided to call the baby and how she found the whole process. This would lead naturally into open questions about how she has been feeling and why she had asked for an urgent appointment.

COMPLETING THE TASKS

You are asked to review this patient. This sounds 'vague' but it gives you the opportunity to interview the patient and address her concerns and main problems. Before you even see the patient you should already be considering whether her anxiety has worsened, if she has 'baby blues' or postnatal depression/psychosis.

Take a history of recent events and in particular how her anxiety and mood have been over the last 2 weeks. Enquire fully about her anxiety symptoms and whether she feels they have worsened since the baby. If you identify an area of concern e.g. anxiety, then probe further (refer to anxiety station). Enquire about the delivery and any complications, prenatally, perinatally or immediately postnatally – is she still in pain. Any physical illness? Screen for depression and psychotic features – if positive for any, continue as for puerperal psychosis or postnatal depression.

Ask if she has been prescribed anything from the GP or whether she has purchased anything over the counter.

Ask about alcohol and illicit drugs.

Enquire about biological features. Reduced sleep and excessive tiredness associated with a new baby is stressful.

Remember risk. Risk to self and others – ask direct questions relating to her baby's safety.

Is anyone with her and providing support? Enquire about her ability to look after the baby, whether she has a partner/parent around. Does she have a health visitor and/or support from antenatal peers? Many mothers find breastfeeding difficult and need help and encouragement. Failure to breastfeed easily can be associated with guilt feelings and frustration for some mothers.

It's useful to 'normalize'. Acknowledge that many of her anxieties are understandable and that many women experience similar feelings.

The actor is primed to give you a history and features of 'blues' in this case: 'Tearfulness, low mood, emotional lability, confusion', a few days after delivery.

Management

Support and reassurance. You should reassure her that:

> This usually resolves within a few days.

> Up to half of all mothers are affected.

> It's normal to feel tearful and down in the days after the birth and for these feelings to pass off after a short period. This phase is often called 'the baby blues'.

Biological

> It is worth delaying medication if her symptoms fit with 'baby blues'.

> Any signs of depression and medication will need to be considered.

> Consider medication if anxiety is debilitating and unresponsive to CBT.

> If Mrs Gray is breastfeeding she will need to be informed about the risks of infant drug exposure.

Psychological

Considering her history, it would be sensible to follow her up either in your clinic or at home.

There could be a role for a CPN to visit in addition to a health visitor.

The psychologist may be able to provide further top-up sessions considering her positive response.

Social

Plan to talk to the health visitor if she has one or other professional involved.

Offer to meet with her family to discuss further.

Postnatal support group.

Provide with more information (leaflets/telephone contact/web).

PROBLEM SOLVING

It can feel awkward attempting to demonstrate familiarity with someone you have never met before – but in the scenario are supposed to know. Candidates who practise these sorts of situations come across far more naturally in the real exam. You do not want to appear sheepish or uneasy – but calm and confident.

ADDITIONAL POINTS

Postnatal depression is different from 'the blues' which is a brief period of low, irritable and fluctuating mood (feel a bit weepy), occurring about 3–5 days after giving birth, in up to half of new mothers. It does vary in intensity and duration, but is transient and considered a normal process.

Little/no support from partner or family may play a major role in poor adjustment to new life circumstances.

FURTHER READING

Welford, H. (2001) *Feelings after birth: the NCT book of postnatal depression*. London: NCT Publishing.

Chapter 11

Addictions

Dr Virupakshi Jalihal

O LINKED STATION 1

1a.

Mr Smith, a 22-year-old man, has been referred to you by his probation officer (PO) for help with his illicit drug use. You are assessing him in an outpatient clinic.

Evaluate Mr Smith for illicit drug use.

Please make notes if you wish as in the next station you will be discussing Mr Smith's problems and treatment with the probation officer.

1b.

You are meeting Mr Smith's probation officer to discuss his treatment options. You have already assessed Mr Smith and taken consent to discuss his treatment.

O LINKED STATION 2

2a.

Mr Johnson, a 25-year-old man, has been brought to the Section 136 Suite at a psychiatric unit. The police who detained him report that he appeared confused and was found wandering on the streets. He is unable to provide any sensible information but is settled enough to allow a physical examination. There are no informants to obtain collateral history. Do not elicit a history from the patient.

Carry out a physical examination for signs and symptoms of drug intoxication/withdrawal state.

Make notes if you wish as in the next station you will be discussing Mr Johnson's differential diagnosis and immediate management plan with the consultant psychiatrist over the phone.

2b.

You are about to speak to the on-call consultant psychiatrist over the phone.

Discuss the differential diagnosis and immediate management.

O LINKED STATION 3

3a.

You are the junior doctor working in an inpatient unit where Mr Mark Roberts, a 19-year-old man, was recently admitted and diagnosed with schizophrenia. You are exploring factors that were relevant in the onset of the illness and suspect that illicit drug use may have contributed to it. Mr Roberts is reluctant to talk about this. His mother is visiting the unit and wants to speak to you. Mr Roberts has consented for you to meet his mother and share information about him.

Gather information on Mr Roberts's illicit drug use history from his mother.

Make notes as required as you will be meeting Mr Roberts in the next station.

3b.

You meet Mark Roberts, a 19-year-old man, on the ward. You are familiar with him and know that he has been diagnosed with schizophrenia. He is no longer displaying any active symptoms of schizophrenia and you are working towards a discharge plan. He had been reluctant to speak about his illicit drug use despite his urine drug screen being positive for cannabis. You have met his mother and discussed his cannabis use.

Educate him about the effects of cannabis on schizophrenia.

SINGLE STATIONS

4.

You have been asked to assess Mr Jones, a 35-year-old man who was admitted to an acute medical assessment unit for severe stomach pain 2 days ago. His stomach pain has subsided and he is feeling better. The physical examination and routine investigations are essentially normal except for slightly raised mean corpuscular volume (MCV) and gamma glutamyl transferase (GGT). The medical team suspect alcoholic liver disease secondary to excessive alcohol consumption and are suggesting that he undergo further tests. He is agitated, anxious, reluctant to have any more tests and keen to leave the unit. The medical staff are concerned and want you to assess him. He has agreed to speak to you.

Evaluate Mr Jones for alcohol dependence, take an alcohol history and provide feedback to him.

5.

A 45-year-old engineer has come to see you as he was found drunk on duty and his employer wants feedback on this individual. You have obtained the history which reveals that he has been drinking over a bottle of spirits every day for the last year, started drinking during his lunch break 6 months ago and more recently he started drinking in the mornings. He experiences withdrawal symptoms if he does not drink, craves alcohol and has gradually increased his alcohol consumption in the last 1–2 years. He blames difficult work conditions and relationship with his partner for his drinking. His employer has warned him that unless he stops drinking he will be dismissed from his job. He wants to stop drinking and wants to know his treatment options. He does not have obvious mental health or physical health problems.

Discuss the treatment of alcohol dependence and any other issues raised by the patient.

6.

A 35-year-old woman who has been suffering from panic attacks and agoraphobia for several years has been referred by her GP for advice regarding prescription of diazepam and temazepam. You are meeting her in the outpatient clinic.

Please discuss with her the management of benzodiazepine use. Do not take a psychiatric history.

7.

A 30-year-old woman was admitted to the acute medical ward following an overdose of prescribed antidepressant medication. At the time of admission she was under the influence of alcohol but 12 hours later she has become sober and has been referred for a psychiatric assessment. You have completed your assessment and found that this patient suffers from depression and has been drinking excessively to cope with stress. You have discovered that being under the influence of alcohol was an important factor in the overdose.

Using motivational interviewing techniques, try to motivate this patient to abstain from alcohol. You are not required to discuss the management of depression.

8.

A 25-year-old woman with a 10-week pregnancy has been referred by the antenatal services for assessment and management of her substance misuse.

Assess her substance misuse history and give advice about substance use in pregnancy and treatment.

STATION 1

1a: Opioid dependence

> **KEY POINTS**
> Communication and empathy
> Details of illicit drug use
> Explore high risk behaviours
> Physical complications
> Psychiatric comorbidity
> Global rating

INTRODUCE YOURSELF

SET THE SCENE

Start the station by thanking the patient for coming to see you. Enquire about reasons for seeking help, whether on his own accord or subject to a Drug Treatment and Testing Order (DTTO) or a Drug Rehabilitation Requirement (DRR). Explain that you will need to ask him details of his legal and illicit drug use and associated problems, if any.

COMPLETING THE TASKS

After the introductions ask what substances he has been using recently, including legal and illicit drug use, type, method of administration, quantity and frequency.

C: 'I understand that you have been using drugs for some time, please can you tell what you have been using recently?'

Pt: 'I have been using heroin.'

C: 'Are you using anything else, for example alcohol or cannabis?'

Pt: 'I drink alcohol occasionally, a couple of pints once or twice a week, and I smoke skunk once in a while.'

One should be familiar with street names of illicit drugs; please refer to the table below.

Common Street Names/Types of Some Illicit Drugs	
Amphetamines	Speed, Uppers
Benzodiazepines	Temazzies & Jellies (Temazepam), Vallies (Diazepam)
Cannabis	Dope, Weed, Skunk, Hash, Grass
Cocaine	C, Charlie, Coke, Snow, Crack & bones (Crack Cocaine)
Heroin	H, Horse, Smack
LSD	L, Acid,
MDMA (Ecstasy)	E, XTC, Hug drug, Adam

C: 'We can discuss use of the alcohol and cannabis later on, but shall we first look into your heroin use? Please can you tell me how much heroin you use and how you use it.'

Ask for details of the amount of heroin used, the frequency of use, the route of administration (whether smoking, snorting or injecting). Some users may not be able to quantify the amount; enquire about the amount of money spent – the street price and the quality of heroin vary and it usually costs about £40 per gram. Many users may smoke (chase) as well as injecting the drug. Ask about first use, pattern of use and any periods of abstinence/treatment.

Explore the following:

- Criteria for dependence: these are the same as for alcohol. The withdrawal symptoms associated with heroin and other opioids are:

  aches and pains, anxiety, stomach cramps, nausea, hot/cold flushes, running nose, yawning, goose flesh, sweating, tremors, dilated pupils, restlessness, tachycardia, diarrhoea, vomiting, muscle twitches.

- Use of other illicit drugs and alcohol.
- Medical complications: any accidental overdoses, abscess/infections, blood-borne viral diseases – hepatitis B & C, HIV.
- Psychiatric complications/comorbidity: anxiety, depression, PTSD, etc. When psychiatric symptoms are present, try to establish whether they predate and/or persisted during periods of abstinence. Do not go into details of psychiatric history; remember the task of the station.
- Psychosocial complications: relationships, social and occupational functioning. Briefly explore what are the predisposing, precipitating and maintaining factors.
- Forensic history: the fact that he has been referred by the probation officer indicates involvement with the Criminal Justice System (CJS). Ask how he was funding his drug habit. Often drug users resort to crimes to fund their drug use. Briefly ask about previous offending and criminal records.

PROBLEM SOLVING

Individuals referred by the CJS may have been coerced into treatment; they may view health professionals as part of the CJS. It will be important to emphasize that you are not part of the CJS but will have to work closely with it. If the individual is not motivated one may have to use motivation enhancement techniques to improve this. Use of a non-confrontational approach is essential in dealing with these individuals, who are often complex and difficult to engage.

1b: Discussion with probation officer

KEY POINTS
Consent issues
Dealing with a different profession
Treatment options
Global rating

INTRODUCE YOURSELF

SET THE SCENE

After introductions, thank the PO for coming along and mention that you have the client's consent for sharing information. Enquire whether the PO has any particular question or information before you get into the details. The discussion would be shaped by your earlier assessment and information gathered.

COMPLETING THE TASKS

Outline the principles of opioid dependence treatment, which would include pharmacological and structured psychosocial interventions in a multi-disciplinary setting.

Pharmacological treatment: Opioid detoxification or maintenance; factors that need to be considered are patient choice, motivation and engagement, length and pattern of use, and previous treatments. Detoxification (usually over 2–4 weeks) is usually with gradually tapering doses of the full opioid agonist methadone or partial agonist buprenorphine followed by prescription of opioid antagonists such as naltrexone. Symptomatic and supportive measures, including prescribing of lofexidine (alpha 2 agonist) and non-steroidal analgesics either by themselves or along with the opioid agonist, are an option. If maintenance (substitute prescribing) is chosen then patients are stabilized either on methadone or on buprenorphine and supervised prescription/administration is continued for many years. Regular monitoring via drug testing through urine/salivary analysis is mandatory to prevent misuse of the prescription and detect further use of illicit drugs. The idea behind substitute prescribing is stabilization, prevention of harm associated with injecting, reduction of criminal activity and engaging in treatment.

Psychosocial intervention: Substitute prescribing or detoxification on their own do not have much value; these should be part of a treatment plan which will include structured psychosocial interventions such as individual/group therapy, provision of suitable accommodation, support from family and friends and self-help organizations such as Narcotics Anonymous. Coordination and close working between statutory and non-statutory agencies, including health, Social Services, the Criminal Justice System and the voluntary sector, are essential in order to cater to the needs of these often complex patients. Despite best efforts, a significant number of patients relapse. Needle exchange, education about safe sex and injecting behaviour, screening for blood-borne viruses, vaccination against hepatitis B and nutritional advice are some of the harm minimization strategies for those who continue to use illicit drugs.

FURTHER READING

Department of Health (England) and the devolved administrations (2007) *Drug Misuse and Dependence: UK Guidelines on Clinical Management* (commonly known as the Orange Guidelines). London: DoH.

STATION 2

2a: Physical examination of drug intoxication/ withdrawal state

> **KEY POINTS**
> Communication and empathy
> Sensitivity in conducting examination
> Demonstrate physical examination skills
> Consequences of drug misuse
> Global rating

INTRODUCE YOURSELF

SET THE SCENE

Explain to the patient that you need to carry out an examination on him. If the patient appears confused or seems not to understand your explanation, try again; do not rush into the examination if he resists it.

C: 'I am a doctor and I need to examine you. Is that OK? I would like to check your pulse, blood pressure and temperature first. I'll explain what I'm doing as I go along. You shouldn't experience any discomfort at any time, but let me know if you are uncomfortable at any point. Do you understand me?'

COMPLETING THE TASKS

After explaining the task, proceed to carry out relevant mental state examination (MSE) and systematic physical examination, including general and systems examination.

General examination may include general appearance, behaviour, conscious level (alert, drowsy, confusion), self-care (dress, grooming), movements (voluntary, involuntary) and comprehension.

Systems examination includes:

Cardiovascular:	Pulse, blood pressure, auscultation of precordium.
Respiratory:	Respiratory rate, pattern of respiration (regularity and depth), auscultation of chest (lungs).
Abdomen:	Jaundice, scars, distended veins, tenderness, palpation for mass, liver and spleen.
Nervous system:	Higher mental functions (consciousness, orientation, memory, speech, etc.), cranial nerves (mainly pupils and nystagmus), motor and sensory deficits, coordination, gait.
MSE:	Reaction, evidence of perceptual abnormalities, behaviour suggestive of delusions, mood state.

Be familiar with the features of various drug intoxication and withdrawal states; some of these are summarized below.

Alcohol

Intoxication: tachycardia, hypertension, mydriasis (dilated pupils), skin flushing, slurred speech, impaired coordination, nystagmus, and gait disturbance.

Withdrawal: tremors, sweating, increased temperature, tachycardia, dilated pupils, and diaphoresis. Seizure and delirium tremens are not uncommon.

Look for consequences of long-term excessive alcohol use – virtually any organ in the body could be affected:

GI system: poor nutritional state, anaemia, hepatomegaly, and liver failure signs such as jaundice, oedema and spider naevi.

Nervous system: peripheral neuropathy, Wernicke's encephalopathy (ataxia, nystagmus and confusion), Korsakoff syndrome (memory impairment).

Cardiovascular: higher blood pressure, alcoholic cardiomyopathy.

Musculoskeletal: proximal myopathy (proximal muscle weakness, shoulder and hip).

Opioids

Intoxication: varying degrees of clouded consciousness, pinpoint pupils, and respiratory depression.

Withdrawal: sweating, nausea, vomiting, diarrhoea, abdominal cramps, myalgia, bone pains, dilated pupils, rhinorrhoea, insomnia.

Stimulants (cocaine and amphetamines)

Intoxication: euphoria, agitation, increased pulse and blood pressure, sweating, tremors, confusion, dilated pupils, hyperactivity, seizures, stroke, cardiac arrhythmias (irregular heart beats), and sudden death can occur.

Withdrawal: dysphorea (crash), anxiety, hypersomnolence, paranoid ideation, hallucinations.

Benzodiazepines

Intoxication: drowsiness, ataxia, dysarthria, nystagmus, and hypothermia.

Withdrawal: irritability, anxiety, insomnia, hypersensitivity to stimuli, tremor, hypotonia and hyporeflexia, seizures.

Cannabis

Intoxication: dry mouth, red eyes, impaired perception and motor skills, decreased short-term memory, paranoia, mood swings, and rarely hallucinations.

Lysergic acid diethylamide (LSD)

Intoxication: dilated pupils, higher body temperature, increased heart rate and blood pressure, sweating, loss of appetite, sleeplessness, dry mouth, tremors, flashbacks, perceptual abnormalities.

Look for factors associated with use of illicit drug use such as needle track marks, thrombosed veins, perforated nasal septum.

PROBLEM SOLVING

This will be a challenging station. You will need to be selective in your assessment and focus on the task.

If the patient is uncooperative, try to carry out as much of the examination as possible. Try Kirby's examination of an uncooperative patient.

General reaction, attitude, posture, hygiene, dressing, behaviour towards staff, symptoms and signs of resistance, evasiveness, irritability/apathy, movements (retardation/overactivity), facial expression and conscious level (alert, attentive, placid, vacant, aversive, perplexed, distressed), emotional state and indication of mood fluctuations (tears/smiles), eyes (open or closed, if open, do they follow the examiner's movements or are they fixed, any eye contact? and if closed, does the patient resist attempts to open the eyes?), pattern and content of speech (mute, slow/retarded, over talkative, relevance, coherence), reaction to what is said or done, muscular reactions (rigidity, resistance).

2b: Discussion with the consultant

> **KEY POINTS**
> Effective communication of key findings
> Differential diagnosis
> Management plan
> Global rating

INTRODUCE YOURSELF

'Hello, my name is Dr____. Am I speaking to the on-call consultant?'

SET THE SCENE

'I am the doctor on call, I am sorry to disturb you. I need to discuss a patient whom I have assessed....' The discussion would be shaped by your findings from the previously carried out assessment.

COMPLETING THE TASKS

Try to present the findings in a systematic way; when prompted, discuss the differential diagnosis with points for and against. Explain that if possible you will try to obtain further information (from staff/professionals, family/friends if and when they are identified and from the patient himself if he becomes communicative) and attempt tests such as urine and other body fluid drug screen, routine bloods (be prepared to justify any of the investigations). Be familiar with the management of illicit drug and alcohol intoxication and withdrawal states, including management of overdoses and complications such as delirium and seizures.

Consider the management in the short, medium and longer term.

A discussion of risk is likely to ensue, as will issues of disposal and whether the patient is likely to need further assessment and/or treatment under the Mental Health Act.

FURTHER READING

Department of Health (England) and the devolved administrations (2007) *Drug Misuse and Dependence: UK Guidelines on Clinical Management* (commonly known as the Orange Guidelines). London: DoH.

STATION 3

3a: Cannabis and schizophrenia: discussion with family

KEY POINTS
Communication and empathy
Details of illicit drug use
Associated problems
Sensitive to the needs of carer
Global rating

INTRODUCE YOURSELF

SET THE SCENE

Start the station by thanking the mother for coming to the ward and speaking to you. Inform her that her son has consented to the meeting. Enquire about her views on his current state, treatment, and the effects of the illness on herself and other carers (family/friends).

COMPLETING THE TASKS

After setting the scene you might say:

C: 'This must be a difficult time for you. Have you been told about your son's diagnosis?' If not, be prepared to explain to her. 'Today I want to find out more about the things that may have had a role in Mark becoming unwell. There are a number of risk factors for the development of schizophrenia. One such risk factor is use of illicit drugs. Mark has been reluctant to talk about it, but I wonder whether you know anything about his drug use....'

M: 'Well, doctor, as far as I know Mark does not use drugs ... except for cannabis.'

C: 'Actually, did you know that cannabis is an illicit drug and can contribute to the development of mental health problems? Please can you tell me about Mark's use of cannabis?'

M: 'I caught him smoking cannabis soon after his 14th birthday; I was not happy about it but didn't say much as many kids nowadays smoke the stuff.'

C: 'We know that quite a few people use cannabis but that does not make it any less harmful. There is increasing evidence that it causes mental health problems. Do you know when Mark started using cannabis and how often he used it?'

Obtain illicit drug and alcohol consumption details as outlined in the Opioid Dependence and Alcohol Dependence Stations.

M: 'I didn't know that cannabis caused so many problems. If I had only known these things before, I could have done something about it.'

C: 'Please don't be hard on yourself; as you said, you did not know these things and probably even Mark himself didn't know about it. The important thing is how we can help Mark to get better and remain well. It will be important for him to stay clear of all illicit drugs. Now I know that he regularly smoked cannabis from a young age, I can talk to him about it.'

PROBLEM SOLVING

The carers may feel guilty about their role in the causation of the condition, be it genetics, family environment, lack of supervision, etc. It is important to acknowledge these feelings, and to educate and empower them so that they can contribute constructively to the care and treatment of the affected individual.

ADDITIONAL POINTS

There can be similar scenarios involving the role of genetics (family history of similar illness), compliance with medication, and illicit drugs in a relapse of schizophrenia, etc. The key skills would be about obtaining collateral history from carers and being sensitive to their needs.

3b: Cannabis and schizophrenia

KEY POINTS
Communication and rapport
Empathy
Explaining cannabis's links to illness
Educating patient
Global rating

INTRODUCE YOURSELF

SET THE SCENE

C: 'Hello Mr Roberts, I am Dr_____, the ward doctor; we have met a few times in the last few days, and it is good to see you doing well. I think you will soon be ready for discharge. There are a few important things that we need to talk about today. We need to discuss your cannabis use and be sure that you understand its effects.'

If the patient were to deny use of cannabis you might have to mention the positive urine drug screen and collateral history from his mother. However, it is important not to be confrontational and you may use the motivational interviewing techniques as outlined in the Motivational Interviewing Station.

COMPLETING THE TASKS

Pt: 'Cannabis helps me to relax, most of my friends use it....'

C: 'Cannabis helps some people to relax but it also causes a number of problems. Are you aware of these?'

Pt: 'I am not sure....'

C: 'Cannabis users are known to experience higher rates of anxiety, depression, paranoia and psychosis. The heavier and longer the use, the higher the chance of someone developing mental health problems. For example, the risk of schizophrenia and psychosis doubles in regular cannabis users, especially, as in your case, if they started using it before the age of 15 years.'

Use an interactive approach to explain and educate about the role of cannabis in the causation of schizophrenia and the higher risk of relapse with continued use. You may suggest alternative ways to cope with difficulties and to 'relax'.

PROBLEM SOLVING

Many individuals may have a history of poly-substance misuse. Be familiar with the role of stimulants in the causation of schizophrenia/psychosis.

FURTHER READING

Cannabis and mental health leaflet (with references) published by the Royal College of Psychiatrists (available from http://www.rcpsych.ac.uk).

STATION 4: Alcohol dependence history

KEY POINTS
Communication and empathy
Details of alcohol consumption
Explore the criteria for dependence
Associated problems
Psychiatric comorbidity
Feedback to patient

INTRODUCE YOURSELF

SET THE SCENE

Thank the patient for agreeing to speak to you and acknowledge his anxiety and any distress. Ask if it would be OK to talk about what had been happening (open question to start).

COMPLETING THE TASKS

After the introductions you might say:

C: 'I heard that your physical examination was OK but some of your blood tests were abnormal. What you think might be the reason?'

Pt: 'I don't know.'

C: 'The commonest reason for these tests to be abnormal is excessive alcohol consumption.'

Pt: 'I do not drink excessively.'

C: 'Shall we look at what it is you drink? Please can you tell me what you drink each day?' 'Thank you for that, what about the weekends?'

Ask the patient what he drinks each day, including the brand and quantity of the alcoholic beverage. As individuals often minimize their alcohol consumption, ask them: 'Are there times and days when you might drink more than the usual amount?' It would look impressive (although not necessary), once the patient has given the details of his consumption, to calculate the units by multiplying the volume in mL by the alcohol by volume (ABV) and dividing the result by 1000; one 500 mL can of 5 per cent lager would be 2.5 units. Most often people consume a mixture of alcoholic beverages, in which case you should calculate units for each beverage and add them up to arrive at the total. The following is a table of commonly used quantities of beverages and approximate units of alcohol:

Beverage	Quantity	Units
Ordinary beer (3–4%)	1 pint (568 mL)	2
Strong beer (8–9 %)	1 pint (568 mL)	4.5
Wine (12 %)	1 glass (175 mL)	2
Spirits (40%)	1 pub measure (25 mL)	1

Do not get bogged down with numbers and percentages; you should get an idea of quantity of alcohol being consumed and demonstrate that to the examiner. 'So you are telling me that in a week you consume about 2 litres of vodka and 10 pints of lager, that's approximately 100 units per week, which is far in excess of the recommended maximum of 21 units per week for men.'

After eliciting the alcohol consumption details, including the age of first drink, lifetime pattern of drinking, and any previous periods of abstinence/treatment, focus on the following:

• Criteria for dependence: Check for cravings, loss of control, tolerance, withdrawal symptoms, salience and excessive use despite knowledge of harmful physical or mental health consequences.

- Medical complications: Seizures, delirium tremens, head injury, liver damage, etc.
- Psychiatric complications/comorbidity: Anxiety, depression, post-traumatic stress disorder (PTSD), etc. When psychiatric symptoms are present, try to establish whether the psychiatric conditions are primary by enquiring whether these symptoms predated and/or persisted during periods of abstinence. Do not go into details of psychiatric history; remember the task of the station.
- Psychosocial complications: Relationships, social and occupational functioning, forensic history.
- Time allowing, you could provide feedback of your assessment to the patient. You might say: 'You have told me that on average you have been drinking 100 units of alcohol per week for the last 2 years, you crave alcohol and experience shakes and sweats in the morning. Without alcohol you feel anxious about facing people. You have been warned at your workplace for being drunk on duty and your wife is threatening to leave you if you don't stop drinking. I think you are dependent on alcohol and it has caused you a number of problems. I think you need to do something about it.'

Pt: 'What can I do about it?'

C: 'Ideally you should stop drinking and there is help available for you to achieve this. You are possibly suffering from withdrawal symptoms, which is why you are uncomfortable and may be your reason for wanting to leave. You can be prescribed medication to avoid these withdrawal symptoms. You might also need help with some of the problems associated with alcohol dependence. I will give you information on how you can access our service and also give you some leaflets. You can look through these and I'll be happy to discuss any issues with you another time. In the meantime it's important that you undergo further tests and assessments that have been recommended to you.'

PROBLEM SOLVING

Individuals who consume alcohol excessively can be defensive and minimize their alcohol consumption. A gentle and non-confrontational approach often succeeds in building rapport and eliciting details of alcohol consumption and problems associated with it. Be prepared to have a more detailed conversation about treatment options, including inpatient detoxification.

Features of the alcohol dependence syndrome (more information below)

Stereotyped pattern of alcohol consumption

Salience of drinking behaviour

Compulsion to drink

Increased tolerance to alcohol

Repeated withdrawal symptoms on reduction of alcohol intake

Relief/avoidance of withdrawal symptoms with alcohol intake

Reinstatement after abstinence

ADDITIONAL POINTS

Harm minimization if patient not willing to stop drinking.

Identify predisposing, precipitating and maintaining factors for alcohol dependence.

⇧ **Features of the alcohol dependence syndrome – more information**

1 Non-dependent drinkers drink in accordance with a variety of cues whereas the dependent drinker drinks to avoid symptoms of withdrawal. The drinking repertoire is therefore narrowed.

2 The dependent drinker will continue to drink even though there are several negative consequences such as financial, familial and physical.

3 The individual knows that taking a drink is irrational and the action is resisted but as in the case of compulsions in obsessive–compulsive disorder (OCD), further drink is taken.

4 Physiological and neurochemical changes (more alcohol is required to achieve the same effect). In the later stages, tolerance develops, often with loss of control over alcohol intake.

5 Shaking, trembling, anxiety, physiological craving, vomiting, seizures.

6 Can drink throughout the night and on waking in severe cases.

7 For severe dependants, following a period of abstinence, the previous high levels of alcohol intake and tolerance can be achieved within a number of days.

FURTHER READING

Edwards, G. & Gross, M. (1976) Alcohol dependence: provisional description of a clinical syndrome. *British Medical Journal*, *1* (6017), 1058–61.

STATION 5: Alcohol dependence management

KEY POINTS
Communication and empathy
Treatment options
Confidentiality
Answering other questions
Global rating

INTRODUCE YOURSELF

SET THE SCENE

C: 'I am glad that you have come to see me today about your drinking and that you want to address it. I think we should discuss the options for treatment. How does this sound?'

COMPLETING THE TASKS

Enquire about the aims and goals of treatment, i.e. abstinence or reduced and controlled drinking. Discuss the treatment options, including the medical and psychosocial interventions, both in the short term and in the long term (bio-psychosocial approach).

Short term – The rationale and principles of medically assisted withdrawal from alcohol (detox):

- Management of withdrawal symptoms – Most commonly with benzodiazepines. Chlordiazepoxide is the most widely used medication; dose can vary considerably depending on the severity of dependence, physical health, etc., but the usual starting dose is 20–40mg qds and tapered down and stopped over 7–10 days. 'Front loading' and symptom-triggered therapy are alternatives but not commonly used. The aim is to minimize the discomfort of withdrawal symptoms and prevent serious complications such as withdrawal seizures and/or delirium tremens. Lorazepam or oxazepam is used in those with hepatic failure. Chlormethiazole and carbamazepine are other options but are not commonly used in the UK.
- Vitamin supplements – Mainly thiamine and other vitamin B preparations, often by parenteral route. Pabrinex, a preparation with thiamine, riboflavin, pyridoxin, ascorbic acid and nicotinamide, is administered by the intramuscular (i.m.) route for 3–5 days; intravenous (i.v.) preparation can be used in suspected cases of Wernicke's encephalopathy (WE). Vitamin supplements are administered to replenish body stores and to prevent WE and Korsakoff's syndrome.
- Management of comorbid medical and psychiatric conditions.
- Psychological support prior to and during the detox.
- Setting – Planned treatment works better. Community setting for those with less severe dependence, no significant physical or psychiatric comorbidity and good social support, inpatient setting for complex cases or failed community detox.

Long term – Aim to maintain abstinence; psychosocial interventions, including relapse prevention, motivational enhancement and cognitive behavioural therapy (CBT) in individual or group settings, are the mainstays of treatment. Pharmacological treatments can supplement psychosocial interventions and these may include acamprosate, naltrexone and disulfiram. Self-help organizations such as Alcoholics Anonymous can benefit many individuals. Measures such as suitable accommodation, debt counselling, employment, and family work are often necessary to rehabilitate and integrate the individual with the family and society.

C: 'You seem to have been dependent on alcohol for about a year, you do not have any physical or mental health problems and have a supportive family, hence I think you can be detoxed at home. I will explain and provide some leaflets about the treatment process. Detox is only a small part of giving up alcohol; it will be important for you to look into the reasons for your drinking and how to avoid drinking again and this can be achieved through psychological help.'

C: 'What we have discussed is confidential. Your employer may ask us for a report or an opinion about your suitability to return to work, etc., and we can only provide information to your employer with your consent. If you were to object to information being shared with your employer we would not do so; however, that might adversely affect your employment.'

PROBLEM SOLVING

As with other substances of addiction, relapse rates for alcohol dependence are high. Many individuals are able to achieve abstinence only after several treatment episodes. Consider residential rehabilitation for those who find it difficult to stop drinking. Consider harm minimization strategies such as reduced drinking, improved nutrition, vitamin supplements and social support for those who do not want to stop drinking.

Although management of delirium tremens or Wernicke's encephalopathy might be an unlikely Clinical Assessment of Skills and Competencies (CASC) scenario, it would still be advisable to familiarize yourself with these topics.

FURTHER READING

Lingford-Hughes, A.R., Welch, S. & Nutt, D.J. (2004). Evidence-based guidelines for the pharmacological management of substance misuse, addiction and comorbidity: recommendations from the British Association for Psychopharmacology. *Journal of Psychopharmacology*, *18*, 293.

Scottish Intercollegiate Guideline Network (2003, September) *The management of harmful drinking and alcohol dependence in primary care.* Clinical Guideline No 74.

STATION 6: Benzodiazepine (BZD) misuse

KEY POINTS
Communication and empathy
Details of drug use/misuse
Management of BZD use/misuse
Global rating

INTRODUCE YOURSELF

SET THE SCENE

C: 'Your GP has requested we discuss your medication, particularly the diazepam and temazepam. Would that be OK? Before I can make any suggestions I need to ask you about your use of these medications, so please can you tell me about it.'

COMPLETING THE TASKS

Enquire about the dose and duration of the BZD use and whether all the medication is prescribed by the GP or she gets some/all of it from 'the street'. Enquire about use of other illicit drugs and alcohol. You may need to enquire briefly about the anxiety symptoms, whether the BZD use predated the panic attacks and agoraphobia and if there were any periods in which she was free of the anxiety symptoms. What was the pattern of her BZD use? Similarly, how were the anxiety symptoms during the BZD-free period, if any?

It can often be useful to summarize, particularly towards the end of the station.

C: 'So you are telling me that you started having panic attacks about 3 years ago and started drinking excessively (alcohol), but you soon realized the dangers of drinking after you were caught drink driving. About a year ago your GP prescribed you some diazepam as you found it difficult to go out of the house, but you soon started taking more than was prescribed, and you sometimes bought diazepam and temazepam from "the street".

In the last few months you have been taking 30–40mg of diazepam and 10–20mg of temazepam per day and you experience panic attacks if you can't take the BZD. What do you want to do about it?'

Pt: 'I don't want to take the diazepam or the temazepam, but I get horrible panic attacks, I can't go out of the house, and I can't sleep without these, I feel so anxious without them, the very thought of not taking them makes me anxious.'

C: 'BZDs are very good at providing short-term relief but you soon develop tolerance and need more and more of them. Soon you can end up becoming dependent on them. I understand you experience significant anxiety and panic but in the long run BZDs are not the answer to these.'

Pt: 'What do you suggest?'

C: 'The panic attacks and agoraphobia are best managed with another medication which is not addictive and there is good evidence that CBT is more effective than medication alone in the long run. A combination of these two is quite effective, which leaves us with what to do about your BZD prescription.'

Pt: 'How can I stop the BZD?'

Outline the principles of medically assisted BZD withdrawal:

- Transfer all BZD & Z drug prescriptions to a long-acting preparation such as diazepam (refer to the table below for equivalent doses).

Approximate equivalent doses to diazepam 5mg	
Chlordiazepoxide	15mg
Lorazepam	0.5mg
Clonazepam	0.25mg
Nitrazepam	5mg
Oxazepam	15mg
Temazepam	10mg
Zopiclone	7.5mg
Zolpidem	10mg

- If on large doses of BZD or concomitant use with methadone/alcohol dependence, consider BZD withdrawal in an inpatient setting.
- Taper down the dose of diazepam gradually – an individual approach is needed as patient sensitiveness can differ; in an outpatient setting the GP can consider decreasing it by 10–25 per cent per fortnight.
- Be cautious and seek expert advice if there are more complex psychiatric and/or physical comorbidities such as epilepsy.
- Supportive counselling/groups along with treatment of underlying conditions such as panic attacks and agoraphobia as in this patient is required.
- Urine drug screens to monitor misuse of other drugs and prevent diversion of the prescribed medication.

PROBLEM SOLVING

At times it may be better to prescribe/stabilize some individuals on a small dose of diazepam if they cannot be successfully withdrawn from BZD. The aim here would be to stabilize the individual's life and prevent their dealing in the illicit drug market.

FURTHER READING

Department of Health (England) and the devolved administrations (2007) *Drug Misuse and Dependence: UK Guidelines on Clinical Management* (commonly known as the Orange Guidelines). London: DoH.

Lingford-Hughes, A.R., Welch, S. & Nutt, D.J. (2004). Evidence-based guidelines for the pharmacological management of substance misuse, addiction and comorbidity: recommendations from the British Association for Psychopharmacology. *Journal of Psychopharmacology*, *18*, 293.

STATION 7: Motivational interviewing (MI)

KEY POINTS
Communication and empathy
Assess stage of motivation
Demonstrate MI skills
Answering other questions
Global rating

INTRODUCE YOURSELF

SET THE SCENE

C: 'We have talked about what happened, and how you got to be here, and part of it seems to be due to alcohol. I guess what I'd like to know is, what are the things you like about alcohol? What's really good about drinking for you?'

COMPLETING THE TASKS

After setting the scene you might try to assess the patient's views on excessive alcohol consumption, whether she recognizes it to be a problem and if so whether she wants to address it. If she wants to address her drinking, what does she want to do? The discussion would depend upon her current stage of motivation. Described below are the stages of motivation for change and suggested tasks relevant to the stage.

Stage of Motivation for Change	Suggested Task
1. Pre-contemplation: Does not consider the possibility for change.	Raise doubt. Increase patient's perception of risks and problems with current behaviour. (Excessive alcohol consumption worsening the depression).
2. Contemplation: Ambivalence, considers change and rejects it.	Tip the balance, evoke reasons to change, risks of not changing, and strengthen self-efficacy. (Increased risk of self-harm while intoxicated).

3. Preparation: Determination, considers various strategies for change.	Help patient determine best course of action (reduced drinking or abstinence).
4. Action: Engages in particular actions designed to bring about change.	Help patient to take steps toward change. (Engage with treating team for depression and alcohol consumption.)
5. Maintenance: Strives to sustain changes made in action phase.	Help patient identify and use strategies to prevent relapse. (Effective treatment of depression, coping with stress.)
6. Relapse: May have minor slips or major relapses.	Help patient renew process of contemplation, determination and action, without becoming stuck or demoralized due to relapse (re-engagement with treatment).

In the current scenario the patient is likely to be in one of the first three stages.

C: 'Do you think the overdose might have happened even if you hadn't been drinking? Or do you think that really had to do with the alcohol?'

Pt: 'I think I just lost control for a minute, I wouldn't have lost that control if I had been sober.'

The principles of motivational interviewing include the following.

Express empathy

Expression of empathy is critical to the MI approach. When patients feel that they are understood, they are more able to open up to their own experiences and share those experiences with others. Importantly, when patients perceive empathy, they become more open to gentle challenges by the interviewer about lifestyle issues and beliefs about substance use.

Support self-efficacy

Patients' belief that change is possible is an important motivator to succeeding in making a change. Patients are responsible for choosing and carrying out actions to change in the MI approach. The interviewer focuses his/her efforts on helping the patients stay motivated, and supporting their sense of self-efficacy is a great way to do that.

Roll with resistance

In MI, the interviewer does not fight client resistance, but 'rolls with it'. Statements demonstrating resistance are not challenged. Instead the interviewer uses the patients' resistance to further explore their views. MI encourages individuals to develop their own solutions to the problems that they themselves have defined; the interviewer should not impose his/her ideas.

Develop discrepancy

Motivation for change occurs when people perceive a discrepancy between where they are and where they want to be. When individuals perceive that their current behaviours are not leading towards some important future goal, they become more motivated to make important life changes.

C: 'We have talked about your alcohol consumption and how it adversely affects your mood and makes you impulsive, but you feel it helps you cope with the stress.'

Pt: 'I know I shouldn't be drinking, especially when I am on an antidepressant. My key worker and my family have been telling me not to drink but I was ignoring them, I guess this overdose changes that. I will have to stop drinking and look at other ways of handling the stress in my life.'

C: 'What do you think you can do?'

Pt: 'I will discuss with my key worker a group programme she was talking about. She was telling me that it helps people stop drinking. I think I will attend that group, and I will also attend the sessions about handling stress so that I am less likely to drink.'

C: 'These seem to be good ideas. You have been managing your home, looking after kids and supporting your mother. You have been under a lot of stress and turned to drink. I think you are a capable person and you will able to stop drinking, which might help improve your depression....'

PROBLEM SOLVING

If the patient denies problems and does not wish to change anything, do not become despondent, but try to provide information, educate about the link between worsening depression and alcohol consumption. Use open-ended questions and MI principles.

> **FURTHER READING**
> Sciacca, K. (1997) Removing barriers: dual diagnosis and motivational interviewing. *Professional Counselor*, *12* (1), 41–6.

STATION 8: Substance misuse management in pregnancy

> **KEY POINTS**
> Communication and empathy
> Elicit history
> Effects on the unborn baby
> Treatment options
> Confidentiality
> Global rating

INTRODUCE YOURSELF

SET THE SCENE

Thank the patient for coming to see you, and enquire about her understanding of the referral. State that you want to enquire about her use of illicit drugs and alcohol.

COMPLETING THE TASKS

Obtain the history as outlined in the Alcohol History and Opioid Dependence stations. Specifically ask about the quantity and duration of substances she has been using during the pregnancy. Tactfully ask whether it was a planned pregnancy and who the father might be. A difficult issue is asking about a history of prostitution and this would best be done by normalizing e.g. 'Sometimes I see people who have had to fund their habit by sleeping with men for money. Has anything like this happened to you?' Do not spend too much time on history as the scenario has other tasks as well.

An example scenario might be as follows:

C: 'You have been telling me that you have used heroin and alcohol daily in the last 6 months and at times taken diazepam as well. What do you want to do about it?'

Pt: 'I am not sure, the pregnancy was unexpected, and I am not sure whether the baby is affected. What might have been the effects on the baby?'

Briefly explain the effects of the substances on the foetus; the higher the doses and duration of substance intake, the greater is the risk to the foetus.

Substance	Main effects on unborn baby
Smoking (Tobacco)	Miscarriage, low birth weight, sudden infant death syndrome (SIDS), congenital defects.
Alcohol	Miscarriage, foetal alcohol syndrome – low birth weight, cognitive deficits, facial abnormalities and failure to thrive.
Opioids	Low birth weight, pre-term delivery, SIDS.
Benzodiazepines	Cleft palate, reduced growth and brain development.
Cocaine	Miscarriage, placental abruption, stillbirth, neonatal death and SIDS.

C: 'Alcohol and drugs can affect the baby throughout the pregnancy, so the sooner you stop, the less will be the effect on the baby. Continuing use of alcohol or drugs increases the risks of complications to you as well.'

Treatment principles – these are broadly similar to non-pregnant drug users; some of the additional and specific requirements are:

- Substance misuse treatment to be fast tracked.
- Close coordination of treatment between various agencies including antenatal, substance misuse, paediatric, social services and the family.
- Support to stop smoking (tobacco), alcohol and all illicit drugs.
- Psychosocial interventions (PSI) for tobacco smoking cessation, nicotine replacement therapy in those who do not succeed with PSI.
- No safe limit for alcohol consumption in pregnancy. If detox is required, inpatient setting preferred with least effective doses of BZD; benefits of detox with BZD outweigh risk of continued alcohol use.
- Stabilize opioid users on methadone. The dose may need to be increased in the third trimester due to increased metabolism; the risks to the mother and the unborn baby are least on methadone. If detoxification is planned, carry this out with caution in the second trimester, usually 2–3mg every 3–5 days.
- If BZD dependent, prescribe least effective dose of diazepam.
- Illicit drugs such as cocaine, amphetamines and cannabis can be safely stopped, no pharmacological intervention needed. Monitor drug use through regular screening.

- Immunize against hepatitis B and counsel about risk of blood-borne viral infections to the baby during pregnancy, childbirth and breastfeeding.
- Effective pain relief during childbirth and management of neonatal withdrawal symptoms, if any.
- Psychosocial interventions are of paramount importance; most often pregnant users have substance misusing partners, so consider family/couples therapy.

PROBLEM SOLVING

Some women worry that their baby may be 'taken into care' because they use drugs. Substance misuse in itself is not a reason to involve the Social Services or to assume that these individuals cannot care for their baby. However, if there is concern about the safety or welfare of the child, their involvement will be necessary. This is true for everyone, whether they use substances or not.

FURTHER READING

Department of Health (England) and the devolved administrations (2007) *Drug Misuse and Dependence: UK Guidelines on Clinical Management* (commonly known as the Orange Guidelines). London: DoH.

Lingford-Hughes, A.R., Welch, S. & Nutt, D.J. (2004). Evidence-based guidelines for the pharmacological management of substance misuse, addiction and comorbidity: recommendations from the British Association for Psychopharmacology. *Journal of Psychopharmacology*, *18*, 293.

○ LINKED STATION 1

1a.

This is Mrs Arnold, a 53-year-old married woman, who has been seeing a counsellor in primary care as she is stressed and anxious most of the time. The patient does not feel that the sessions have been helpful and the general practitioner (GP) phones you and describes her being persistently anxious with little let-up in symptoms. He has tried to identify triggers without success and hopes you will be able to advise further.

She attends with her husband and you see them together with her consent.

Assess this woman and consider the differential diagnosis.

1b.

Mr Arnold asks if he can see you alone for a moment. His wife agrees and is happy for you both to discuss her case. He explains that he has little understanding of what it all means and wants to know what causes someone to be 'like this'. He acknowledges that she has always been a little cautious about things, but that it had become so much worse over the last few years. He had hoped she would be able to 'pull herself together' rather than having to see a psychiatrist.

Explain to Mr Arnold what causes this condition.

SINGLE STATIONS

2.

This 28-year-old taxi driver has a painful tooth but is refusing any dental intervention. He has not been to a dentist for 15 years.

Explain how you intend to help him.

3.

You have just finished a discharge planning meeting for a patient with obsessive–compulsive disorder (OCD). There were a number of healthcare professionals present, including some students. One of the student nurses asks if you had a moment to answer some questions. Although you are busy, you agree to spend a few minutes teaching.

She asks you how you make a diagnosis of OCD and what the future holds for this patient.

STATION 1

1a: Generalized anxiety disorder

KEY POINTS
Communication and rapport
Empathy
History taking
Differential diagnosis
Explanation of preferred diagnosis
Risk

INTRODUCE YOURSELF

'Hello, my name is Dr_____, I'm one of the psychiatrists.'

SET THE SCENE

Thank the couple for coming to see you today. Direct your questioning to the patient but keep the husband involved in the dynamic.

'I'd like to ask you what's been happening and I've been told you're comfortable to talk with your husband here? I understand that you've been feeling anxious – is that correct? Could you tell me what things make you feel anxious? What does the anxiety feel like?' Start with open questions as usual and then become more focused in your approach.

COMPLETING THE TASKS

Assess this woman and consider the differential diagnosis.

Your thoughts should turn to generalized anxiety disorder (GAD) from the history provided but you are to consider the differential:

Normal worry: People with GAD tend to have more worries. There is also little reprieve from the anxiety. Often they will report a history of longstanding worry as reported here. The worry is all-consuming and it is difficult to focus on other issues. It is ruminative and uncontrollable, with individuals unable to stop themselves worrying despite an acknowledgement that they worry too much. In GAD there are also the manifestations of continuous tension (psychological e.g. irritability, nervousness, and physical e.g. muscle tension, headache). These features are often enough to cause significant disruption to social and employment activities.

Medical: Ask about features of hyperthyroidism and other chronic physical ill health. Examples include:

Cardiovascular – angina, arrhythmias, heart failure

Endocrine – hyperthyroidism, carcinoid, adrenal gland dysfunction

Neurological – encephalopathies, head injury, intracerebral lesions

Respiratory – asthma, COPD, hypoxia

Mental illness: Consider and attempt to exclude:

Anxiety related to psychosis, depression, dysthymia and personality disorders (anxious and dependent).

GAD, OCD, panic disorder, agoraphobia, social phobia, specific phobia, post-traumatic stress disorder (PTSD), and adjustment disorder.

Medication: Stimulants – amphetamines, aminophylline

Anticholinergics – benztropine, procyclidine

Sympathomimetics – ephedrine (cold remedies), epinephrin

Antipsychotics – related to akathisia

Others – levodopa, bromocriptine, baclofen

Substance misuse: The use of amphetamines, cocaine, hallucinogens, alcohol and sedative hypnotics can lead to anxiety.

Withdrawal – benzodiazepines, alcohol, narcotics, hypnotics, barbiturates.

Diet – caffeine intake, monosodium glutamate, vitamin deficiencies.

RISK

GAD is often associated with depression. These patients tend to be more treatment resistant and comorbid depression increases the suicide risk.

PROBLEM SOLVING

Differentiating GAD from dysthymia can be clinically challenging. Both are associated with dysphoric mood and patients with GAD often present initially with depression as a consequence of their anxiety. Unlike PTSD and adjustment disorders in GAD, there is usually the absence of a significant life event or trauma. Unlike specific phobias, the anxiety is broad and persistent.

ADDITIONAL POINTS

GAD diagnostic guidelines (ICD-10):

Primary symptoms of anxiety are present most days for at least several weeks at a time and usually several months. Symptoms usually involve:

- apprehension – worries of future misfortune, feeling on edge, difficulty concentrating;
- motor tension – fidgeting, tension headaches, trembling, unable to relax;
- autonomic overactivity – sweaty, tachycardic, tachypnoeic, dizzy, dry mouth.

GAD is a common form of anxiety, particularly in primary care. It affects women more than men (2:1) and is commonly associated with other psychiatric morbidity. It is a chronic condition and up to one-quarter of sufferers will develop panic disorder.

In DSM-IV, the distinction between GAD and normal anxiety is explained by anxiety that is excessive, difficult to control, with significant impairment or distress.

FURTHER READING

Massion, A.O., Warshaw, M.G. & Keller, M.B. (1993) Quality of life and psychiatric morbidity in panic disorder and generalized anxiety disorder. *American Journal of Psychiatry*, *150*, 600.

World Health Organization (1992) *The ICD-10 classification of mental and behavioural disorders; clinical descriptions and diagnostic guidelines.* Geneva: WHO.

1b: Generalized anxiety disorder – aetiology

KEY POINTS
Communication and empathy
Exploring any sensitive issues
Aetiological formulation
Explanation in lay terms
Answering related questions

INTRODUCE YOURSELF

The link here would not demand an introduction but to pick up on the situation as the wife exits the scenario.

SET THE SCENE

'You asked to talk about how this could have happened to your wife. Tell me what it is you would like to know and I'll do my best to answer your questions.'

'Was there a specific reason you didn't want Mrs Arnold to be here?' 'Sometimes it is difficult to discuss things openly with loved ones. Was there anything that you thought might upset her?'

COMPLETING THE TASKS

Explain to Mr Arnold what causes this condition

'As I explained to you both, I believe your wife has a condition called generalized anxiety disorder. This belongs to a family of anxiety disorders. These conditions are common and widespread but we are still not exactly sure what causes GAD or other anxiety disorders. I'll explain to you what the current thinking is on how these conditions develop and if at any time you have questions or don't understand, please interrupt me.'

In lay terms try to explain the following.

Biological

Genetic: There is little evidence for genetic influence in GAD and it is unlikely to have a specific genetic or familial basis. Studies have shown that children of GAD mothers were no more likely to be anxious than counterparts with unaffected mothers. However, other studies have shown higher rates of GAD in families, but this may reflect the influence of a shared environment.

Pathophysiological: Neurotransmitter systems have been implicated, including serotonin, noradrenaline, glutamate, GABA and cholecystokinin. Currently there is limited evidence for one neurotransmitter having a dominant role in GAD. The benzodiazepine receptor has also been implicated.

Other: There are no consistent neuroimaging findings in GAD. There are some suggestions that the hypothalamic–pituitary–adrenal axis changes in functionality, which has a role in the stress response. There may be chronically increased cortisol levels in GAD.

Psychosocial

Cognitive–behavioural theory – according to this school of thinking, people with GAD respond inappropriately to perceived dangers. They selectively attend to negative stimuli around them and doubt their own ability to cope with them. Other cognitive models include worry as a cognitive avoidance, beliefs about the benefits of worry (worrying leads to avoidance of danger) and low self-efficacy (anxiety due to the belief that one is unable to exercise control over events).

Psychodynamic – No specific model has been developed for GAD and the theorists believe that anxiety in general is a symptom of unresolved conflicts.

Childhood: There is some evidence that early loss or separation from a parent is seen more than would be expected in GAD cases. Individuals with GAD have described the relationships with their parents as overprotective, controlling, rejecting and dysfunctional. However, these are not specific to GAD.

Life events: Despite the usual gradual onset of GAD, increased stress and life events can be a precipitant.

RISK

As part of your assessment in the previous station you will probably have enquired about suicidal ideation. You could follow that up here with the husband, but could also discuss the risks associated with comorbid depression, alcohol or substance misuse, if appropriate. Similarly risks associated with benzodiazepine (BZD) dependence could come up if treatment issues are raised by Mr Arnold.

PROBLEM SOLVING

Mr Arnold is looking for answers and the lack of definite causality might leave him feeling disgruntled. You should explain that whilst the research evidence does not allow us to be certain of what causes GAD, we have a good understanding of the condition itself and how we should treat people. This might lead him to ask about management.

ADDITIONAL POINTS

Little is known about its precise aetiology. There may be a common vulnerability shared with other anxiety and affective disorders.

The earlier GAD is treated the more effective therapy is likely to be. Unfortunately, most people tolerate the anxiety for years before they come to the attention of healthcare professionals. By this time the condition is usually severe, disabling and frequently associated with other psychiatric morbidity. The treatment is a combined psychological and pharmacological approach.

⇧ **FURTHER READING**

Cowley, D.S. & Roy-Byrne, P.P. (1991) The biology of generalized anxiety disorder and chronic anxiety. In R.M. Rapee & D.H. Barlow (eds), *Chronic anxiety. Generalized anxiety disorder and mixed anxiety-depression*. New York: Guilford Press, pp. 52–75.

STATION 2: Specific phobia

KEY POINTS
Empathy and rapport
Communication – lay terms
Differential diagnosis
Diagnosis – explanation
Management plan
Treatment options
Risk issues

INTRODUCE YOURSELF

'Hello, my name is Dr____, I'm one of the psychiatrists.'

SET THE SCENE

'I'm sorry to hear that you're in some discomfort with your tooth. Can you tell me what happened? Why haven't you seen a dentist for so long? What do you think would happen if you saw a dentist?'

COMPLETING THE TASKS

Explain how you intend to help him.

This is a management station but establishing the diagnosis and understanding the nature of his avoidance will allow you to plan his treatment appropriately. It is important therefore to ask screening questions for evidence of psychosis, affective, neurotic and somatoform disorders. Enquire about any previous or current psychiatric ill health. Ask whether he has any physical health problems e.g. thyroid dysfunction, and about caffeine and substance misuse. Ask if he would allow you at some point in the future to speak with his partner/family/friend for more information.

It is important to tease out what the anxiety relates to. In the dental situation, is it the fear of a specific dental procedure, needles, blood, pain, anaesthesia, choking, losing control, acquired infections such as HIV? Does it relate to the dentist, white coat, equipment or chair?

You quickly identify that this gentleman has a specific dental phobia related to a fear of needles. You need to explain in lay terms what you think is happening and how you suggest he is treated.

'Based on what you have told me today I believe you have what we call a specific phobia. This means that you are not usually anxious about things in your day-to-day life, but are worried specifically about the needles dentists sometimes use. Some people are petrified of spiders and this is the same sort of thing. Because we dislike spiders or needles we'll do anything to avoid them. Even the thought of it can make people feel anxious and panicky and sometimes when confronted by the object they can have panic attacks. Specific phobias are not uncommon; some suggest that about one in ten of us are affected at some point in our lives. The good news is that we can help and the most effective form of treatment is a psychological approach.'

Management: remember to use lay terms to explain the following.

Psychological

Behavioural approaches are generally accepted as the most effective approach, although cognitive therapy is also used on occasion.

Exposure-based treatment:	usually involves gradual exposure in vivo. The patient is exposed to various aspects and parts of the feared object or situation in an organized hierarchy of increasing difficulty. So initially the patient might be shown pictures of a dentist and syringe and then videos with situations of increasing use of the object. The next step might be to visit the dentist and once again grade the exposure from the waiting area until the patient is able to sit in the dentist's chair. The anxiety response should eventually habituate.
Systematic desensitization:	is seldom used today and involves using imagination to picture the feared object or scenario whilst undergoing progressive muscle relaxation. This technique uses the mechanism of reciprocal inhibition.
Modelling:	is employed by many therapists alongside exposure-based treatment, where they will demonstrate how to manage the exposure to the feared object or situation. They might, for example, hold a syringe and then ask the patient to do the same.

Medication

The role of medication is limited and no drug can be confidently recommended, particularly for regular treatment. Where psychology has failed or when patients have associated anxiety disorders, selective serotonin reuptake inhibitors (SSRIs) can have a role. BZDs should be used with caution because of the high risk of dependence, but are given for time-limited relief of severe and disabling anxiety. In flying phobia, for example, they can be used with good effect for essential journeys.

RISK

The risk in this scenario relates to his oral hygiene and how a prolonged and serious neglect of his dentition could put his health at risk.

PROBLEM SOLVING

Should, following your consultation, he decline assistance, the concern would be that any future dental work would be more complicated. Clearly the earlier he attends the better. The use of motivational interviewing techniques here can be helpful in preventing resistance.

ADDITIONAL POINTS

Ungraded exposure or flooding is thought to be as effective as graded exposure but is more unpleasant for people and thus used less frequently.

According to the ICD-10 diagnostic guidelines, a specific (isolated) phobia requires all of the following for a definite diagnosis:

1 The psychological or autonomic symptoms must be a primary manifestation of anxiety, and not secondary to other symptoms such as a delusion or obsessional thought.

2 The anxiety must be restricted to the presence of the particular phobic object or situation.

3 The object or situation is avoided whenever possible.

There is usually an appreciation that the fear or phobia is irrational and exposure precipitates anxiety which can lead to a panic attack.

FURTHER READING

Strauss, C.C. & Last, C.G. (1993) Social and simple phobias in children. *Journal of Anxiety Disorders*, 2, 141–52.

World Health Organization (1992) *The ICD-10 classification of mental and behavioural disorders; clinical descriptions and diagnostic guidelines.* Geneva: WHO.

STATION 3: OCD

KEY POINTS
Dealing with a junior colleague
Explanation of diagnosis
Prognosis
Teaching skills
Answering other questions
Risk issues

INTRODUCE YOURSELF

'Hello, I'm Dr_____, I didn't catch your name at the meeting.'

SET THE SCENE

'I'd be delighted to talk to you about obsessive–compulsive disorder. It's great that you've shown an interest. You had some specific questions which we'll talk about. Please feel free to interrupt or ask questions as we go along. Tell me, do you know anything about OCD already?'

COMPLETING THE TASKS

How do you make a diagnosis of OCD?

As its title suggests, OCD is characterized by obsessions and compulsions. This takes the form of obsessional thoughts and compulsive acts together with anxiety, depression and depersonalization in varying proportions.

Obsessions can present as:

- obsessional thoughts – repetitive intrusive words, ideas or beliefs. Usually unpleasant;
- obsessional ruminations – repetitive, circular internal debates often over simple issues;
- obsessional imagery – imagined visualized scenes, often repulsive or sexual;
- obsessional doubts – about actions not having been adequately performed e.g. closing a door or switching off gas stove;
- obsessional impulses – to carry out socially unacceptable acts e.g. shouting in public areas.

The individual will usually consider their obsessions to be illogical or 'ego-dystonic'. It is important diagnostically to explore whether thoughts are overvalued or delusional.

Compulsions present as:

- overt behaviours that the individual feels driven to do in response to an obsession;
- repetitive, stereotyped and seemingly purposeful actions.

Compulsions are repetitive behaviours or unobservable mental acts performed in response to an obsession, often according to strict rules. There are attempts to resist as they are recognized as irrational. Commonly they involve checking, cleaning and counting. As with obsessions, compulsions are ego-dystonic, persistent and intrusive. Compulsions can be associated with a sense of relief but this is short lived, so the act is repeated over.

ICD10

According to the diagnostic guidelines, a definitive diagnosis of OCD requires the following:

> Obsessional symptoms or compulsive acts, or both, on most days for at least 2 weeks, which must be distressing and interfere with activities.

> Obsessional symptoms should have the following characteristics:

- Must be recognized as the individual's own thoughts or impulses.
- At least one thought or act that is still resisted unsuccessfully.
- The thought of carrying out the act must not in itself be pleasurable.
- The thoughts, images or impulses must be unpleasantly repetitive.

What does the future hold for an OCD patient?

OCD tends to be a chronic illness for the majority of people. There are three generally agreed outcomes:

- a fluctuating course with lifelong remissions (complete or partial) and relapses (reports of 2–45 per cent);
- constant largely unchanging chronic course (15–60 per cent);
- progressive, deteriorating course (5–15 per cent).

Spontaneous and lasting remissions are rare. Some studies have even shown that after a 10–20-year remission people can still relapse. It follows that it is a condition that rarely affords complete recovery but lies dormant. Stressful life events are likely to contribute to relapses.

Despite this, some longitudinal studies have shown improvement in severity of OCD in approximately two-thirds of cases. Seventy per cent of 'mild' cases improve after 1–5 years; 33 per cent of severe (hospital admitted) patients improve after 1–5 years.

Poor prognosis is associated with:

- longer duration of illness;
- greater initial severity of illness;
- early age of onset;
- unmarried;
- presence of obsessions and compulsions;
- marked magical thinking;
- delusions;
- poor social adjustment and social skills.

Better prognosis associated with:

- short duration of illness;
- clear precipitating event;
- mild symptoms;
- absence of childhood symptoms or abnormal personality traits;
- absence of compulsions.

RISK

Often patients with OCD are secretive about their symptoms and do not seek psychiatric input for years, sometimes decades. Approximately one-third of OCD patients have comorbid depression, and severe depression is associated with higher relapse rate. There is an associated suicide risk with OCD.

PROBLEM SOLVING

It is important to mention that in making the diagnosis of OCD one has to exclude other psychiatric illness where OCD symptoms may be a feature:

- depression;
- phobias;
- personality disorder (anankastic);
- schizophrenia;
- Tourette's syndrome.

ADDITIONAL POINTS

Obsessions are usually described as recurrent thoughts, impulses and/or images that are experienced as uncontrollable. They are associated with significant distress so the individual is desperate to deal with them in some way.

Mental (covert) compulsions usually involve silent counting, use of numbers/calculations, imagining a certain situation or repeating a particular thought a certain number of times. Prevention of harm to themselves is a common explanation for mental compulsions.

If asked about demographics;   65 per cent, onset   < 25 yrs

15 per cent   > 35yrs

According to psychodynamic theory, OCD is a regression from the oedipal to the anal phase of development.

FURTHER READING

Goodman, W.K. (1999) Obsessive-compulsive disorder: diagnosis and treatment. *Journal of Clinical Psychiatry*, *60* (Suppl. 18), 27–32.

Veale, D. (2007) Cognitive behavioural therapy for obsessive compulsive disorder. *Advances in Psychiatric Treatment*, *13*, 438–46.

World Health Organization (1992) *The ICD-10 classification of mental and behavioural disorders; clinical descriptions and diagnostic guidelines.* Geneva: WHO.

○ LINKED STATION 1

1a.

This is Miss Anderson, a 22-year-old woman with an established diagnosis of anorexia nervosa (AN) who has been admitted to hospital with significant weight loss and hypokalaemia.

You are seeing her on the medical ward where you have been asked to:

Find out about her current and past episodes of anorexia nervosa.

Ask about her physical symptoms.

1b.

The ward sister asks to talk to you. She has never managed a patient with anorexia nervosa before.

She wants to know what they should do about feeding her and how the staff should engage with the patient.

SINGLE STATIONS

2.

This 18-year-old dancer has been referred by the liaison psychiatry team. She has a 3-year history of low weight and stopped menstruating 12 months ago. Last week she was admitted overnight with gastritis and mild haematemesis. She was seen by the duty psychiatrist as the medical team were concerned about her weight.

Find out about her dietary and weight history.

3.

You have been asked to see a 34-year-old woman, referred to your team by her general practitioner. The patient has been concerned about her weight for many years and believes she is overweight. As a teenager her school teacher told her parents he was concerned she might have anorexia nervosa, but she was never formally diagnosed and did not receive any specialist treatment. She is a now a successful barrister, working in a high-pressure job which appears to have led to an abnormal eating pattern.

Her husband has asked to see you first, alone. He wants to know if she is bulimic and if so what caused it and what can be done to help her.

Assume the patient has given consent to discuss her care.

STATION 1

1a: History of anorexia nervosa

KEY POINTS
Empathy/rapport
Weight and dietary history
History of episodes
History of treatment and contact with eating disorder (ED) services
Physical complications

INTRODUCE YOURSELF

'Hello, my name is Dr_____, I'm one of the psychiatrists.'

SET THE SCENE

'I've been told you've come into hospital because of your weight and blood results. Have you been told your blood results?' (If not, explain about her potassium.) 'How have you been in the run-up to being admitted?'

'I'd like to ask you about your eating and weight over the years. Would that be OK?'

COMPLETING THE TASKS

Enquire about the following.

Current episode

Features of anorexia nervosa (ICD-10/DSM-IV).

Her current weight and ideal weight.

Does she know her body mass index (BMI)? If not, what is her height?

How much weight loss over what period of time? Rapid weight loss more dangerous than gradual loss.

Ask about purging and bingeing (associated with medical complications and electrolyte abnormalities).

Has she been in touch with the eating disorders team in the community? If so, by whom and how often?

What treatment has she been receiving? How has she found this?

Has she been involved in psychological therapy and was she able to employ any techniques she has learnt, recently?

Have there been any new or worsening stressors at home or in her private life recently?

Past episodes of anorexia nervosa

When diagnosed?

Main features?

Least/most she's ever weighed?

Restricting or binge-eating/purging type

Avoidance of food types, calorie counting

Associated methods used to lose weight (e.g. exercise, drugs)

When did she come to the notice of mental health services?

Cooperation with community/outpatient treatment?

Any significant environmental psychosocial stressors contributing to relapses?

History of treatment:

- Pharmacological – physical and psychiatric?
- Psychological – family therapy, CBT, interpersonal therapy?
- Psychiatric admissions, inpatient regime, nutritional rehabilitation, treatment of core symptoms, enforced feeding? Length of admissions?
- Medical admissions (for physical manifestations)? Length of admissions?
- Psychiatric comorbidity. Has she been diagnosed with an affective disorder, for example?

Enquire about substance misuse.

Physical symptoms (refer to Chapter 14, Eating Disorder station)

Patients often describe cold intolerance, light-headedness, constipation and abdominal discomfort. If she was hypokalaemic she might have felt lethargic, common with electrolyte disturbance and dehydration. Similarly, if cardiovascular function is impaired or she is clinically depressed, energy levels would also be reduced. However, generally in AN, despite malnutrition, they are extremely active. Ask screening questions to cover cardiovascular, gastrointestinal, neurological, endocrine, musculoskeletal, reproductive, dermatological and dental problems.

RISK

AN has the highest mortality rate amongst psychiatric illnesses. The mortality rate for women is 0.56 per cent per year. There is also a high associated suicide rate. Poorer prognosis is associated with low serum albumin, poor social functioning, length of illness, purging and bingeing, substance misuse and comorbid affective disorders.

PROBLEM SOLVING

The likeliest problem in this station would be a reluctance by the patient to disclose information about her eating disorder. If you are empathetic and patient, 'the actor' will tell you the information you require. You are not asked about management issues here, so should not run into trouble with discussions about psychiatric admission and potential use of the Mental Health Act, but this could arise in related stations.

ADDITIONAL POINTS

AN usually presents in adolescence. It is often a chronic illness characterized by relapses. The majority of sufferers actively binge or purge and many will move diagnostically from the restricting type of AN to the binge/purging type or to bulimia nervosa (BN) with the passage of time.

Fewer than 50 per cent recover fully, 33 per cent improve and 20 per cent remain chronically unwell.

FURTHER READING

Birmingham, C.L. & Beumont, P.J.V. (2004) *Medical management of eating disorders.* London: Cambridge University Press.

1b: AN on the medical ward

KEY POINTS
Dealing with a colleague
Providing adequate professional support
Advice on immediate medical and psychiatric management
Unified nursing approach
Further management and transfer arrangements
Risk issues

INTRODUCE YOURSELF

'Hello, my name is Dr____, I'm one of the psychiatrists. Can I ask your name?'

SET THE SCENE

'I've just seen Miss Anderson, the lady admitted with hypokalaemia and weight loss in the context of AN.'

'Am I right in saying that you wanted some advice on how to manage her?'

COMPLETING THE TASKS

If the staff are uncomfortable with the patient being on a general medical ward, you should suggest that her hypokalaemia needs to be corrected first. You want to know what other investigations the medical team have requested and once the results confirm she is medically stable you would ideally like her to be transferred to an eating disorders unit (EDU). In such a setting they are skilled in the multi-disciplinary management of eating disorders.

Advice for the medical ward

Medical management
Rehydration and electrolyte correction

Nutritional management

Increasing weight should occur with the ward dietician's input – nutritional rehabilitation should begin with 1000–1600 kcal/day. This should be increased slowly, as long as there is no evidence of peripheral oedema or heart failure, up to 3000 kcal/day. Other important complications of overzealous re-feeding include hypophosphataemia, from an increase in metabolic demands, and rarely, but importantly, gastric dilatation, abdominal distension, pain and perforation can occur. It is advisable that feeds are given 6 times a day so the patient is not presented with large amounts of food. Liquid feeds are often used for severely emaciated people, but a soft diet is usually appropriate.

Approach to patient

Such patients can evoke mixed feelings amongst staff, particularly where there is limited experience. Joined-up team working is important, with good communication between nursing staff to avoid splitting and so that consistent care can be provided. You could offer to spend some time talking to staff about AN.

Advise staff to:

Monitor for attempts to purge for up to 2 hours after eating.

The patient should be monitored so that they can't use the bathroom to vomit.

Ensure that the patient does not have access to medications, including diuretics, laxatives or stimulants.

Further psychiatric management

Whilst on the medical ward it would be important to assess her mental state for comorbidity.

In particular, affective disorders, phobic or obsessive–compulsive traits, PTSD, emotionally unstable traits, cluster C (anxious) personality traits and perfectionistic, dependent traits. Ask screening questions for alcohol and substance misuse.

It might help the ward if you mention that you will be asking your team's psychologist to visit her for an assessment for individual therapy if she is well enough and also to advise the staff (psychoeducation).

Consider the need to reinstate/start antidepressant treatment.

Once transferred to the EDU, the specialized multi-disciplinary team (MDT) approach will allow a formalized structured approach to weight restoration.

RISK

It is important that the staff are aware of the patient's mental state and a full risk assessment needs to be conducted. Where it is established that she is a significant suicide risk, this should be addressed. She might need to have a psychiatric nurse present for continuous observations and treatment for depression started if appropriate.

PROBLEM SOLVING

A discussion about what to do if the patient refuses food could ensue. Often patients with AN will refuse food, treatment or hospitalization and where there is a significant risk of medical deterioration as a consequence of malnutrition, use of the Mental Health Act (1983) will apply. If detained, the patient can be treated without her consent and this includes tube feeding, as feeding is ancillary to mainstay of 'treatment for mental disorder'.

ADDITIONAL POINTS

Investigations should include: full blood count (FBC), liver function tests (LFTs), serum creatinine, urea and electrolytes (U&E), calcium, magnesium, phosphate, electrocardiograph (ECG), bone density scan.

The following may necessitate a medical admission in AN:

- cardiovascular, hepatic or renal compromise;
- ECG changes – a variety of ECG changes, including sinus bradycardia, ST depression and a prolonged QT interval;
- reduced pulse (<40bpm), low BP (<90/60) (<80/50 – child);
- low blood glucose, potassium, sodium, phosphate, magnesium;
- high sodium;
- reduced body temperature;
- dehydration, oedema, hypoproteinaemia, profound anaemia;
- rapid weight loss, exhaustion and severe lack of energy.

FURTHER READING

Birmingham, C.L. & Beumont, P.J.V. (2004) *Medical management of eating disorders.* London: Cambridge University Press.

STATION 2: Dietary and weight history (AN)

KEY POINTS
Empathy
Detailed history of weight loss
Dietary history and pattern of eating
Restrictive/bingeing behaviour
Risk issues

INTRODUCE YOURSELF

'Hello, my name is Dr____, I'm one of the psychiatrists.'

SET THE SCENE

'I understand you were in Casualty recently with stomach discomfort. How are you feeling now? One of the doctors who saw you was concerned about your weight, which is why he's asked you to see me today. Does your weight worry you?

COMPLETING THE TASKS

History of weight loss

When did you decide that you wanted to lose weight?

What is the most you have ever weighed?

How tall were you then?

When was that?

Have you been told your BMI (body mass index)?

What was the least you ever weighed in the past year?

When was that?

Have you ever had a stable weight as an adult? Were you restricting at that time?

How much do you think you ought to weigh?

Do you ever take steps to lose weight?

Exercise: How much, how often, level of intensity? How stressed do you feel if you miss a session?

Compensatory behaviours such as bingeing? Frequency, amount, triggers, setting and consequences.

Purging history:

- Use of laxatives, stimulants (amphetamines), diet pills, over the counter medication, complementary medicine.
- Vomiting? Frequency, how long after meals? Is vomiting easy or difficult for her to induce? Some patients drink large quantities of fluid and induce multiple episodes of vomiting to ensure complete emptying.

Psychologically minded questions

Have others ever commented on your weight?

Sometimes significant stress can play a part in people wanting to lose weight. Did anything like this happen to you?

Is there anyone, like a celebrity, whom you aspire to look like?

What do you think you see when you look in the mirror?

Do you perceive yourself as fat or thin?

Do you dislike your body? If so, in what way?

Does she have a distorted body image?

What would happen to her if she couldn't control her weight?

Does anything about her weight loss feel good?

Dietary history

Attempt to outline: Restrictive, avoidant and changed eating patterns.

Current dietary practices: Is she vegetarian or vegan – what does this mean to her?

Ask for specifics about amounts, food groups eaten, preparation time, fluids, restrictions, rituals (cutting, separating, mashing).

Hoarding food?

Take a typical 24-hour diet history – all meals, breakfast etc. (specific details e.g. if she has toast for breakfast, how many slices, does she finish it, plain or with butter or other spread? If using milk in drinks or cereals, what type is it e.g. skimmed?)

Is she missing meals? Does she snack between meals? If so, what does she snack on?

Calorie counting? Does she know the calorific content of her meals? How many calories does she aim for each day?

What happens at meal times? Does she eat alone or with others? Does she prepare meals for others, but not eat with them?

Does she chew food without swallowing?

RISK

Although not specifically asked, consider the risk component in all stations where possible. Does she have insight into the effect her eating restriction is having on her physical health? What does she believe will happen if she continues to lose weight? How does she explain the attendance at A&E? If she appears low in mood, a few screening questions for low mood and suicidality would be prudent.

PROBLEM SOLVING

Some patients will use psychostimulants such as cocaine to help lose weight. It is important to ask about substance misuse in this station, including alcohol. Dependence or intoxication may account for any behavioural change.

ADDITIONAL POINTS

Classic cognitive distortions in the course of the interview in this or other ED stations should be identified and where relevant discussions about CBT may follow. For example:

'If I put on a pound, none of my clothes will fit me' (Magnification)

'If I put on even a pound in weight, I will lose my friends as they'll think I'm ugly' (Catastrophizing).

ICD-10 diagnostic criteria for AN

For a definite diagnosis all of the following are required:

a. body weight 15 per cent below that expected, or a BMI (body mass index) of 17.5 or less;

b. self-induced weight loss by avoiding 'fattening foods'. One or more of the following may also be present: self-induced vomiting, purging, excessive exercise, use of appetite suppressants and/or diuretics;

c. body image distortion;

d. a widespread endocrine disorder involving the hypothalamic–pituitary–gonadal axis (amenorrhoea in women, reduced libido and potency in men);

e. if prepubertal, the sequence of prepubertal events is delayed or even arrested.

FURTHER READING

National Eating Disorders Association: http://www.nationaleatingdisorders.org

STATION 3: Bulimia nervosa

> **KEY POINTS**
> Empathy
> Explanation in lay terms
> Diagnosis explanation
> Aetiology
> Treatment options
> Risk issues

INTRODUCE YOURSELF

'Hello, my name is Dr_____, I'm one of the psychiatrists.'

SET THE SCENE

'Thank you for coming to see me today. I understand that your wife is outside and you wanted to see me first, alone, as you had some specific questions. Is that correct?'

COMPLETING THE TASKS

Does she have bulimia nervosa?

Remember to speak in lay terms. Although her husband will not necessarily know the answers to all of your questions, you could take him through the ICD-10 diagnostic criteria, asking if he recognizes the features as you explain what they mean:

1. Persistent preoccupation with eating and craving for food. Overeating large amounts of food in short periods of time.
2. An attempt to counteract fattening effects of food by one or more of: vomiting, purging, starvation, drugs e.g. appetite suppressants, thyroid analogues, diuretics.
3. Psychopathology: morbid dread of fatness

   Low self-induced weight threshold

   Often history of anorexia nervosa

   Other features of BN can include:

- normal weight (atypical bulimia);
- irregular periods.

You could explain that bulimia refers to episodes of uncontrolled excessive eating or 'binges'. They usually consume a large amount in a relatively short period of time and the person will often describe a lack of self-control during a binge. What follows are actions to counteract the binge, which often involve the person making themself sick and using other methods such as water tablets to lose weight. Often individuals with bulimia are slim or even underweight for their height. Ask him if he recognizes anything in what you have described.

Ask whether he has noticed any of the following characteristics or behaviours associated with BN:

- calorie counting;

- frequently weighing herself;
- feelings of anxiety, loneliness, boredom, depression;
- binges exacerbate self-loathing, disgust, poor self-esteem;
- difficulty eating in front of others.

Aetiology

Explain that you would want to see his wife before you could be certain about the diagnosis and that you would also want to do some tests to exclude a physical cause for her presentation. However, if she does indeed have BN, there are a number of factors thought to increase the risk for development of eating disorders.

Social:	Cultural emphasis on slimness
	Media pressure
	Particular association with certain professions
	Fashion for dieting
	Sense of control over your life when dieting/restricting calories.
Family:	Eating disorders can run in the family. First-degree relatives of individuals with BN have increased risk of an eating disorder.
	Family environment where members of the family have had issues with food or been critical of eating, weight, body shape can often contribute to eating disorders.
Depression:	Often people will turn to food when they feel depressed. It is possible that bulimia starts off in this way, because of feeling unhappy. The guilt associated with bingeing is then associated with vomiting or purging.
Life events:	'Sometimes upsetting events can trigger bulimia, like the end of a relationship.'
	Serious life events can trigger bulimia onset in up to 70 per cent of bulimia cases.
	History of childhood abuse (sexual), parental neglect, loss, indifference or separation have all been suggested as risk factors.
Personality:	'Some of us have parts of our personalities which might make us more likely to develop bulimia.'
	Presence of certain traits or characteristics, including perfectionism, impulsivity, mood lability, thrill seeking, dysphoria associated with rejection, may have a link to eating disorders.

What can be done to help her?

Psychoeducation

Being given information on a number of issues, including the physiological consequences of repeated bingeing and vomiting; use of prescribed and over-the-counter medicines inappropriately and the effects of being underweight.

Advice on how to limit binges through regular eating.

Self-help manuals e.g. 'Getting Better Bit(e) by Bit(e)'.

Psychological treatment

CBT:	The most studied approach and claimed to be the treatment of choice. You could explain the principles of this treatment and the focus of challenging the associated cognitive distortions in an attempt to modify behaviour. An experienced therapist or one specializing in ED is needed in such cases.

ITP: Interpersonal therapy is a short-term focal psychotherapy where the goal is to help patients identify and modify current interpersonal difficulties. It was adapted from the treatment of depression.

Family therapy

Often less useful in BN than AN. It probably has a greater role where patients are of a younger age where family factors are more relevant.

The psychologist might also have ideas on approaches to help with any feelings of loneliness, boredom or anxiety.

Pharmacological treatment

According to the NICE guidelines, psychological treatment is first line and a trial with fluoxetine may be offered as an alternative or additional first step. SSRIs might help by reducing the frequency of binge eating and purging. They are not recommended for the treatment of BN in adolescents.

RISK

Where there is a risk of self-harm or if community treatment has been unsuccessful, a psychiatric admission can be arranged. This is not without risk in itself as patients can sometimes worsen. Admissions are usually therefore kept short.

It is also important to exclude comorbid substance misuse, particularly when considering a treatment plan.

Oesophageal rupture (Boerhaave's syndrome) is a complication associated with vomiting after eating.

PROBLEM SOLVING

Her husband might not know the full extent of her eating behaviour as she is likely to be secretive about it. Certainly she might feel ashamed or guilty about her binges. Gather whatever information he is able to relay.

ADDITIONAL POINTS

Borderline personality traits in BN > AN.

50 per cent of ANs also meet the criteria for bulimia nervosa.

One-third of bulimic patients have a history of AN and one-third a history of obesity.

Benign enlargement of the parotid gland (25 per cent cases of bulimia).

FURTHER READING

Russell, G.F.M. (1979) Bulimia nervosa: an ominous variant of anorexia nervosa. *Psychological Medicine*, 9, 429–48.

Schmidt, U. & Treasure, J. (1993) *Getting better bit(e) by bit(e)*. Mahwah, NJ: Lawrence Erlbaum.

Chapter 14

Physical examination Dr Sangita Agarwal

SINGLE STATIONS

1.

You have been asked to see this man in your clinic. He has been drinking alcohol for many years and would now like help. He has stopped meeting his friends as they also drink heavily and he would like to be 'dry' so that he can get his life back on track.

He saw his general practitioner (GP) who has given him information on local alcohol services and also Alcoholics Anonymous.

As part of your assessment you want to undertake a physical examination.

Examine him for the physical stigmata of chronic alcohol misuse.

2.

This patient has been referred with concerns about her nutritional status. She has been an out-of-work model for some time. When younger, she was told that she was too fat ever to be successful.

She has had a difficult relationship with food for a number of years and heavily restricts her calorific intake.

Her GP has an interest in mental health and believes she has anorexia nervosa (AN). She has been referred to your outpatient clinic.

Examine this patient for the physical manifestations of starvation.

3.

This 28-year-old patient began hearing voices 2 months ago. He was seen by the local community psychiatric service and diagnosed with schizophrenia.

The consultant psychiatrist prefers prescribing the older traditional drugs. He will often quote new research indicating that the atypicals have no advantages and are much more expensive.

Having been given 100mg of chlorpromazine daily he stopped taking it altogether after complaining of uncomfortable legs, stiffness and a feeling of 'unease'. The community psychiatric nurse is concerned that the patient is refusing further treatment and asks you to see him.

Assess this patient for extrapyramidal side effects.

Explain to the patient what has happened and how you will manage him.

4.

Mrs Lloyd has been taking lithium for 12 years. She is an intensive care unit (ICU) charge nurse working in a busy teaching hospital. Her bipolar illness had been poorly controlled prior to this and she was admitted to a psychiatric ward where lithium was commenced. Mrs Lloyd is keen to continue with the lithium treatment as she has been on various treatments which she could not tolerate or were ineffective. Recently she has noticed that her neck has become more prominent and has questioned whether the lithium could be causing this.

She has had some blood tests:

Blood results	
TSH	3.56 (.34–5.6 reference range/value)
Free T4	0.9 (.6–1.6)
Free T3	2.9 (2.5–3.9)
Anti-TPO	435 (<35)
PTH	29 (12–65)
Calcium	9.3 (8.3–10.5)
T3 Total	1.0 (.9–1.8)

Conduct an appropriate physical examination, explain her blood results and discuss how you intend to manage her.

5.

This patient is reporting having lost the ability to walk. There was a recent 'incident' and since this time he has been reporting a loss of function.

The GP made an urgent referral to the neurologist who saw him within 10 days. The neurologist reported that the patient showed 'no obvious course for his functional loss. The pattern of paralysis was not typical and plantar reflexes were present and down going. There is no evidence of muscular atrophy. Of note I believe that the muscles are capable of reacting when the patient's attention is directed elsewhere'. Nerve conduction studies are reported as normal.

Examine this man's lower limbs.

6.

This woman was admitted to the clinical decisions unit at her local hospital. She was brought in by her family who have become concerned that she is unable to move her left arm. The A&E doctor has examined her and performed routine blood tests which are all within normal parameters. You are the psychiatrist on call and have been asked to assess her. Although you are aware that she has already been examined, you are keen to assess her yourself.

Perform a neurological examination of her upper limbs.

7.

Whilst trying to get out of a chair on the ward, this 78-year-old depressed man lost his footing and fell over. The fall was witnessed by nursing staff who observed him hit his head. He was difficult to rouse at first but soon became reorientated. He has a haematoma to his left temple and is complaining of a headache. The staff also report that he appears more irritable following the fall.

Examine this man's cranial nerves.

Do not examine smell; pinprick to face; gag reflex or corneal reflex.

8.

You are called to the psychiatric ICU. This patient, detained under the Mental Health Act, was restrained following aggressive and threatening behaviour that was putting other patients and staff at risk. He has subsequently settled somewhat, with time-out and oral olanzapine and clonazepam, but is now complaining of chest pain. You are called to see him.

Examine this patient's cardiovascular system.

9.

This patient has come back to see you in your outpatient clinic. She has bipolar affective disorder and has been commenced on carbamazepine, as she has a rapid cycling condition and could not tolerate lithium. She is anxious as she has developed blurred vision and occasional diplopia.

Examine her eyes.

10.

You are on call. A nurse bleeps you asking if you could attend to a patient who has collapsed on the ward. When you arrive you are told he is unconscious and does not appear to be breathing. There is no equipment/defibrillator available.

Manage this situation.

General points for the physical stations

A structured approach to the physical stations will help you pass well.

Ask the patient if they would like a chaperone (although in the college exams the answer will invariably be no).

Optimally expose the patient whilst maintaining their decency at the start of the physical examination.

Ideally examine from the patient's right.

Always dress and thank the patient.

Do not make up physical signs. Be honest if unsure of your findings and say that you would ask for further advice (e.g. medical referral).

STATION 1: Alcohol examination

> **KEY POINTS**
> Communication
> Rapport
> Gastrointestinal examination
> Other systems – neurology
> Answering patient's concerns

INTRODUCE YOURSELF
'Hello, my name is Dr____, it's nice to meet you.'

SET THE SCENE
'I'm glad you've decided to come and talk to me today about the drinking. First of all, would it be OK if I examined you?'

'Would you like a chaperone whilst I examine you?'

'Please feel free to ask me any questions you have as I go along.'

COMPLETING THE TASKS
Examine him for the physical stigmata of chronic alcohol misuse.

Gastrointestinal

Abdominal examination is important as gastritis and peptic ulcer disease are common. Liver disease is common (fatty liver, alcoholic hepatitis, cirrhosis, portal hypertension and carcinoma). Alcohol is also the commonest cause of chronic pancreatitis.

Inspection:

- Ask the patient if you can examine his/her 'stomach or tummy'.
- Tell the patient: 'If at any point you are uncomfortable or want me to stop, tell me.'

- Expose the abdomen (and chest if male).
- Look for any obvious abnormalities/clinical signs, e.g. spider naevi, gynaecomastia, tattoos, jaundice (sclera), pigmentation, abdominal distension (ascites).
- Examine the hands for: clubbing, palmar erythema, Dupuytren's contracture, flapping tremor.

Palpation:

- Ask if the patient is comfortable lying flat. Ask that they put their arms by their side.
- Feel the neck and supraclavicular fossae for enlarged lymph nodes (they may be enlarged in carcinoma of the stomach – particularly the left side).
- Light palpation: in all four quadrants. Look at the patient's face and ask if there is any tenderness.
- Deeper palpation: as above, and also midline for possible aortic aneurysm.
- Then examine the main organs individually.
- Liver (start in right lower quadrant and work upwards).
- Spleen (start in right lower quadrant and move across to left upper quadrant).
- Kidneys (bilateral palpation of lateral abdomen).

Percussion:

- From the level of the nipple downwards percuss out both the size of the liver and the spleen.
- Edges of both organs should become apparent.
- Shifting dullness should be demonstrated if ascites is suspected.

Ausculation:

- Bowel sounds.
- Renal artery bruits.

Musculoskeletal

Chronic alcoholic myopathy affects proximal muscles more prominently. Look at muscle bulk and evidence of wasting (e.g. thigh muscles).

Cardiovascular (refer to Cardiovascular station)

Examine for alcohol-associated:

- hypertension;
- arrhythmias;
- cardiomyopathy and related heart failure.

Neurological

Ask some screening questions for cognitive impairment and observe his gait

Wernicke–Korsakoff syndrome (confusion, ataxia, ophthalmoplegia, nystagmus and peripheral neuropathy)

Alcoholic dementia

Cerebellar degeneration (cerebellar signs – intention tremor, dysdiadochokinesis, nystagmus, dysarthria, broad-based gait)

Dermatological

There are a number of skin changes associated with alcohol:

- facial erythema (alcohol-induced vasodilation);
- psoriasis (mainly hands and feet).

PROBLEM SOLVING

As part of a comprehensive physical examination one would also want to examine the male external genitalia and rectum – you could mention that ordinarily this should be done and that his GP could do this.

ADDITIONAL POINTS

Alcohol-related changes to the:

FACE:	Scleral icterus, telangiectasia, xanthelasma
	Cushingoid facies
HANDS:	Clubbing, leuconychia (white nails), palmer erythema
	Dupuytren's contracture
	Hepatic flap (indicating liver cell failure)
SKIN:	Spider naevi, loss of axillary hair
	Jaundice
ABDOMEN:	Hepatomegaly (note that a cirrhotic liver may be dull to percussion and small)
	Splenomegaly (in portal hypertension)
	Ascites
ENDO:	Gynaecomastia, atrophic testes

FURTHER READING

Kelleher, M. (2006) Drugs and alcohol: physical complications. *Psychiatry*, 5 (12), 442–5.

STATION 2: Eating disorder

KEY POINTS
Communication
Rapport
Signs of malnutrition
Signs of purging
Cardiovascular system
Gastrointestinal system
Secondary sexual characteristics

INTRODUCE YOURSELF

'Hello, my name is Dr_____, it's nice to meet you.'

SET THE SCENE

'I've had a letter from your GP. Do you know why your doctor has referred you to see me today?'

'As part of my assessment I would like to check you physically. This will include listening to your heart and examining your tummy. Is that OK?'

'Would you feel more comfortable with a chaperone?'

COMPLETING THE TASKS

Examine this patient for the physical manifestations of starvation

If possible, you should weigh and measure her height.

In AN, body weight 15 per cent below that expected, or a body mass index (BMI) of 17.5 or less (BMI = weight (kg)/height (m)^2).

Cardiovascular: (refer to Cardiovascular station)

There is decreased cardiac muscle, chamber size and output. Examine her cardiovascular system and her pulse, lying and sitting blood pressure.

Bradycardia: <60bpm in 80 per cent of patients

Tachycardia

Hypotension: <90/60 often due to chronic volume depletion

Ventricular arrhythmias: electrolyte disturbances from diuretic/laxative abuse

Cardiac failure: may be terminal event

Electrocardiogram (ECG) changes include: Sinus bradycardia, ST depression and a prolonged QT interval. Regular ECG monitoring is recommended, especially if severely undernourished.

Cachexia

Examine for:

- Loss of body fat. Reduced muscle mass (proximal myopathy – ask about difficulty climbing stairs). Ask the patient to squat and then rise again to an upright position – this will be difficult for her, if present.
- Oedema – may be present as part of malnutrition, although may also be due to electrolyte imbalance.

Ask about: cold intolerance.

Gastrointestinal: (refer to alcohol station)

Conduct an abdominal examination.

Ask specifically about or examine for:

- enamel and dentine erosion if vomiting frequently;
- benign enlargement of the parotid gland;
- mouth – angles of mouth, nutritional deficiency;
- oesophagitis, erosions, ulcers;
- oesophageal rupture (Boerhaave's syndrome) is a complication associated with vomiting after meals (i.e. after bingeing);
- constipation – from inadequate food intake, and fluid depletion from diuretics/laxatives;
- diarrhoea – from stimulating laxatives.

Reproduction

Ask her about: amenorrhoea, delayed sexual maturation. Absence of menses is a defining feature of AN.

Skin

Examine her for: dry skin, lanugo hair or hirsuitism, calluses on her hands (from repeated vomiting), bruising, purpura.

PROBLEM SOLVING

The patient is unlikely to complain of anorexia or weight loss. She may be uncooperative, at least initially. Be supportive and clear why you are asking to examine her. Asking about any problems she has been having, e.g. abdominal pain, bloating or constipation, may be a good way to engage in a dialogue.

ADDITIONAL POINTS

Investigations can be helpful as part of the assessment in anorexia nervosa

FBC:

A pancytopenia is common in severe AN.

Leucopenia in up to two-thirds.

Mild anaemia and thrombocytopenia can occur in up to one-third of patients.

Blood film: There can be morphological changes in red blood cells – acanthocytes (spur cells).

U&Es: Hypokalaemic, hypochloraemic alkalosis, hypomagnesaemia.

Thyroid: Reduced thyroid metabolism (low T3 syndrome).

Sex hormones: Low LH and FSH.

Osteoporosis: Bone density scan (DEXA).

FURTHER READING

Patrick, L. (2002) Eating disorders: a review of the literature with emphasis on medical complications and clinical nutrition. *Alternative Medicine Review*, *7* (3), 184–202.

STATION 3: Extrapyramidal side effects (EPSE)

KEY POINTS
Communication
Empathy
Examination of EPSE
Explanation
Management

INTRODUCE YOURSELF

'Hello, my name is Dr_____, I'm one of the psychiatrists.'

SET THE SCENE

'I'm sorry to hear that you've been having some problems with your legs and some stiffness. Can you tell me a little bit more about this?'

'That sounds very uncomfortable. So that I can try to help you, would you mind if I examined you?'

COMPLETING THE TASKS

Physical examination

Patient should be seated but may be too restless.

Talk the examiner through your examination (based on the Simpson–Angus scale and the Abnormal Involuntary Movement scale).

Start with general inspection and then move from face down the body.

Global
Observe for restlessness, inability to sit/stand still, anxious/tense.

Face inspection

Expression:	Movements of forehead, eyebrows, periorbital area, cheeks, frowning, blinking, smiling or grimacing
Lips/peri-oral:	Puckering, pouting, lip smacking
Jaw:	Biting, clenching, lateral movements
Tongue:	Increased movement in and out
Salivation:	Look under tongue for increased/pooling of saliva
Glabellar tap:	Tap forehead gently with index finger. Parkinsonian patients continue to blink instead of accommodating after several taps.

Upper limbs
- Inspect for abnormal resting movements (choreic/athetoid movements).
- Arm dropping: Ask patient to stand and put arms out to the side, then let them drop.
  You demonstrate for patient.
  In unaffected individuals the arms fall freely with a slap and rebound.

- Elbow rigidity: Place one hand on the forearm and the other at the elbow. Move back and forth. Feel for stiffness and resistance (lead pipe rigidity).
- Wrist rigidity: As above, except examine flexion, extension, lateral, medial and rotational movements (cog wheeling if tremor superimposed).
- Legs: Observe the resting legs (e.g. restlessness). If possible, examine the patient on a couch so that the feet do not touch the ground. Ask the patient to swing their legs (demonstrate if necessary). Look to see if legs swing freely or if there is resistance.
- Gait: Ask the patient to walk 5–10 paces away and then back again. Is there reduced arm swing, stiff gait or a stooped shuffling gait (parkinsonian features)?

Explain what has happened.
This is very likely to be a side effect of the medication, which can sometimes happen. Acknowledge that this can feel very unpleasant. The medication that he has been taking works on brain receptors (dopamine, D2); that helps with their illness but is also

involved in controlling movements. Thank the patient for telling the nurse because it is something you can help with. Explain that the newer medications have less activity against this receptor and are less likely to produce this side effect. Arrange for the nurse to follow up closely over the next few weeks and arrange to see the patient again in outpatients soon.

Management

Further management depends on the type of side effect. It is important to discuss treatment options with the patient.

Dystonic reactions

Unlikely here (usually in early stages of treatment)

Includes oculogyric crisis and torticollis

Anticholinergic treatment (p.o./i.m./i.v.)

Withdraw antipsychotic

Pseudoparkinsonism

Tremor, rigidity, bradykinesia

Can be treated with anticholinergics

Change to an atypical such as quetiapine

Akathisia

Reduce antipsychotic or switch to an atypical such as olanzapine or quetiapine

Responds poorly to anticholinergics

Other treatment options might include propranolol, benzodiazepines, cryptoheptadine, clonidine

Seek senior advice if no improvement

Tardive dyskinesia

Think of risk factors (e.g. female, elderly)

Withdraw any antimuscarinic

Consider withdrawing antipsychotic or changing to an atypical

Consider clozapine if appropriate

Vitamin E, clonazepam, propranolol

PROBLEM SOLVING

Discussion about alternative antipsychotics.

It is important to discuss continued engagement with psychiatric services as the patient will need monitoring.

Ask patient how they feel about these symptoms and enquire about risk (self/others).

It is important that any agitation is not simply attributed to akathisia but that psychosis is considered. Ask how his thoughts have been since stopping the chlorpromazine and whether the voices he used to hear have returned.

ADDITIONAL POINTS

Tardive dyskinesia is difficult to treat and its aetiology is more complex than it appears. Anyone treated with antipsychotics is at risk of developing this condition, although greater risk may occur in those with an affective illness, diabetes, females and the elderly.

FURTHER READING

Gervin, M. & Barnes, T.R.E. (2000) Assessment of drug-related movement disorders in schizophrenia. *Advances in Psychiatric Treatment*, 6, 332–4.

Taylor, D., Paton, C. & Kerwin, R. (2007) *The Maudsley Prescribing Guidelines*, 9th edn. London: Informa Healthcare.

STATION 4: Thyroid dysfunction

KEY POINTS
Communication
Rapport
Examination of thyroid
Thyroid status
Explanation of blood investigations
Differential diagnosis
Management plan

INTRODUCE YOURSELF

'Hello, my name is Dr____, it's nice to meet you. I'm one of the psychiatrists.'

SET THE SCENE

'I understand you've noticed that your neck has changed.'

'When did you first notice this?'

'Would it be OK if I examine you and then we could talk about your blood results?'

'Would you like me to ask for a chaperone?'

COMPLETING THE TASKS

Physical examination

Inspection

> Patient should be sitting with their neck in a neutral or slightly extended position.

> Ask the patient if you can examine her neck.

> Expose the neck.

> Make a show of looking at the thyroid from the front. A goitre or enlarged thyroid nodule may be visible.

To enhance visualization of the thyroid one can extend the neck.

Look at the eyes from the sides and from above.

Next ask the subject to 'Take a sip of water and hold it in your mouth.'

Looking at the neck, 'Now swallow.'

Watch any goitre move upwards as they swallow.

Palpation

Ask the patient if you can feel her neck.

Stand behind her and to the right. This is less threatening than standing directly behind.

With the fingers of both hands, feel the left and right lobes of the thyroid. Ensure the neck is slightly flexed to ease palpation.

Attempt to locate the thyroid isthmus by palpating between the cricoid cartilage and the suprasternal notch.

Move your hands laterally to try to feel under the sternocleidomastoids for the fullness of the thyroid.

Assess hard or soft texture and the presence of any nodules.

Assess the extent of any enlargement.

Again ask the patient to swallow some water whilst feeling a possible goitre move beneath the examining fingers.

Examine local lymph nodes as thyroid carcinoma can spread to local lymphatics.

Percussion

If able to, percuss the manubrium sterni to see if a goitre extends downwards (dullness) into the chest.

AUSCULTATION

If a stethoscope is available, listen to both lobes of the thyroid for bruits.

THYROID STATUS

Examine their hands for tremor (hyperthyroidism), sweaty palms, erythema, thyroid acropachy.

Pulse; rate and rhythm (AF, sinus bradycardia).

Examine for brisk/slowly relaxing tendon reflexes (hyper/hypothyroid respectively).

Examine their eyes specifically for lid retraction (sclera visible above cornea) and lid lag, exophthalmos (sclera visible above the lower lid is a sign of Graves' disease and not related to thyroid status).

Comment on any hair loss, dry flaky skin, lateral loss of eyebrows, hoarse croaky voice, carpel tunnel syndrome (hypothyroidism).

Enquire about intolerance to heat/cold; weight change, appetite.

Ask about increased agitation (hyperthyroid).

PROBLEM SOLVING

Interpretation of results: Feed back to the patient about your findings from the physical examination if you have not already done so.

You will need to explain to her that her thyroid function tests are all within the normal range. However, her thyroid antibodies are high. As a professional colleague, ask her if she has heard of Hashimoto's thyroiditis. It is an autoimmune disease of the thyroid often associated with normal or hypothyroid function. Suggest to her that she needs to be seen by an endocrinologist as a first step. Certainly you would not be suggesting that she discontinues the lithium at this point.

She may need thyroid medication but you will be asking the endocrinologist to advise on further management.

She might ask you about alternative treatments should the physician advise that lithium is withdrawn. This would demand a discussion about the mood stabilizers, including the anticonvulsants and also the antipsychotics.

ADDITIONAL POINTS

You can talk to the patient to describe the physical examination as it is being performed or summarize when the exam is completed. When finished, thank the patient.

Note: An enlarged thyroid is referred to as a goitre. There is no direct correlation between size and function – a person with a goitre can be clinically euthyroid, hypo- or hyperthyroid.

A normal thyroid is estimated to be 10 grams with an upper limit of 20 grams or 2 to 4 teaspoons.

Thyroid nodules are common (prevalence 4 per cent). Half of the thyroid glands examined by ultrasound or direct visualization (surgery or autopsy) have nodules. Less than 5 per cent of all nodules are cancerous.

Differential diagnosis for an enlarged thyroid gland

- Multinodular goitre
- Graves' disease
- Familial goitre
- Hashimoto's thyroiditis
- Painless postpartum thyroiditis
- Malignancy
- Iodine deficiency goitre
- Iodine excess

FURTHER READING

Epstein, O., Solomons, N., Perkin, G.D., Cookson, J. & De Bono. D.P. (2003) *Clinical examination*, 3rd edn. Edinburgh: Mosby.

STATION 5: Lower limbs

KEY POINTS
Communication
Rapport
Inspection
Tone
Power
Reflexes
Coordination
Sensation
Gait

INTRODUCE YOURSELF

'Hello, my name is Dr_____, I'm one of the psychiatrists.'

SET THE SCENE

Be prepared for some hostility as it is clear that he is not keen to see a psychiatrist.

'Thank you for seeing me today. I understand from your GP that you've had some difficulties with your legs. Could you tell me what's been happening?'

'Could you tell me about the "incident" which happened recently?'

'Would it be OK if I examine your legs?'

'Would you like me to ask for a chaperone?'

COMPLETING THE TASKS

Subject should ideally be on an examination couch.

Expose legs, remove any socks.

By explaining what you are doing at each step you are letting the examiner know you are competent.

Inspection

Look for any obvious abnormalities/deformities.

Skin colour/rashes.

Muscle bulk (wasting).

Muscle fasciculation (motor neuron disease).

Restlessness (EPSE).

Tone

'I'm just going to move your legs; let them go all floppy.'

Examine each leg by moving it passively at the hip and knee joints. Roll the leg sideways, bend knees backwards and forwards on the couch/bed. Lift the knee and let it drop. With the legs hanging over the side of the bed, lift the leg and let it drop. Observe natural swing at the knee.

Look in particular for increase/decrease in tone and evidence of cogwheeling or lead-pipe rigidity.

Power

Ask the subject:

1. 'Lift your leg straight up (L1,2), don't let me push it down.'
2. With his knee bent, ask him to 'push against my hand' (L3,4).
3. 'Bend your knee; don't let me straighten it' (L5, S1,2).
4. 'Point your toes up towards your face; don't let me push them down' (L4, 5).

Coordination

Ask the subject to place his heel just below his knee and run it down his shin then back up and down once more. Ask him to repeat with the other foot.

Reflexes

Knee jerk (L3, 4)

Ankle jerk (L5, S1)

Plantar response (start outer part of sole, move inwards towards big toe)

Sensation

Ideally one should test light touch and pinprick in the following areas. Test the same dermatomes on each leg:

Outer thigh (L2)

Inner thigh (L3)

Inner calf (L4)

Outer calf (L5)

Inner foot (L5)

Outer foot (S1)

Vibration sense can be tested in the medial malleoli (if tuning fork is present), as can joint position sense (up and down).

Gait

Ask if subject is OK to walk for you.

Observe his normal gait.

Then ask him to walk heel to toe (ataxia).

Romberg's Test

Feet together, arms outstretched, closed eyes.

Stand in front of the patient with your own arms outstretched to ensure they do not fall.

PROBLEM SOLVING

For the purposes of the exam you will probably not be expected to examine pinprick sensation. Examining light touch using either cotton wool, or asking the patient to close their eyes and say 'yes' when they feel you touching them with a finger, should suffice.

ADDITIONAL POINTS

Romberg's is only positive if the subject is more unsteady with eyes closed.

A positive Romberg's indicates a loss of proprioception (e.g. subacute combined degeneration of the cord, tabes dorsalis).

FURTHER READING

Epstein, O., Solomons, N., Perkin, G.D., Cookson, J. & De Bono. D.P. (2003) *Clinical examination*, 3rd edn. Edinburgh: Mosby.

STATION 6: Upper limbs

KEY POINTS
Communication
Rapport
Inspection
Tone
Power
Reflexes
Coordination
Sensation

INTRODUCE YOURSELF

'Hello, my name is Dr_____, I'm one of the psychiatrists.'

SET THE SCENE

'I know that you've already seen one of the doctors, but could I ask you to briefly tell me what has been happening with your arm?'

'Would it be OK if I examine you?'

'Would you like me to ask for a chaperone?'

COMPLETING THE TASKS

Subject should ideally be on an examination couch and optimally exposed.

By explaining to the patient what you are doing at each step you are letting the examiner know you are competent.

Inspection

Look for any obvious asymmetry/deformities in the arms and hands.

Skin colour.

Muscle bulk (wasting).

Muscle fasciculation (motor neuron disease).

Tremor (EPSE, Parkinson's disease).

Tone

'I'm just going to move your arms; let them go floppy.'

Examine each arm by passively bending the elbow joint to and fro. Flex and extend the hand at the wrist and rotate the hand, to detect cog-wheel rigidity (Parkinson's disease).

Power

Demonstrate movements to make instructions easier.

Ask the patient to:

1. Put arms at right angles to their body, 'don't let me push them down' (deltoid, C5).
2. Bend elbow, 'don't let me straighten it' (biceps, C56).
3. Push each arm out straight, against your resistance (triceps, C7).
4. 'Squeeze my fingers', offer two fingers (C8, T1).
5. Keep fingers straight, 'don't let me bend them' (motor C7, radial).
6. Spread your fingers out, 'don't let me push them together' (dorsal interossei – ulnar).
7. Point your thumb to the ceiling, 'don't let me push it down'.
8. Put your thumb and little finger together, 'don't let me pull them apart'.

Coordination

1. 'Tap quickly on the back of your hand' (demonstrate).
2. Touch my finger touch your nose – test.

Reflexes

Biceps jerk (C5, C6)

Triceps jerk (C7)

Supinator (C5, C6)

Sensation

Ideally one should test light touch and pinprick in the following areas (although for the purposes of the exam a light touch using either cotton wool or a finger should be adequate). Ask the patient to close their eyes and tell you when they feel something. Reassure them that you will be gentle.

Shoulder (C4, C5)

Upper arm (C5, C6)

Forearm (C6, C7, T1)

Hand (C6, C7, C8)

Vibration and joint position sense can also be tested.

PROBLEM SOLVING

Once the physical examination is complete, help the patient get dressed, thank her and explain your findings. If your examination is normal and there is time, a conversation about psychological contributory factors may ensue. Take care not to upset the patient if possible, as this will be an unsatisfactory end to the station. Establish whether she believes her presentation could have a psychological component. The use of normalization here is very helpful.

ADDITIONAL POINTS

A discussion related to management may follow and you should explain that you have only had time to conduct a physical examination. You would want to look at her health records, speak to the GP and invite her back for a consultation where you would take a thorough history of recent and past events that could account for her presentation.

FURTHER READING

Epstein, O., Solomons, N., Perkin, G.D., Cookson, J. & De Bono. D.P. (2003) *Clinical examination*, 3rd edn. Edinburgh: Mosby.

STATION 7: Cranial nerves

KEY POINTS
Communication
Rapport
CNII to XII examined
Technique

INTRODUCE YOURSELF

'Hello, my name is Dr____, it's nice to meet you. Can I ask your name?'

SET THE SCENE

'I was told about your fall. Can you remember what happened?'

'How is your head now? Do you have any concerns at the moment?'

'Do you feel confused? Or feel sick at all?'

'I would like to examine you. This will involve looking at your eyes and testing your hearing, would that be OK?'

COMPLETING THE TASKS

Ask the patient if you can examine him.

Tell him to 'let you know if he's uncomfortable at any point'.

Patient should be sitting.

CN

(I)	'Do you have any problems with your sense of smell?'
(II)	'Do you have any problems with your eyesight?'
	Ask to put on glasses if normally wears them
	'Can you see that clock on the wall (or similar distant object)?'
	'What does it say?'
(II)	Visual fields
	Use your finger or red-headed pin if available.
	'Keep looking at my nose.' Ask subject to cover one eye.
	'Tell me when you see the pin.' Map out their field of vision.
	Light reflex and accommodation – convergence reflex (with your finger close to their nose ask them to look at an object in the distance and then at your finger).
	Fundoscopy (refer to Eye station)
(III, IV, VI)	Eye movements
	'Can you see my finger? Keep looking at it whilst it moves.'
	Move in the shape of a cross.
	At the extremes of their gaze, ask whether they can see one or two fingers (i.e. double vision). Also look for nystagmus.
(VII)	Facial movement
	'Raise eyebrows, screw eyes up tight, puff out cheeks, whistle, show me your teeth.'
(V)	'Clench your teeth'; as they do, feel masseter and temporalis.
	'Open your mouth and stop me closing it.' Gently try to close chin.
(IX, X)	Palate and gag reflex
	'Open your mouth and say aah.' Look at back of throat.
	Gag reflex – touch back of throat both sides with an orange stick.*
(XII)	Tongue
	Ask to stick out. Observe for deviation to left/right.
	Observe resting tongue for wasting and fasciculation.
(XI)	Accessory nerve
	'Shrug your shoulders and don't let me push them down.'
	'Turn your head to the right' (feel left sternomastoid) 'and to the right' (feel right side).
(VIII)	Hearing
	'How is your hearing?'
	Can they hear you rubbing your index finger against your thumb in each ear?
(V)	Trigeminal – sensation
	'Can you feel me when I touch here?' Use finger/cotton wool. Examine ophthalmic, maxillary and mandibular territories (corneal reflex*)

---

*Will often be asked to omit pin-prick, corneal, and gag testing – but be able to do them in practice.

PROBLEM SOLVING

Should be able to assess all nerves within 7 minutes.

ADDITIONAL POINTS

Smell and taste (I, VII, IX)

Visual acuity (II)

Visual field (II)

Eye movements (II, IV, VI)

Nystagmus (VIII and cerebellum)

Ptosis (III, sympathetic)

Pupils (III)

Discs (II)

Facial movements (V, VII)

Palatal movements (IX, X)

Gag reflex (IX, X)

Tongue (XII)

Accessory (XI)

Hearing (VIII)

Facial sensation (V)

Corneal reflex (V)

FURTHER READING

Epstein, O., Solomons, N., Perkin, G.D., Cookson, J. & De Bono. D.P. (2003) *Clinical examination*, 3rd edn. Edinburgh: Mosby.

STATION 8: Cardiovascular

KEY POINTS

Communication

Rapport

Inspection

Palpation

Percussion

Auscultation

INTRODUCE YOURSELF

'Hello, my name is Dr____, I'm one of the doctors.'

SET THE SCENE

'I understand you've had some chest pain. When did it start?'

'Can you tell me what it feels like?'

'Where is the pain now?'

'Is the pain travelling anywhere or is it only in your chest?'

'I need to examine your heart, would that be OK?'

'Would you like a nurse chaperone?'

COMPLETING THE TASKS

Remember inspection, palpation, percussion and auscultation.

Expose the patient's chest; lying at 45° on the bed.

Explain that if he feels uncomfortable at any point to let you know.

Whilst explaining the above, look for features of anxiety or shortness of breath.

HANDS:	Sweaty, hot/cold, erythematous/cyanosed Nails for splinter haemorrhages/clubbing.
RADIAL PULSE:	Rate, rhythm (tell patient, e.g. 80bpm – regular).
BLOOD PRESSURE:	Sitting (tell patient reading).
JVP:	Lie patient at 45 degrees and observe.
INSPECTION:	Chest Observe breathing pattern.
PALPATE:	Feel for the apex beat and for any heaves or thrills.
AUSCULTATE:	Listen to the heart sounds. Try to pick up any abnormal flow murmurs at apex (mitral – 4th intercostal space (IC)). Listen at 2nd IC space (pulmonary artery – left, aortic – right). Listen over the carotids.
LUNGS:	Listen to the lung bases for any inspirational crepitations (CCF).
OEDEMA:	Check ankle for pitting oedema. If present, how extensive? Press gently.

PROBLEM SOLVING

The patient may be anxious or distressed and need reassurance. A discussion about how you intend to manage him is possible. Offer some analgesia/aspirin if appropriate. If you believe the pain to be cardiogenic, explain the need for further investigations (bloods, ECG, chest X-ray (CXR)). If you are concerned that he has had a myocardial infarct, immediate management and emergency transfer will need to be organized.

ADDITIONAL POINTS

Remember to dress the patient and thank them when you have finished your physical examination. Explain your findings.

FURTHER READING

Epstein, O., Solomons, N., Perkin, G.D., Cookson, J. & De Bono. D.P. (2003) *Clinical examination*, 3rd edn. Edinburgh: Mosby.

STATION 9: Eye examination

> **KEY POINTS**
> Communication
> Rapport
> Visual acuity
> Eye movements
> Reflexes
> Fundi

INTRODUCE YOURSELF

'Hello, nice to see you again. I'm sorry to learn you've had some problems with your eyes.'

SET THE SCENE

'Could you tell me how your vision has been since we last met?'

'I would like to examine your eyes. Would that be OK?'

'Part of the examination will involve shining a light into your eyes, so let me know if it is uncomfortable at any point.'

COMPLETING THE TASKS

You are asked to examine her 'eyes' so remember to perform a complete eye examination, i.e. CNII–VI , not just fundoscopy.

Visual acuity

Monocular i.e. test each eye individually. Finger count: 'How many fingers do you see?'

Visual fields

Monocular: Ask the patient to cover one eye; you cover your eye on the opposite side so that you are comparing the patient's visual fields to your own. 'Keep looking at my eye.'

Test the patient's upper and lower temporal quadrants by moving your wagging finger from the periphery to the centre. Ask them to say 'yes' when they see your finger moving. To test their nasal fields you need to swap hands. Any area of field defect will become obvious by comparing the patient's visual fields to your own. Do the same for the other eye.

Eye movements (ocular palsy, nystagmus, lid lag)

Binocular i.e. both eyes together. 'Follow my finger with your eyes.'

Move your finger in the shape of an 'H' from side to side, then up and down at the extremes. Ask if they can see one finger clearly; does it change?

Reflexes

First accommodation – convergence reflex:

'Look into the distance.'

'Now look at my finger.' Place your index finger close to the patient's nose; if normal, pupils will constrict.

Light reflex:

Pick up the ophthalmoscope, switch on and check that it works. Shine the light into each eye twice to check direct and consensual reflexes.

Fundoscopy

Hold on to the ophthalmoscope to examine the patient's fundi. 'I'm going to look at the back of your eyes now. I will need to get quite close – please let me know if it is too uncomfortable and I will stop.' Tell the patient to fixate on a distant target. Examine the patient's right eye with your right eye and then her left eye with your left eye. Sit at arm's length opposite the patient. Aim to find the optic disc and comment on this and the appearance of blood vessels around it. Come away from the fundus once you have had a good view.

Optic disc
Locate and bring into focus.

Look for: size; blurred disc edge; cupping (glaucoma); new vessels (diabetic retinopathy); pale disc (e.g. optic atrophy).

Blood vessels
Arteries are narrower and brighter and have a reflective pale streak.

Start at the disc and follow the vessels out to look for hypertensive changes (A–V nipping) and atherosclerotic changes.

The fundus
Look for: haemorrhages; exudates; cotton wool spots; new vessel formation; micro-aneurysms.

Ask the subject to look straight at the light to examine the macula.

Be familiar with the basic appearance of:

Papilloedema: blurred disc edge, haemorrhages, hard exudates (late feature), cotton wool spots (due to retinal infarction)

Diabetic retinopathy: microaneurysms, small haemorrhages, exudates, cotton wool spots, new vessel formation (proliferative diabetic retinopathy)

Hypertensive retinopathy: silver wiring, A–V nipping, haemorrhages, cotton wool spots, disc swelling if malignant

Glaucoma: optic disc enlargement, undermining of the disc margins and blood vessel bowing (advanced)

Photocoagulation (laser) scars

Optic atrophy.

PROBLEM SOLVING

If faced with a mannequin in the exam – treat it as you would a real patient.

ADDITIONAL POINTS

Describe any features with reference to a clock face and optic disc size, i.e. 'there are soft exudates at 3 o'clock, two disc diameters away from the disc'.

Explain that ideally you would like to examine the retinas in a dark room or dilate the pupils to get a better view (1 per cent cyclopentolate).

FURTHER READING

Epstein, O., Solomons, N., Perkin, G.D., Cookson, J. & De Bono. D.P. (2003) *Clinical examination*, 3rd edn. Edinburgh: Mosby.

STATION 10: BLS

KEY POINTS
Communication
Information gathering
Requesting assistance
Risk consideration
BLS algorithm

INTRODUCE YOURSELF

The patient is unconscious and non-responsive. There is also a member of staff in this scenario.

SET THE SCENE

'Hello, I'm the on-call doctor, Dr____. Could you quickly tell me what happened and how long he's been like this?'

COMPLETING THE TASKS

You will most likely be presented with a Resuscitation Annie. Do not stop to have a chat with the nurse, but talk to her as you are assessing the patient. (Based on the Basic Life Support algorithm, Resuscitation Council UK, 2005.)

1. Ensure safety of the patient and yourself.
2. Check patient and see if they respond. Gently shake shoulder and ask loudly 'Are you OK?'
3. If he does not respond:
   Shout for help from a nurse.
   Turn the patient onto his back and open the airway by gently tilting the head back and chin lift.

4. Keeping the airway open, look, listen and feel for breathing.
   Look for chest movement, listen for breath sounds.
   Feel for air on your cheek.
   Spend no more than 10 seconds deciding if patient is breathing normally.

5. If not breathing:
   Send someone for help (999, crash team, or resuscitation trolley).
   If on your own, leave the patient for shortest possible time to get help.
   Start chest compressions:
   - Do not apply pressure over the lower tip of the sternum or upper abdomen. Depress the sternum 4–5cm during a compression.
   - After each compression, release all the pressure on the chest, but don't let go of your hands.
   - Repeat at a rate of about 100 times a minute (a little less than 2 compressions a second).

6. Combine chest compression and rescue breaths
   After 30 compressions open the airway again using head tilt and chin lift.
   Give 2 slow, effective rescue breaths each of which should make the chest rise and fall:
   - Ensure head tilt and chin lift.
   - Pinch nose closed with finger and thumb of hand on forehead.
   - Open mouth a little (maintain chin lift).
   - Take deep breath, place lips around their mouth, make sure you have a good seal.
   - Blow steadily for approx 2 seconds and watch chest rise.
   - Continue with chest compressions and rescue breaths in a ratio of 30:2.
   - Stop to recheck the patient only if he starts breathing normally, otherwise continue resuscitation.

7. Continue resuscitation until:
   Help arrives and can take over.
   Victim starts breathing.
   You become exhausted.

PROBLEM SOLVING

Ideally you would want to protect yourself by using a reservoir bag and mask for ventilation, rather than 'mouth to mouth'. Ask the nurse whether the patient has any known infectious diseases.

Dilated pupils are an unreliable sign so continue cardiopulmonary resuscitation (CPR) if present.

Mouth-to-nose ventilation can be used if, for example, mouth obstruction cannot be relieved.

Ask the nurse if there is any resuscitation equipment available. Explain that you want to use the resuscitation trolley to get a cardiac tracing and start defibrillation if required.

Ask the nurse to call for help early on in the scenario, especially if no equipment is available.

ADDITIONAL POINTS

Once you establish that the person is not breathing and is unresponsive, start immediate resuscitation.

Get as much history from the nurse as possible; for example, is this a drug overdose or suicide attempt? Can you initiate pharmacological treatment, e.g. flumazenil in BZD overdose? Ask about other vital signs.

Ask if the nurse has been trained in CPR, as this could allow you to examine the patient more thoroughly whilst he or she continues chest compressions.

If cervical spine is damaged, as in a hanging attempt, care must be taken to maintain alignment of the head, neck and chest. Use minimal head tilt when opening airway.

FURTHER READING

Resuscitation Council (UK): http://www.resus.org.uk. Check this website for more information and any updates to guidelines.

Investigations and procedures

SINGLE STATIONS

1.

You are the ward doctor on an acute adult inpatient ward. You have been asked to see a 30-year-old university student who has a history of cannabis abuse but recently tried injecting himself with heroin. He was found collapsed in the street and was transferred to the psychiatric ward after being stabilized medically. He is worried about the risks of injecting and is seeking further advice. He is anxious and has a number of questions for you.

Answer his questions and give him information on harm minimization and injection techniques should he continue to use.

What infections could I get from intravenous heroin use?

Are any medical conditions associated with intravenous heroin use?

What do you think would happen if I continued with intravenous heroin use?

2.

In your role as a liaison psychiatrist you have been asked to see a man who was admitted for treatment of delirium tremens. The 50-year-old homeless man is thought to be mentally unwell and you have been asked to transfer him to the local psychiatric hospital. During your initial review of the hospital notes you note the following blood results taken earlier today:

Albumin = 21g/L   (35–50g/L);
Bilirubin = 250 μmol/L   (3–20 μmol/L);
GGT (gamma-glutamyltransferase) = 600 IU/L   (<60 IU/L);
ALP (alkaline phosphatase) = 300 IU/L   (30–130 IU/L);
ALT (alanine aminotransferase) = 55 IU/L   (0–45 IU/L);
AST (aspartate aminotransferase) = 170 IU/L   (10–50 IU/L);
MCV (mean cell volume) = 150 fL   (80–100 fL).

You have an extremely inquisitive fourth-year medical student with you who asks you a number of questions:

1 How do you interpret the liver function tests?

2 What other validated markers of alcoholism are there?

3 What are the clinical signs and symptoms of alcohol withdrawal?

4 What are you going to say to the ward staff?

3.

You are on call in the local A&E and are asked to see a 'difficult' 18-year-old patient who was brought in by her parents with whom she lives. Her worried mother had informed the A&E doctor that her daughter had not been eating for some time as she feels that she is too fat. The mother further stated that her daughter, a ballet dancer, spends hours doing exercises, and appears to have stopped menstruating. You note from the A&E clerking that no physical examination has been performed, as the patient is refusing a physical examination as well as blood tests. You are also informed that the patient has been waiting to see you for three and a half hours and that she will soon 'breach' the four-hour waiting period.

Her mother, a university lecturer, believes her daughter has anorexia nervosa (AN) and has a number of questions for you:

1 **What eating disorders are there and what are their features?**
2 **What are the differential diagnoses of anorexia nervosa?**
3 **What symptoms may be reported in anorexia nervosa?**
4 **What are the possible medical complications of anorexia nervosa?**

4.

As part of the clerking of a newly admitted patient on the ward you are covering on your week of nights, you have been asked to perform an electrocardiogram (ECG) and report your findings to the notoriously pedantic but supportive on-call consultant. You note that the patient, a 55-year-old female, who has a history of anxiety in the context of a dependent personality disorder, is cooperative, has a Glasgow Coma Scale (GCS) of 15/15, appears slightly anxious and sweaty but is otherwise unremarkable. The patient is not on any regular medication. Unfortunately, the nurse on the ward has not done the ECG course and is therefore unable to help you.

You manage to perform the ECG by following the instructions on the machine. You note that the ECG printout reports the following parameters:

'Sinus Rhythm but otherwise normal ECG'
HR   110
PR   150
QTc   429

The consultant has turned up on the ward and uses the opportunity to cross-examine you on your ECG knowledge.

Questions
1 **What anatomical positions do the different leads of the ECG represent?**
2 **How do you know that the electrodes have been correctly applied to the patient and that the ECG trace is accurate?**
3 **How is sinus rhythm represented on the ECG?**
4 **What is the QTc interval? What psychotropics may be associated with prolongation of the QTc interval?**
5 **If the patient were being treated on clozapine, what ECG changes might you see?**

5.

You are the junior doctor on a busy, general adult ward and have been asked by the departing locum consultant to commence clozapine on a 29-year-old patient with newly diagnosed schizophrenia. The patient has been on olanzapine for 8 months but this was changed to modecate (fluphenazine) depot due to variable compliance which the patient attributed to side effects.

A student nurse is in the management round and keeps firing questions at you.

Questions

1 **When should clozapine be considered?**
2 **What are the life-threatening side effects of clozapine?**
3 **What other adverse effects of clozapine are there?**
4 **What blood tests are needed for clozapine and when?**
5 **What are the grounds for discontinuing clozapine?**
6 **Are there any protocols when commencing clozapine?**

6.

You have been asked to review some blood results for a patient in her fifties who was recently admitted after concerns by her husband that she had become increasingly listless and 'odd'. She has stopped going out for walks, had become increasingly forgetful and complained of feeling tired all the time.

The ward doctor noted that she had no previous psychiatric or medical history and had been gaining weight and complaining of constipation. He also noted a hoarse voice and a slow heart rate.

Her husband is a psychologist and wants to understand her test results. He asks:

1 **What blood tests are done and why?**
2 **You perform a number of tests and find that the serum thyroid stimulating hormone (TSH) is 120 mU/L (normal range approximately 0.3 – 0.4 mU/L) and the serum-free thyroxine (T4) is 4 pmol/L (normal range approximately 9–26 pmol/L). How do you explain these results to the husband?**
3 **In general terms, how will she be managed?**
4 **What are the clinical signs and symptoms of hypothyrodism?**

7.

One of the local general practitioners (GPs) has referred a 32-year-old lawyer with a history of bipolar affective disorder (BAD) to your hospital outpatient clinic after recently commencing him on lithium. The patient had previously been discharged from an out-of-area psychiatric hospital and is reported to be intelligent, insightful and willing to comply with treatment so that he can get back to work. He is also said to be interested in learning more about lithium, and has been told by the GP that you are the expert in this! The GP has done blood levels, and noted that the level after 4 days was 0.2 mmol/L. No other information has been supplied.

He asks a number of questions:

1 **What are the clinical uses of lithium?**
2 **What are main side effects of lithium?**
3 **What is the plasma reference range of lithium?**
4 **What are the signs of toxicity and how do these relate to plasma level?**
5 **Are there any additional blood tests that should be done in a patient on lithium?**

8.

You are phoned by a work colleague who is the psychiatrist on call. He has been called by the A&E registrar concerning a Mr Z, an obese 44-year-old man who has presented to A&E saying he feels 'unwell' though only describes vague physical symptoms.

Although apparently stable from a mental state point of view, the registrar wants a review as the patient is known to have a diagnosis of schizophrenia and has been on olanzapine for some years. He also wants the patient transferred to the local psychiatric hospital as soon as possible. He has not performed any blood tests and has done only a brief physical examination as the patient is 'psychiatric' and 'bizarre'. The registrar does not further define this but feels that the patient is acutely psychiatrically unwell and in urgent need of sectioning.

A urine dipstick suggested microalbuminuria, but the registrar does not feel that this is significant. There was also evidence of hypertension, but again this was dismissed.

Your colleague calls for help as he thinks he might have the metabolic syndrome and wants your thoughts on the matter.

Questions

1 **What important metabolic side effects of antipsychotics do you know about?**
2 **What are the clinical symptoms of metabolic syndrome?**
3 **What are the clinical signs of metabolic syndrome?**
4 **What is the major differential diagnosis of metabolic syndrome?**
5 **What general approaches may be used to manage metabolic syndrome in a patient receiving antipsychotics?**

9.

During a night on call you are called to one of the wards to see a patient that the nurses are worried about. This is a 35-year-old man who was recently re-commenced on antipsychotic treatment, with lithium recently added due to an apparent history of bipolar affective disorder. The nurses inform you that the patient looks 'unwell', and is agitated and sweaty, although not aggressive or hypomanic. He has a temperature, but is not complaining of any pain.

They have done some basic observations, and let you know that his pulse rate is 120/minute, his respiratory rate is 24/minute and his blood pressure is 160/110.

You are concerned and call the on-call medical team. They want to know more about his presentation and likely diagnosis.

Questions

1 What are possible differential diagnoses?
2 What is NMS (neuroleptic malignant syndrome)?
3 What are the clinical signs and symptoms?
4 What medications are implicated in NMS?
5 What immediate action needs to be taken on the ward?
6 What additional measures may be useful in treatment of NMS?
7 What laboratory tests, if any, are useful for diagnosis and monitoring of NMS?
8 What is the prognosis of NMS?

10.

You have been called to A&E to see Mr Richards, a 46-year-old man, who has been 'medically cleared'. He was assessed by one of the psychiatric liaison nurses (PLNs) who noted that he was confused, and appeared sweaty. She is concerned that he might be medically unwell and feels that a doctor's opinion is needed. The patient had apparently been taking a herbal medication, which the nurse thinks may be St John's wort. The helpful GP has confirmed that Mr Richards has a history of amphetamine abuse and had been prescribed a selective serotonin reuptake inhibitor (SSRI) due to depression but appears to have been non-compliant. When you see him you note that he is confused, agitated and appears to be shaking.

The PLN asks you the following questions.

Questions

1 What are the possible differential diagnoses?
2 What is serotonin syndrome?
3 What are the clinical signs and symptoms?
4 What immediate action needs to be taken?
5 What additional measures may be useful in treatment of the syndrome?
6 What laboratory tests, if any, are useful for diagnosis and monitoring of serotonin syndrome?
7 What is the prognosis of serotonin syndrome?

STATION 1: Advising an intravenous drug user (IVDU) on injection technique and risk minimization

> **KEY POINTS**
> Communication and empathy
> Recognition of risks of injecting drugs
> Patient education
> Answering other questions

INTRODUCE YOURSELF TO THE PATIENT

SET THE SCENE

Explain that you have been asked to see him. Try to get some background history of the events leading up to his collapse. Explain that you have not been able to speak to the nursing staff as yet or had access to his notes or other sources of information. Try to briefly get an idea of his current and recent history of illicit drug use.

COMPLETING THE TASKS

What infections may be associated with intravenous heroin use?

You would need to explain the following in lay terms, perhaps explaining the risks at the injection site and those affecting the 'whole body'.

These may be divided into systemic and local.

Systemic infections may result from direct transmission into the bloodstream of a number of organisms, for example:

Type of Organism	Name of Organism	Notes
Bacteria	Clostridium spp.	May cause myonecrosis; tetanus relatively uncommon due to vaccination
	Mycobacterium tuberculosis	Tuberculosis may occur in malnourished/ immunosuppressed individuals
	Staphylococcus aureus	Causes tricuspid (right-sided) endocarditis, especially in patients with HIV
	Streptococcus spp.	Can cause septicaemia and endocarditis, especially left-sided
Fungi	Candida spp.	Can cause endocarditis, CNS infections, endophthalmitis, disseminated candidiasis
	Aspergillus spp.	Pulmonary aspergillosis may occur
	Rhizopus spp.	Mucormycosis may occur, especially in neutropenic patients. May present with orbital cellulitis, pain and vascular thrombosis
Parasites	Malaria	More common in tropical areas of the world
Viruses	Hepatitis A	May be spread via contaminated drugs themselves or water used in injection

⇧	Hepatitis B Hepatitis C	Viruses transmitted via shared needles
	HIV	May be asymptomatic for many years and then present with opportunistic infections e.g. tuberculosis or *Pneumocystis carinii* pneumonia

Note that atypical pathogens may be implicated, as can the effects of 'poly-infection' with a number of pathogens. Systemic infections may also affect the nervous system, producing cerebral abscess, infarction or meningitis.

Local infections may result from skin flora such as *Staphlococcus* species such as *aureus* or *epidermidis* and include abscess, cellulitis, necrotizing fasciitis, thrombophlebitis or tissue necrosis ('gas gangrene'). Infections may also result from foreign bodies such as broken needles remaining in situ or following use of contaminated drugs/water. Infections of joints and bones have also been reported, and chronic use can lead to 'stigmata' such as fibrosis, bruising, skin discolouration, granulomata and chronic phlebitis.

What other medical conditions may be associated with intravenous heroin use?

These may be divided into drug-related and non-drug-related factors. Examples of the former include sequelae of the drug itself (such as irritant effects leading to thrombophlebitis, thromboembolism), injection with adulterants added to the drug mixture (with variable effects), from drug overdose (such as heart failure, pulmonary embolism, respiratory arrest), or drug withdrawal.

Medical effects of intoxication include the following:

System	Condition	Notes
Cardiovascular	Cardiac arrhythmia	Bradycardia may occur in intoxication, tachycardia may occur in withdrawal
	Endocarditis	May be right- or left-sided
Dermatological	Abscess, cellulitis, necrotizing fasciitis, thrombophlebitis or tissue necrosis; 'stigmata' may also be seen with chronic use	Common findings, see above
Endocrine	Hyperglycaemia	Rare, but may occur in heavy, chronic use
	Hyperprolactinaemia	Rare, but may occur in heavy, chronic use or following head trauma or seizures
	Thyroid dysfunction	Raised T4 levels may occur, may not be clinically significant
Gastrointestinal	Abnormal liver function	Non-specific changes in LFTs may be seen
Pancreatitis	May occur following consumption of large doses	

⇩

⇧

Haematological	Eosinophilia	May occur in up to one quarter of addicts
	Lymphocytosis	Common occurrence
	Thrombocytopenia	May occur due to contaminants
Metabolic	Hypocholesterolaemia	Decreased cholesterol levels sometimes seen
	Hypoxia	Occurs with high/toxic doses
Musculoskeletal	Rhabdomyolysis	May occur in infection or in toxic doses
Neurological	Acute transverse myelitis	May arise due to hypoxia and increased blood pressure
	Cerebral infarction	
	Encephalopathy	
	Parkinsonism	
	Peripheral neuropathies	May be related to trauma
Pulmonary	Emboli	May be secondary to injected, non-dissolved substances
	Pneumonia	Usually bacterial
	Pulmonary granuloma	May be secondary to injected, non-dissolved substances
Renal	Myoglobinuria	Occurs in association with rhabdomyolysis
	Nephropathy	May be due to contaminants

What non-medical risks are associated with intravenous heroin use?

These can be classified as risk to self and risk to others. Amongst risks to self are:

- violence associated with drug use;
- psychiatric sequelae (lability of mood, personality changes, cognitive impairment, psychosis, mania);
- economic and social costs (debt, homelessness, loss of employment, relationship difficulties).

Risk to others:

- violence;
- social costs (disruption of relationships);
- economic costs (increased crime, increased costs of policing, providing healthcare).

Harm minimization

Recognizes that certain individuals cannot or will not stop using drugs and therefore aims to minimize the harmful sequelae of drug taking. A number of interventions have been described, including:

Methadone maintenance programmes

Counselling

Supplying clean equipment (e.g. alcohol swabs, sterile containers or filters for mixing drugs, sterile needles, sterile water)

Educating users in order to try to minimize risk of infection

Using non-injecting means of administration

Supervised injection (controversial)

Discouraging poly-substance use

Administering drug in presence of others

Education regarding safer injecting techniques

Education regarding disposal of used equipment

Using low initial 'test dose' to gauge strength of drug

What advice regarding injection technique can you suggest?

Try to inject when sitting or lying down.

Try to inject in the presence of others.

Use of sterile, single-use only needles and syringes.

Never share needles.

Pay attention to hygiene such as washing hands and injection site, possibly by using alcohol wipes.

Use of sterile water for injection, or, failing this, tap water that has been boiled for at least five minutes.

Allow heated drug mixture to cool prior to injecting.

Avoid use of lemon juice to dissolve heroin and using safer alternatives such as citric or ascorbic acid.

Filter drug mix prior to injection via use of sterile, single-use filters.

Use a small-bore needle.

Use a vein that is less likely to be painful or inaccessible; the cubital fossa is generally recommended.

After drawing up drug tap syringe to remove air bubbles.

Gently push syringe plunger to expel air.

Rotate injection sites to allow veins to heal.

Do not over-tighten tourniquet or leave in place for too long.

Ensure that needle faces the same direction as the blood flow.

After needle is in the vein, pull back to ensure blood appears in the syringe to confirm that the needle is actually in the vein.

Remove tourniquet prior to injecting.

After removing needle apply clean tissue or cotton wool to puncture site to stop bleeding.

Dispose of used needles and syringes carefully.

ADDITIONAL POINTS

Clinical features of opiate intoxication/complications

Mental effects: Anorexia, decreased activity, diminished libido, drowsiness, euphoria, personality change;

Physical effects: Bradycardia, constipation, miosis, nausea, pruritis.

Features of withdrawal

Abdominal cramps, agitation, craving, diarrhoea, diaphoresis, mydriasis, piloerection, restlessness, tachycardia, yawning.

FURTHER READING

Foster, R. (2008) *Clinical laboratory investigation and psychiatry: a practical handbook.* London: Informa Healthcare.

Hutin, Y., Hauri, A., Chiarello, L. et al. (2003) Best infection control practices for intradermal, subcutaneous, and intramuscular needle injections. *Bulletin of the World Health Organization*, *81* (7), 491–500.

Theodorou, S. & Haber, P.S. (2005) The medical complications of heroin use. *Current Opinion in Psychiatry*, *18* (3), 257–63.

Zollner C. & Stein, C. (2007) Opioids. *Handbook of Experimental Pharmacology*, *177*, 31–63.

STATION 2: Abnormal blood results in an alcoholic patient

KEY POINTS
Communication and empathy
Knowledge of basic liver function tests
Knowledge of clinical features of alcohol use/withdrawal
Answering other questions

INTRODUCE YOURSELF TO THE MEDICAL STUDENT

SET THE SCENE

Ask if the medical student has ever seen anyone with delirium tremens before. You could go on to explain that when seeing any patient in a liaison setting it is helpful to determine first what has been done to investigate and treat the patient, given that delirium tremens is a medical emergency and often patients can be sedated or be in receipt of ongoing medical treatment and thus may not be immediately amenable to proper psychiatric assessment. You can explain that it is useful to check whether the PLN has seen the patient and whether the patient is medically stable or requires further input.

COMPLETING THE TASKS

1 How do you interpret the above results?

All results are above the normal range, suggesting that they are abnormal. Looking at the liver function tests, the raised GGT is consistent with chronic alcohol use as it is raised in roughly two-thirds of such patients. Although ALP and AST are non-specific markers of liver disease, the ratio of AST/ALT is >2, confirming liver disease – a ratio >3 is suggestive of myocardial infarction. The ratio of GGT/ALP is 2, suggesting alcoholic liver disease – a ratio >3.5 is considered by some authorities to be diagnostic. The raised bilirubin suggests an obstructive pattern, such as that found in cirrhosis, and the decreased albumin is probably due to decreased synthesis, as occurs in liver disease. ALP is a non-specific marker of liver disease.

2 What other validated markers of alcoholism are there?

Carbohydrate-deficient transferrin (normal range approximately 1.9–3.4g/L) is increasingly being used, especially in monitoring abstinence from alcohol. It is a form of iron-transport protein that also increases in liver diseases such chronic active hepatitis, autoimmune hepatitis and primary biliary cirrhosis.

Mean cell volume is a measure of the average size of red cells (normal range approximately 80–100 fL) and increases in alcoholism and various forms of anaemia. Mood stabilizers such as carbamazepine, lamotrigine and valproate may cause an increased MCV.

Alcoholic cirrhosis may be monitored by measuring a specific plasma peptide (procollagen type III), although raised levels are also seen in infection, inflammation and tissue necrosis.

3 What are the clinical signs and symptoms of alcohol withdrawal?

Withdrawal syndromes may be considered depending on the period of time elapsed from the last use of alcohol.

Short-term (within 24 hours of stopping use):

There are a wide range of possible signs and symptoms, including: convulsions (grand mal), depression, diaphoresis, hallucinosis (auditory, transient), hyperacusis, itching, muscle cramps, nausea, tinnitus, vomiting; can last for several days.

Medium-term (within 1–3 days of stopping use):

Delirium tremens: agitation, autonomic overactivity, confusion, delusions, hallucinations (visual), sleeplessness; delirium tremens constitutes a medical emergency and patients should be treated in a medical facility which has appropriate resuscitation facilities as mortality is approximately 10 per cent.

Longer-term (variable length of time after stopping use):

Wernicke–Korsakoff syndrome.

Alcoholic hallucinosis: auditory hallucinations in clear consciousness, usually resolves within a week but rarely may progress to amnesic, cognitive impairment or schizophreniform syndromes.

4 What are you going to say to the ward staff?

After reviewing the notes and seeing the patient (where you perform a full history, mental state examination and, if possible, a physical examination) you will decide whether the patient is acutely unwell psychiatrically or remains physically unwell with liver cirrhosis. You might need to discuss the case with a senior colleague and then explain to the ward staff that the patient does/does not merit admission to an acute psychiatric ward. If not, you will agree to continue to provide liaison psychiatric input as required.

ADDITIONAL POINTS

The clinical associations of chronic alcohol use

These are numerous, including:

Cardiovascular:	angina, arrhythmias, cardiomyopathy
Endocrine:	pseudo-Cushing's syndrome, hypogonadism
Gastrointestinal:	alcoholic cirrhosis, hepatitis, gastritis, carcinoma, pancreatitis
Haematological:	anaemia (macrocytic, iron deficiency, sideroblastic)
Musculoskeletal:	myopathy
Neurological:	Korsakoff's syndrome, seizures

FURTHER READING

Foster, R. (2008) *Clinical laboratory investigation and psychiatry: a practical handbook.* London: Informa Healthcare.

Mannelli, P. & Pae, C.U. (2007). Medical comorbidity and alcohol dependence. *Current Psychiatry Reports*, 9 (3), 217–24.

Marshall, W.J. (1995) *Clinical chemistry*, 3rd edn. London: Mosby.

STATION 3: Physical examination and laboratory investigation of eating disorders

KEY POINTS
Communication and empathy
Knowledge of eating disorders
Knowledge of physical complications of AN
Metabolic changes in AN
Answering other questions

INTRODUCE YOURSELF TO STAFF/PATIENT

SET THE SCENE

Apologize for the delay in getting to see her. Explain that you understand that she must be extremely concerned about her daughter. Find out what she knows about eating disorders. Make sure that you consider issues of patient confidentiality if you discuss issues relating to her daughter. Has the daughter consented to her case being discussed with her mother?

COMPLETING THE TASKS

Remember to discuss in lay terms.

1 What eating disorders are there and what are their features?

Although there is some disagreement, five major groupings of eating disorders may be identified: obesity, anorexia nervosa, bulimia nervosa, pica and eating disorder not otherwise specified (EDNOS).

Obesity:

Obesity may be defined as a body weight exceeding 120 per cent of the accepted average for age, gender and height in a given culture or setting. It may be further defined using the Quetelet's Body Mass Index (BMI): [weight in kilograms] divided by [height in metres]^2.

Anorexia nervosa (ICD Code F50.0):

Time frame: None specific

Features:

1. Weight loss of at least 15 per cent below the expected weight for height and age.
2. Weight-loss is self-induced.
3. Perception/dread of being too fat leading to a self-imposed desire for low weight.
4. Multiple endocrine effects on hypothalamic–pituitary–gonadal axis leading to alterations in sexual potency and amenorrhoea.

Bulimia nervosa (ICD Code F50.2):

Time frame: Specific features (recurrent over-eating) at least twice a week for at least three months

Features:

1. Recurrent episodes of over-eating (large amounts of food eaten in short periods of time).
2. Preoccupation with eating with compulsion/craving to eat.
3. Manoeuvres are undertaken by the patient to counteract the effects of eating by at least one of self-induced vomiting/purging, alternating episodes of fasting/starvation, use of drugs such as appetite suppressants, thyroid preparation, diuretics and insulin.
4. Fear of and self-perception of being fat.

2 What are the main differential diagnoses of anorexia nervosa?

Important differentials include:

Psychiatric: Depression, OCD, psychotic disorders, schizophrenia; note that individuals with eating disorders may have comorbid personality disorders.

Medical:

Endocrine: Diabetes mellitus, hypopituitarism, thyrotoxicosis
Gastrointestinal: Malabsorption
Other: Neoplasia, reticulosis

3 What symptoms may be reported in anorexia nervosa?

Often patients do not complain of symptoms, although universally they report thinking they are fat. Careful questioning may elicit the following:

Psychiatric symptoms – biological symptoms of depression, compulsions, low mood, obsessions, psychotic symptoms.

Physical symptoms – abdominal pain (possibly secondary to acute pancreatitis), amenorrhoea/menstrual dysfunction, constipation, erectile dysfunction/loss of libido (males), hypothermia, increased urinary frequency (may be secondary to diabetes insipidus or renal failure), muscle cramps, tiredness, vomiting.

4 What are the possible metabolic complications of anorexia nervosa?

There are many of these, including:

Domain	Condition
Metabolic	Acid–base disturbance (metabolic acidosis/alkalosis)
	Azotaemia
	Hypercholesterolaemia
	Hypertriglyceridaemia
	Hypoglycaemia
	Hyponatraemia
	Hypokalaemia
	Hypoalbuminaemia
	Hypocalcaemia
	Hypomagnesaemia
	Hypophosphataemia
	Osteoporosis
Endocrine	Diabetes insipitus
	Thyroid abnormalities (e.g. hypothyroidism, sick euthyroid syndrome: $\downarrow$T3)
	Menstrual disturbance/amenorrhoea
	$\uparrow$ GH, $\uparrow$ cortisol
Haematological	Anaemia
	Coagulopathies
	Leukopenia
	Lymphocytosis
	Thrombocytopenia
Gastrointestinal	Abnormal LFTs (hepatitis, steatohepatitis)
	Pancreatitis ($\uparrow$ plasma amylase)
	Nutritional deficiencies

ADDITIONAL POINTS

Eating disorders, especially anorexia nervosa, are complex conditions that require a multi-disciplinary perspective due to the large number of associated medical, metabolic and psychiatric complications.

The disorder is more common in females (female:male = 10:1) and young females appear more susceptible. Higher social classes are over-represented, as are athletes, ballet dancers and gymnasts.

⇧ Comorbid psychiatric diagnoses are common (especially major depression and possibly personality disorders).

Laboratory investigations should be guided by clinical presentation and it is always advisable to seek expert advice when requesting these.

Management involves correction of medical/metabolic complications with efforts to promote weight gain important.

Prognosis is usually worse with an older age of onset, comorbid personality disorders, long duration of illness (>5–6 years), male gender and previous history of obesity.

FURTHER READING

Berkman, N.D., Bulik, C.M., Brownley, K.A. et al. (2006) Management of eating disorders. *Evidence Report/Technology Assessment (Full Report)*, *135*, 1–166.

Herzog, W., Deter, H.C., Fiehn, W. & Petzold, E. (1997) Medical findings and predictors of long-term physical outcome in anorexia nervosa: a prospective, 12-year follow-up study. *Psychological Medicine*, *27* (2), 269–79.

Van Binsbergen, C.J., Odink, J., Van den Berg, H., Koppeschaar, H. & Coelingh Bennink, H.J. (1988) Nutritional status in anorexia nervosa: clinical chemistry, vitamins, iron and zinc. *European Journal of Clinical Nutrition*, *42* (11), 929–37.

STATION 4: Basic ECG interpretation

> ### KEY POINTS
> Communication
> Knowledge of basic ECG interpretation
> Knowledge of psychotropics that alter specific ECG parameters
> Answering other questions

INTRODUCE YOURSELF TO YOUR COLLEAGUE

SET THE SCENE

You can explain to the consultant why you decided to perform the ECG and what your findings are.

COMPLETING THE TASKS

1 What anatomical positions do the different leads of the ECG represent?

Standard leads:

The **left lateral surface** of the heart is looked at by leads **VL, I, II**.

The **inferior surface** of the heart is looked at by leads **VF** and **III**.

The **right atrium** is looked at by **VR**.

'V' Leads:

The **right ventricle** is looked at by **V1** and **V2**.

The **intra-ventricular septum** and **anterior wall of the left ventricle** are looked at by leads **V3** and **V4**.

The **anterior and lateral walls of the left ventricle** are looked at by **V5** and **V6**.

2 How do you know that the electrodes have been correctly applied to the patient and that the ECG trace is accurate?

Many machines now give real time interpretations, but with older machines the following rules of thumb are helpful to confirm correct lead placement in a normal ECG:

Lead	Overall direction of QRS complex
I	Mainly **up**wards
II	Mainly **up**wards
III	Mainly **up**wards
VR	Mainly **down**wards

3 How is sinus rhythm represented on the ECG? What conditions may be associated with a sinus tachycardia (heart rate>100 bpm)?

Sinus rhythm is indicated by a P wave occurring before a QRS complex. Sinus rhythms may be fast (>100 bpm = tachycardia) or slow (<40 bpm = bradycardia).

Sinus tachycardia may be associated with medical and non-medical conditions, for example:

Medical: anaemia, bleeding, cardiac failure, catacholamine-secreting tumours (rare, e.g. phaeochromocytosis), fever, hypovolaemia, pain, thyrotoxicosis

Non-medical: anxiety, drug intoxication/withdrawal, exercise, extreme emotion (release of catecholamines), fear, psychotropics.

4 What is the QTc interval? What psychotropics may be associated with prolongation of the QT interval?

The QTc interval is the time between the initial deflection of the P wave and the end of the T wave that is corrected for heart rate. It is normally less than 450 ms in men although may be slightly higher in women (up to 470 ms).

Psychotropics commonly associated with QTc prolongation include: chloral hydrate, chlorpromazine, citalopram, haloperidol, lithium, pimozide, sertindole, tricyclic antidepressants (TCAs), ziprasidone.

5 If the patient were being treated on clozapine, what ECG changes might you see?

Clozapine may cause myocarditis or cardiomyopathy, which may be heralded by non-specific symptoms such as chest pain, fever, shortness of breath, sweating and tachycardia. In some cases there may be no changes, although the following may occur:

On ECG, myocarditis may cause a tachycardia and non-specific, transient ST waves. It may also resemble an MI, with Q waves and lack of R waves in the anterior leads.

Cardiomyopathy may show non-specific ST and T wave changes in association with arrhythmias, such as atrial fibrillation or ventricular tachycardia.

ADDITIONAL POINTS

If asked to report the ECG it should be done systematically. You should have a scheme in mind, such as the following:

This is the ECG from [name of patient] a 55-year-old [ethnicity] female who was admitted with [brief history].

The ECG was taken on [date] and [time].

The rate is...

The axis is [normal, shows right/left axis deviation].

The rhythm is [sinus rhythm, atrial fibrillation, atrial flutter, etc.].

The PR interval is [normal, shows first/second/third degree heart block].

The QRS width is [normal, prolonged].

The QRS height is [normal, high].

There are/are no q waves.

The QT interval is [normal, prolonged].

The ST segment [is normal, is elevated/depressed in leads...].

The T waves are [normal, peaked, flattened].

There are/are no U waves.

In summary, this is a 12-lead ECG of a 55-year-old which is normal/shows the following abnormalities...

Interpreting an ECG is often difficult, and if there is any doubt the opinion of an experienced physician should be sought. When performing an ECG the patient is instructed to remain still during the recording in order to minimize any artefacts. Note that serial ECGs may be required, and that most modern ECG machines will try to interpret the trace, often inaccurately.

As you may have forgotten how to interpret an ECG, perusal of a suitable reference text (such as 'The ECG Made Simple' is suggested). Although a basic investigation, its interpretation is complex and if uncertain, it is always best to be honest and admit this!

FURTHER READING

Demangone, D. (2006) ECG manifestations: noncoronary heart disease. *Emerging Medical Clinics of North America, 24* (1), 113–31.

Goodnick, P.J., Jerry, J. & Parra, F. (2002) Psychotropic drugs and the ECG: focus on the QTc interval. *Expert Opinion in Pharmacotherapy, 3* (5), 479–98.

Hampton, J.R. (1994) *The ECG made easy*, 4th edn. London: Churchill Livingstone.

Mackin, P. (2008) Cardiac side effects of psychiatric drugs. *Human Psychopharmacology, 23* (Suppl. 1), 3–14.

Merrill, D.B., Dec, G.W. & Goff, D.C. (2005). Adverse cardiac effects associated with clozapine. *Journal of Clinical Psychopharmacology, 25* (1), 32–41.

Taylor, D., Paton, C. & Kerwin, R. (2007) *The Maudsley Prescribing Guidelines*, 9th edn. London: Informa Healthcare.

STATION 5: Initiation and monitoring of clozapine

KEY POINTS
Communication
Knowledge of clozapine pharmacology
Awareness of laboratory aspects of clozapine – therapeutic blood monitoring, metabolic side-effects, NICE guidelines
Answering other questions

INTRODUCE YOURSELF TO THE MEMBER OF STAFF

SET THE SCENE
Ask if they have ever seen clozapine used before and, if so, what they know about it. Explain that you will need to obtain appropriate background information about the patient, including details of all previous treatments, how long the patient was on them and why they were stopped. The views of the patient should also be canvassed.

COMPLETING THE TASKS

1 When should clozapine be considered?
Clozapine is an 'atypical' antipsychotic which is used in the treatment of schizophrenia in patients who have either not responded to two full courses of other antipsychotics (one of which should be an 'atypical') or who are intolerant of conventional antipsychotic agents (e.g. suffer from severe extra-pyramidal side effects or severe tardive dyskinesia).

Clozapine is contraindicated in patients with myeloproliferative disorders, active/progressive cardiac, hepatic and renal disease, and individuals with uncontrolled epilepsy.

2 What are the life-threatening side effects of clozapine?

Important life-threatening side effects of clozapine	
Agranulocytosis	Incidence around 0.8 per cent, risk of fatal agranulocytosis estimated at 1 in 5,000; women/older age may be risk factors
Pulmonary embolism	Rare, risk estimated at 1 in 2,000–6,000; may be more likely in early stages of treatment (first three months)
Myocarditis/Cardiomyopathy	Risk variable (from 1 in 1,300 up to 1 in 67,000) and may be more likely in early stages of treatment (first 2–3 months)
Seizures	Incidence around 3 per cent, risk is dose-related and may require use of prophylactic valproate

3 What other adverse effect of clozapine are there?

Agranulocytosis, which occurs in about 1 per cent of patients thus requires regular, mandatory monitoring of FBC.

4 What blood tests are needed for clozapine and when?

Blood tests should be done prior to, and following, initiation. As agranulocytosis (white cell count $< 2 \times 10^9$/L) is a major risk, full blood count (FBC) should be regularly monitored. *Weekly* full blood counts are required for the first 18 weeks, then *two-weekly* until one year; if blood counts remain stable, then *four-weekly* thereafter (including four weeks post-discontinuation). There is a traffic-light system for clozapine FBC monitoring, with red = stop clozapine immediately; amber = repeat FBC and proceed with caution; green = safe to continue.

Additional laboratory monitoring with clozapine	
Regular monitoring	FBC
Three-monthly	HbA1C, Lipid profile
Six-monthly	U&Es, LFTs, Lipid profile*
Other	CPK (if NMS suspected); other parameters as based on clinical suspicion (see table below)

Regular laboratory monitoring of laboratory parameters is suggested below:

5 What are the grounds for discontinuing clozapine?

If white cell count $< 2 \times 10^9$/L;

Suspected myocarditis or other cardiovascular dysfunction;

Suspected neuroleptic malignant syndrome;

Eosinophilia (above 3.0×10^9/L);

Thrombocytopenia when platelet count $< 50 \times 10^9$/L;

---

*Especially advised when specific risk factors present

6 Are there any protocols when commencing clozapine?

All patients should be registered with a clozapine monitoring service. Prior to commencing clozapine the patient should be warned about the risk of side effects and should be instructed to notify their key worker in the event of any sign of infection (sore throat, fever, etc.). Close collaboration between the patient, the GP and secondary mental health services is important, and may be incorporated into a formal, 'shared care' agreement.

ADDITIONAL POINTS

The accepted reference range for clozapine is **350–500 µg/L**. Blood should be collected for **trough** levels (i.e. just before the dose) in a plain tube. It should be noted that the time to steady-state is approximately three days, and levels may be lower in males, especially those who are younger and smoke.

FURTHER READING

Foster, R. (2008) *Clinical laboratory investigation and psychiatry: a practical handbook.* London: Informa Healthcare.

Raggi, M.A., Mandrioli, R., Sabbioni, C. & Pucci, V. (2004). Atypical antipsychotics: pharmacokinetics, therapeutic drug monitoring and pharmacological interactions. *Current Medicinal Chemistry*, *11* (3), 279–96.

Rostami-Hodjegan, A., Amin, A.M. et al. (2004) Influence of dose, cigarette smoking, age, sex, and metabolic activity on plasma clozapine concentrations: a predictive model and nomograms to aid clozapine dose adjustment and to assess compliance in individual patients. *Journal of Clinical Psychopharmacology*, *24* (1), 70–8.

Taylor, D., Paton, C. & Kerwin, R (2007) *The South London and Maudsley 2007/8 Prescribing Guidelines*, 9th edn. London: Martin Dunitz.

STATION 6: Interpreting thyroid function tests

KEY POINTS
Communication and empathy
Knowledge of thyroid function tests
Knowledge of psychotropics that affect the thyroid
Answering other questions

INTRODUCE YOURSELF TO HER HUSBAND

SET THE SCENE

Remember to consider issues of patient confidentiality and whether the patient has capacity and consents to your discussing her case. In order to understand the blood results, further information about the patient is needed. This can be obtained from ward staff and reading the hospital notes. You will be particularly interested in the history of presenting complaint and medication history, further details of which may be obtained from the husband or GP.

COMPLETING THE TASKS

1 What blood tests are done and why?

The above information suggests a possible organic disorder, although a full history, mental state examination, physical examination and appropriate, additional investigations need to be performed.

Suitable first-line screening tests will be guided by the important differentials, in this case, hypothyroidism. Thus thyroid function tests, a full blood count, urea and electrolytes will be the usual first-line tests.

2 You perform a number of laboratory investigations and find the following abnormal results:

MCV = 106 fL (normal range approximately 76–96 fL)

Serum TSH = 120 mU/L (normal range approximately 0.3–0.4 mU/L)

Serum free T4 = 4 pmol/L (normal range approximately 9–26 pmol/L).

How do you explain these results to the husband?

The high TSH is suggestive of the diagnosis of hypothyroidism, as is the low free T4. The presence of a macrocytic anaemia is consistent with this diagnosis.

3 In general terms, how will she be managed?

The main treatment of hypothyroidism is with thyroxine replacement, which should be initiated either by the GP or after referral to an endocrinologist. Although the main treatment is with thyroxine (T4) replacement, T3 may be used in patients with ischaemic heart disease. An open and clear dialogue with the patient and her husband will be helpful to allay possible fears or concerns.

4 Psychiatric manifestations of hypothyroidism?

Symptoms that have been reported include: anhedonia, delirium (rare), dysphoria, irritability, mania, personality changes, psychomotor agitation or retardation, psychosis (rare, may occur in long-standing, untreated individuals), slowing of cognitive function, sleep disturbance, suicidality.

5 Clinical signs and symptoms of hypothyrodism?

Clinical signs: bradycardia, cerebellar ataxia (rare), congestive cardiac failure, dry/cool skin, facial swelling, goitre, hair loss, hoarse voice, non-pitting oedema, slowed muscle reflexes (pseudomyotonia), slowed speech, tongue thickening, weight gain.

Clinical symptoms: cold intolerance, constipation, cramps, deafness, fatigue, menstrual disturbances, muscle pain, weakness.

ADDITIONAL POINTS

Psychiatric manifestations of hyperthyroidism

Psychiatric symptoms: anxiety, cognitive decline, delirium, depression, emotional lability, feeling of apprehension, irritability, nervousness, psychosis (rare)

Clinical signs and symptoms of hyperthyrodism

Clinical symptoms: fatigue, heat intolerance, menstrual irregularities, weakness

⇑ Clinical signs: agitation, atrial fibrillation, dermopathy (pretibial myxoedema, pruritis), diaphoresis, diarrhoea, dyspnoea, eye signs (exophthalmos, 'lid lag'), goitre, hair loss, palpitations tachycardia, thyroid bruit, tremor, weight loss

Both hyper- and hypothyroidism are associated with changes in mental state and many signs and symptoms may be elicited, not all of which are clinically significant. It is always advisable to seek the advice of a physician in order to provide optimal management for such patients.

FURTHER READING

Costa, A.J. (1995) Interpreting thyroid tests. *American Family Physician*, 52 (8), 2325–30.

Davis, D. & Tremont, G. (2007) Neuropsychiatric aspects of hypothyroidism and treatment reversibility. *Minerva Endocrinologica*, 32 (1), 49–65.

Foster, R. (2008) *Clinical laboratory investigation and psychiatry: a practical handbook.* London: Informa Healthcare.

STATION 7: Interpretation of lithium levels

KEY POINTS
Communication and empathy
Knowledge of lithium side effects and plasma concentrations
Knowledge of NICE guidelines
Answering other questions

INTRODUCE YOURSELF TO THE PATIENT

SET THE SCENE

Briefly try to obtain some details about the patient's history. Ask what, if anything, he knows about lithium and how he has been in himself since commencing this treatment.

COMPLETING THE TASKS

Remember to talk in lay terms.

1 What are the clinical uses of lithium?

1. Prophylaxis and treatment of bipolar affective disorder
2. Prophylaxis of recurrent depression, especially as an adjunct in refractory depression
3. As an adjunct to antipsychotics in the treatment of schizoaffective disorder
4. In the treatment of aggressive or self-mutilating behaviour

2 What are main side effects of lithium?

Early side effects of lithium are dose-related and include gastrointestinal side effects (nausea, vomiting, diarrhoea), tremor (may manifest as intention tremor) and dry mouth.

Later side effects amenable to laboratory measurement are more numerous and appear at higher plasma concentrations).

Later side effects of lithium which may affect laboratory parameters:

System	Condition	Laboratory tests
Endocrine	Hypothyroidism	TFTs
	Hyperparathyroidism (both increased)	Calcium, parathyroid hormone
	Nephrogenic diabetes insipidus	U&E
	Raised levels of ADH	U&E, urine osmolality, urine sodium
Haematology	Leucocytosis	FBC
	Thrombocytosis	
Metabolic	Hypercalcaemia (may cause cardiac arrhythmias)	Calcium
	Hypokalaemia (may cause cardiac arrhythmias)	U&E
Renal	Nephropathy	eGFR, U&E, urinalysis
		Renal failure
Immune	SLE	Autoantibody screen
	Myasthenia gravis	Acetylcholine receptor antibodies; Tensolon (Edrophonium) test

3 What is the plasma reference range of lithium?

Approximately 0.6–1 mmol/L.

4 What are the signs of toxicity and how do these relate to plasma levels?

Severe toxicity may occur at levels >1.5 mmol/L and death may occur at higher levels (>2.0 mmol/L), although toxicity has also been reported at only mildly elevated serum concentrations.

Lithium has a narrow therapeutic index and has a number of important adverse effects in overdose, which may be fatal; these include neurological effects (tremor, ataxia, nystagmus, convulsions, confusion, slurred speech, coma) as well as renal impairment

5 Are there any additional blood tests that should be done in a patient on lithium?

Prior to commencing lithium, the following baseline tests should be considered:

Baseline laboratory measurements for patients initiating lithium	
Clinical biochemistry	eGFR, U&E, calcium, creatinine, TFTs.
Haematology	Full blood count

Additional, regular laboratory monitoring of laboratory parameters is suggested below:

Additional laboratory monitoring with lithium	
After seven days	Plasma lithium levels then **weekly** until the required level is reached (between 0.6 and 1.0 mmol/L)
Three-monthly	U&Es, plasma lithium levels
6–12 monthly	eGFR, U&Es, calcium, TFTs
Other	CPK (if NMS suspected)
	Calcium if hyperparathyroidism suspected
	U&Es if patient dehydrated/vomiting/having diarrhoea
	Other parameters as based on clinical suspicion.

ADDITIONAL POINTS

NICE recommends the following laboratory monitoring for lithium at three months after initial screening:

Laboratory parameter	Notes
Lithium levels	3 times over 6 weeks following initiation of treatment and 3-monthly thereafter.
U&E	U&E may be needed more frequently if patient deteriorates or is on ACE inhibitors, diuretics or NSAIDs.
TFTs	Thyroid function, for individuals with rapid-cycling bipolar disorder; thyroid antibodies may be measured if TFTs are abnormal.
Glucose	As based on clinical presentation.

FURTHER READING

Bazaire, S. (2003) *Psychotropic drug directory 2003/04*. Salisbury, Wilts: Fivepin Publishing.

Foster, R. (2008) *Clinical laboratory investigation and psychiatry: a practical handbook*. London: Informa Healthcare.

http://www.nice.org.uk/nicemedia/pdf/Bipolar_2ndconsultation_full.pdf

Taylor, D., Paton, C. & Kerwin, R (2007) *The South London and Maudsley 2007/8 Prescribing Guidelines*, 9th edn. London: Martin Dunitz.

STATION 8: Interpretation of laboratory results (metabolic syndrome)

KEY POINTS
Communication with clinical colleagues
Knowledge of diagnosis of metabolic syndrome, including screening laboratory tests

INTRODUCE YOURSELF TO YOUR COLLEAGUE

SET THE SCENE

You will need to obtain any additional appropriate background information about this patient, including details of all previous treatments, how long the patient was on them and why they were stopped.

COMPLETING THE TASKS

1 What important metabolic side effects of antipsychotics do you know about?

Antipsychotics have a number of metabolic side effects, including those comprising the metabolic syndrome; these include disturbed glucose metabolism (raised fasting plasma glucose), abnormal insulin metabolism (hyperinsulinaemia) and dyslipidaemia (reduced high-density lipoprotein (HDL), hypertriglyceridaemia). Microalbuminaemia may also occur, but this is variable.

2 What are the clinical symptoms of metabolic syndrome?

Frequently there may be none in early stages, while in later stages they are those of the underlying disorder such as glucose intolerance/diabetes mellitus or hyperlipidaemia.

3 What are the clinical signs of metabolic syndrome?

These may include obesity, hypertension, and signs of associated disorders such as acanthosis nigricans, haemochromatosis or polycystic ovary syndrome.

4 What is the major differential diagnosis of metabolic syndrome?

The major differential is diabetes mellitus.

5 Are there any other medications associated with metabolic syndrome?

Apart from antipsychotics, stavudine, steroids and zidovudine have been associated with development of metabolic syndrome.

6 What general approaches may be used to manage metabolic syndrome in a patient receiving antipsychotics?

This will depend on both clinical presentation and severity and may include general and specific interventions. Interventions will require a multi-disciplinary focus. General interventions may include lifestyle modification (increased exercise, weight loss) and dietary changes, while specific interventions may include aspirin prophylaxis for pro-thrombotic states, anti-hypertensive treatment, pharmacological treatment aimed at lowering blood cholesterol and oral hypoglycaemics or insulin.

Regular monitoring of blood sugar via urine dipstick, 'near patient' blood sampling or laboratory testing (fasting glucose, HbA1c) is required, and it may be appropriate to switch to another class of antipsychotic. In all cases expert advice is required.

PROBLEM SOLVING

The first task is to try to find out any additional information about the patient. Advise that your colleague obtain collateral information from the CMHT (if there is one) or the GP. He will need to perform a proper history, mental state and physical examination to determine whether this man is acutely psychiatrically unwell or is in need of immediate medical attention. In his history he will need to specifically ask about any psychiatric history, medical history and medication history, as you are concerned about the microalbuminuria, which you recall may be associated with renal toxicity of some medications.

He will need to ask the A&E team to perform a thorough physical examination and request appropriate blood tests in order to rule out an organic cause for this man's presentation.

Laboratory features of the metabolic syndrome:

Feature	Laboratory Investigation	Notes
Disturbed glucose metabolism Disturbed insulin metabolism	Random blood glucose, HbA1c, glucose tolerance test, plasma insulin	May manifest as any of hyperinsulinaemia, impaired glucose tolerance, insulin resistance or diabetes mellitus
Obesity	None specific	Particularly abdominal distribution
Dyslipidaemia	Plasma cholesterol/ triglycerides	Decreased HDL cholesterol and/or hypertriglyceridaemia
Hypertension	None specific	May not have any obvious clinical manifestations in early stages
Microalbuminuria	Urinalysis	May not be present, absence does not preclude the diagnosis

ADDITIONAL POINTS

Definition:	Metabolic syndrome, also called syndrome of insulin resistance, syndrome X and Reaven's syndrome, consists of the association of central obesity with two or more of the four key features of the disorder (hypertension, hypertriglyceridaemia, raised fasting plasma glucose, reduced HDL). The World Health Organization guidelines also include the feature of microalbuminuria.
Incidence:	Controversial; in schizophrenic patients treated with antipsychotics the published ranges vary between 22 and 54.2 per cent.
Psychiatric associations:	Psychotic illnesses (especially schizophrenia); treatment with antipsychotic medication (especially atypicals); note that other medications have been associated with the development of metabolic syndrome including some anti-retrovirals (stavudine, zidovudine) and steroids.

FURTHER READING

De Hert, M.A., van Winkel, R., Van Eyck, D., Hanssens, L., Wampers, M., Scheen, A. & Peuskens, J. (2006) Prevalence of the metabolic syndrome in patients with schizophrenia treated with antipsychotic medication. *Schizophrenia Research*, 83 (1), 87–93.

Grundy, S.M., Cleeman, J.I., Daniels, S.R., Donato, K.A., Eckel, R.H., Franklin, B.A., Gordon, D.J., Krauss, R.M., Savage, P.J., Smith, S.C., Jr, Spertus, J.A. & Costa, F. (2005) Diagnosis and management of the metabolic syndrome. *Circulation*, *112*, 2735–52.

Haddad, P., Durson, S. & Deakin, B. (eds) (2004) *Adverse syndromes and psychiatric drugs – a clinical guide.* Oxford: Oxford University Press.

Taylor, D., Paton, C. & Kerwin, R. (2007) *The Maudsley Prescribing Guidelines*, 9th edn. London: Informa Healthcare.

STATION 9: Diagnosis and management of neuroleptic malignant syndrome

> **KEY POINTS**
> Communication with colleagues
> Longer-term problems with management
> Immediate medical management
> Immediate and longer-term 'crisis' management
> Recognition of signs/symptoms of NMS
> Answering other questions

INTRODUCE YOURSELF

SET THE SCENE

It is important to let the medics know that this is a possible NMS, which is a medical emergency. Let them know that he needs transfer to a medical setting for further management. Remember to talk in clear, calm and polite terms and be prepared to explain how you intend to manage the situation acutely. If your colleague refuses to accept the patient you should explain that you will have to call for an ambulance as there is a significant mortality associated with this condition.

COMPLETING THE TASKS

1 What are possible differential diagnoses?

Medication-related:	Lethal catatonia, lithium toxicity, malignant hyperthermia, serotonin syndrome, severe EPSE.
Drug-related:	Acute intoxication (amphetamine, cocaine); toxicity (anaesthetics, anticholinergics, monoamine oxidase inhibitors (MAOIs)), withdrawal (alcohol, anti-Parkinsonian medications, benzodiazepines).
Organic:	Cerebral tumours, cardiovascular attack (CVA), dehydration, delirium, heat exhaustion, myocardial infarction, phaeochromocytoma, seizures, sepsis (encephalitis, encephalomyelitis, HIV, systemic), systemic lupus erythematosus (SLE), thyrotoxicosis, trauma.
Psychiatric:	Mania, severe psychosis.

2 What is NMS?

Neuroleptic malignant syndrome (NMS) is a rare, idiosyncratic and life-threatening condition which is thought to be related to use of medications which block dopamine receptors and thereby induce sympathetic hyperactivity.

3 What are the clinical signs and symptoms?

Core features: Behavioural change, diaphoresis, hyperthermia, impaired consciousness, labile blood pressure, tachycardia.

Associated features: Akinesia, dystonia, sialorrhoea, tachypnoea, tremor.

4 What medications are implicated in NMS?

Antidepressants: e.g. Monoamine oxidase inhibitors, tricyclic antidepressants (TCAs).

Antipsychotics: All, possible increased risk with clozapine and risperidone.

Others: Metoclopramide, reserpine, tetrabenazine, lithium, especially in combination with antipsychotics.

Discontinuation of: Amantadine, bromocriptine, levodopa.

5 What immediate action needs to be taken on the ward?

Ensure patient and staff safety.

Perform rapid primary survey, ensuring adequate airway, breathing and circulation.

Stop putative offending agent.

Insert venflon.

Monitor observations (temp, pulse, respiratory rate, blood pressure, O_2 saturation).

Perform ECG if possible.

If in any doubt transfer patient to general hospital.

Ensure good communication with ward staff, on-call senior and receiving hospital.

Once patient is stabilized:

Ensure that appropriate documentation occurs.

Ensure that ward staff feel supported.

Ensure that the ward consultant is notified.

6 What additional measures may be useful in treatment of NMS?

Monitor and correct metabolic imbalances.

Monitor temperature and cool the patient as required.

Medications such as benzodiazepines, thiamine, dextrose and/or naloxone may be needed.

Monitor kidney function and urine output.

ECT may be helpful in some patients.

7 What blood/laboratory tests, if any, are useful for diagnosis and monitoring of NMS?

Possible laboratory abnormalities in NMS:

Domain	Parameter	Notes
Clinical biochemistry	Blood gases	May reveal anoxia and/or metabolic acidosis
	Creatine phosphokinase	Elevated levels may be seen, reflecting myonecrosis from sustained muscle contractions (rhabdomyolysis)
	LFTs	Raised liver enzymes (LDH, ALP, AST) may be seen
	U&Es	May reflect altered renal function
	Urinalysis	May reveal myoglobinuria (rhabdomyolysis)
Haematology	FBC	May reveal leucocytosis

8 What is the prognosis of NMS?

Mortality: Between 5 and 12 per cent, due to cardiac arrhythmia, DIC, respiratory failure, renal failure, shock.

Morbidity: Variable, better outcome in younger people and early intervention: arrhythmias, aspiration pneumonia, DIC, respiratory embarrassment, rhabdomyolysis, renal failure, seizures.

PROBLEM SOLVING

Remember that NMS and its differentials are potentially life-threatening conditions, and prompt action is always required. Ensure that staff are aware of the urgency of intervention and have appropriate equipment to hand and that the crash team has been alerted. There must be no delay in seeing the patient, and it is advisable to ring for an ambulance at the earliest opportunity, ensuring that the receiving hospital is also warned about the patient. A copy of the current drug chart and psychiatric notes is always helpful, as is a transfer letter.

Prior to transfer to A&E, basic interventions (airway, breathing, circulation) and basic observations should be performed, with additional input given where the doctor in charge deems this appropriate.

ADDITIONAL POINTS

In normal practice 'heroic' interventions are not appropriate on the ward, and although you have a duty of care towards your patient, performing interventions which you are not adequately trained or experienced in is never appropriate. Management of medical emergencies is best performed in A&E.

FURTHER READING

http://www.nice.org.uk/nicemedia/pdf/CG38fullguideline.pdf

Schweyen, D.H., Sporka, M.C. & Burnakis, T.G. (1991) Evaluation of serum lithium concentration determinations. *American Journal of Hospital Pharmacy*, 48 (7), 1536–7.

Taylor, D., Paton, C. and Kerwin, R. (2007) *The South London and Maudsley 2007/8 Prescribing Guidelines*, 9th edn. London: Informa Healthcare.

STATION 10: Diagnosis and management of serotonin syndrome

> **KEY POINTS**
> Communication and empathy
> Longer-term problems with management
> Immediate medical management
> Immediate and longer-term 'crisis' management
> Recognition of signs/symptoms of serotonin syndrome
> Answering other questions
> Serotonin syndrome

INTRODUCE YOURSELF TO THE NURSE

SET THE SCENE

The current scenario should set alarm bells ringing as it implies a medical emergency that requires immediate medical input. Try to get more of a handover from the nurse and explain that you do not want to delay seeing the patient. Ask what she knows about his history, physical examination and any investigations.

COMPLETING THE TASKS

1 What are possible differential diagnoses?

Psychiatric:	Catatonia.
Medication-related syndromes:	Malignant hyperthermia, neuroleptic malignant syndrome.
Drugs/medication intoxication:	Anticholinergics, amphetamine, cocaine, lithium, MAOIs, salicylates.
Drug withdrawal:	baclofen (acute withdrawal).
Other:	Encephalitis, hyperthyroidism, meningitis, non-convulsive seizures, septicaemia, tetanus.

2 What is serotonin syndrome?

Serotonin syndrome is a disorder caused by the over-stimulation of serotonergic receptors following administration of a number of medications, especially antidepressants, including SSRIs, MAOIs and TCAs. It is a rare and idiosyncratic disorder which is nearly always observed following administration of a serotonergic agent. Clinical features are based on the triad of autonomic, cognitive/behavioural and neurological symptoms.

3 What are the clinical signs and symptoms?

Clinical features of the serotonin syndrome	
Autonomic	Blood pressure lability
	Diaphoresis
	Dyspnoea
	Fever
	Tachycardia
Cognitive/behavioural	Changes in mental state (confusion, possible hypomania) and behaviour (agitation, insomnia) may be seen
Neurological	Akathisia
	Hyperreflexia
	Impaired coordination
	Myoclonus
	Tremor

4 What immediate action needs to be taken?

Severe serotonin syndrome, as appears to be the case with this patient, is a medical emergency. Thus the medical team should be made aware immediately. Attention should be paid to airways, breathing and circulation, with supportive measures such as cooling, muscle paralysis and intubation initiated to prevent complications such as rhabdomyolysis, renal failure and disseminated intravascular coagulation (DIC). It would be prudent to cease any putative contributory agents and if necessary seek advice from the local poisons unit.

5 What additional measures may be useful in treatment of serotonin syndrome?

Some authorities suggest the use of serotonin antagonists, and cyproheptadine and chlorpromazine have both been used.

6 What laboratory tests, if any, are useful for diagnosis and monitoring of serotonin syndrome?

Whilst the diagnosis is primarily clinical, based on the presence of autonomic, cognitive/behavioural and neurological symptoms, there are no specific diagnostic laboratory investigations. Rather, any investigations are aimed at evaluating and monitoring associated morbidity:

Possible laboratory changes in serotonin syndrome:

Domain	Parameter	Notes
Clinical biochemistry	Bicarbonate	Decreased levels seen
	Creatine kinase (total)	Elevated levels seen
	Transaminases	Elevated levels seen
	Metabolic acidosis	May be seen
Haematology	Leucocytosis	May be seen
	Disseminated intravascular coagulation	May be seen

7 What is the prognosis of serotonin syndrome?

Although severe serotonin syndrome is a medical emergency, it is rarely life threatening with appropriate treatment.

ADDITIONAL POINTS

In normal practice 'heroic' interventions are not appropriate on the ward, and although you have a duty of care towards your patient, performing interventions which you are not adequately trained or experienced in is never appropriate. Management of medical emergencies is best performed in A&E.

Two separate sets of clinical features have been proposed to assist in the diagnosis of serotonin syndrome.

The Hunter Serotonin Toxicity Criteria provide a series of 'decision rules', with spontaneous clonus in the presence of a serotonergic agent or the presence of induced clonus with other features (agitation, sweating) or ocular clonus with other features (agitation, sweating) or tremor/hyperreflexia or hypertonia/ hyperthermia/clonus (ocular or induced).

The Sternbach Criteria include: agitation, alteration in mental state (confusion, hypomania), diarrhoea, fever, hyperreflexia, incoordination, myoclonus, shivering, sweating and tremor.

FURTHER READING

Dunkley, E.J., Isbister, G.K., Sibbritt, D. et al. (2003) The Hunter Serotonin Toxicity Criteria: simple and accurate diagnostic decision rules for serotonin toxicity. *Quarterly Journal of Medicine, 96*, 635–42.

Isbister, G.K., Buckley, N.A. & Whyte, I.M. (2007) Serotonin toxicity: a practical approach to diagnosis and treatment. *Medical Journal of Australia, 187* (6), 361–5.

Sternbach, H. (1991) The serotonin syndrome. *American Journal of Psychiatry, 148* (6), 705–13.

Taylor, D., Paton, C. and Kerwin, R. (2007) *The South London and Maudsley 2007/8 Prescribing Guidelines*, 9th edn. London: Informa Healthcare.

Chapter 16

Miscellaneous

Dr Justin Sauer

SINGLE STATIONS

1.

This is Michael Green, a 28-year-old who lives with boyfriend Steve. He is seeking comprehensive female gender reassignment and has been considering travelling to Thailand for surgery. Steve is not keen on the idea and would prefer that he receive treatment within the NHS.

Mr Green, who likes to be known as 'Lesley', has had some feminizing hormone treatment privately. He would now like to join an NHS programme, which is why he has come to see you.

Manage this situation, taking a relevant history and explaining what such a programme is likely to involve.

2.

This 29-year-old woman, who lost her husband 7 months ago to cancer, has been attending the general practitioner (GP) regularly with multiple non-specific complaints and it often ends up as a counselling session.

He has been seeing her but has not been providing any formal psychological treatment or medication. She will call the surgery often, asking to speak her doctor, and has also asked him to visit her at home on a number of occasions.

The GP has noticed that she continues to grieve and is unsure whether this is normal. In her medical history she has asthma and psoriasis. There is no past psychiatric history. Her brother has an autistic spectrum disorder, but lives independently.

She is close to her mother, with whom she speaks almost every day.

Assess this woman's response to the loss of her husband.

3.

This woman attends the community clinic wanting to speak to her husband's psychiatrist. She is angry that their sex life has deteriorated as a result of him taking a selective serotonin reuptake inhibitor (SSRI) antidepressant.

She has had plans to start a family. It is reported through correspondence from the GP that she may have advised her husband to stop the medication.

Speak to this woman.

4.

Assess this patient who feels that his eyes are too widely spaced apart and is seeking corrective surgery.

Explain your diagnosis and how you plan to help.

5.

You have been asked to assess this 32-year-old gentleman. He has been to his GP on and off for 5 years complaining of changes in his sleep pattern and mood. One year, whilst working abroad during the winter, he did not complain of low mood.

The GP informs you that he is noticeably more depressed between October and April, when he will sleep excessively and put on weight. As spring arrives he can become mildly elated and irritable. His partner is finding his unpredictability difficult to manage.

The GP referred him for psychotherapy but this did not help. He wonders whether excessive travelling is responsible for his unstable mental state.

What is the differential diagnosis – explain your rationale for each.

Give him advice on what can be done to help.

STATION 1: Gender reassignment

> **KEY POINTS**
> Empathy and rapport
> History of gender dysphoria
> Diagnostic clarification
> Details of the programme
> Management

INTRODUCE YOURSELF

'Hello Lesley, my name is Dr____, I'm one of the psychiatrists.'

SET THE SCENE

'I understand you're not happy living as a man, is that correct? Could you tell me more about this?'

'When did these feelings begin?'

'When did you seriously consider having surgery?'

COMPLETING THE TASKS

It would be useful to let the examiner know that you understand the distinction between the gender identity disorders.

In transsexualism there is a desire to live as a member of the opposite sex. There is often a feeling of discomfort or uneasiness with one's own anatomy and a strong desire to have this corrected with hormonal and surgical interventions. According to the ICD-10 diagnostic criteria, the person should have been behaving as a member of the opposite sex persistently for at least 2 years. Their beliefs about their gender should not be a symptom of another illness such as schizophrenia or associated with structural or genetic abnormalities.

Relevant history

Sense of gender dysphoria

Dressing as a woman – for how long – ? in childhood

Feelings towards own gender-specific features – sexual organs

Tendency to behave as a member of the opposite sex

Fantasies about normal vaginal intercourse

Evidence of transsexualism rather than transvestism

It is important to establish whether there is a physical abnormality, such as intersex, contributing to the presentation.

Management

Psychiatric management involves the identification and treatment of any underlying psychiatric illnesses (e.g. schizophrenia, delusional disorder, affective disorder).

Investigations and physical examination of the external genitalia and genetic testing (if necessary).

Practical support such as counselling or more formal psychological input during the gender transition process.

Prior to surgery, living as a woman for a minimum of 2 years for male to female transsexuals. Help can be given with this process, including learning mannerisms, cosmetic procedures, e.g. depilation.

Hormone treatment to induce secondary sexual characteristics (female sex hormones, anti-testosterone drugs).

If the adjustment goes well, then they will proceed to the transgender surgery – penis dissection and vaginal fashioning.

RISK

Men who take oestrogen should be fully informed of the changes that will occur physically but also of the adverse effects. Patients should be monitored for hyperglycaemia, hypertension, liver function and thrombo-embolic events.

Post surgery – and particularly if the results are unsatisfactory – patients may be low and have been known to self-harm or attempt suicide.

PROBLEM SOLVING

Expert help will be needed to assist with the practicalities of a gender change, including changing one's name, passport and other documentation.

This is a sensitive station in which candidates can feel embarrassed. This will only make the patient uncomfortable. Remaining confident and unfazed will put everyone at ease.

ADDITIONAL POINTS

The differential diagnoses will include: dual-role transvestism (wearing clothes of the opposite sex, to temporarily enjoy the experience being a woman/man, but without sexual excitement or the wish for a permanent change); and fetishistic transsexualism (wearing clothes of the opposite sex mainly to obtain sexual excitement).

Gender reassignment surgery is permanent and not reversible.

FURTHER READING

World Health Organization (1992) *The ICD-10 classification of mental and behavioural disorders; clinical descriptions and diagnostic guidelines.* Geneva: WHO.

STATION 2: Grief reaction

KEY POINTS
Communication and rapport
Empathy
History of grief
Features of abnormal grief
Explanation of diagnosis and management

INTRODUCE YOURSELF

'Hello, my name is Dr_____, it's nice to meet you.'

SET THE SCENE

'I am sorry to hear about your recent loss.'

'How have you been since this happened?'

COMPLETING THE TASKS

Try to elicit the features of grief in your history.

A normal grief reaction can include the following:

Preoccupation with the deceased (occurs in all cases of grief).

Pining or searching for the deceased.

Somatic responses e.g. crying, insomnia, reduced appetite.

Mummification; where the survivor preserves the deceased's belongings or room, exactly as it was before their death.

Hallucinations or illusions of the deceased; common in normal individuals and considered to be part of the normal grieving process. Can occur in any of the sensory modalities, but usually auditory.

Guilt.

Resolution follows.

Abnormal grief reaction:

Grieving process longer than 6 months (although this is not universally accepted).

Grieving process delayed for more than 2 weeks.

General inability to function.

Excessive hallucinatory experiences (bizarre and varied hallucinations).

Protracted mummification – a whole house may be left unchanged, with a place set for the deceased at meal times.

Thoughts of self-harm or suicide, beyond what might be expected in a normal reaction.

Other features can include:

Acquiring features or symptoms of the deceased's final illness (indeed this patient has taken on some of her late husband's symptoms).

Retaining an idealized view of the deceased.

Management

Explain to the patient what you think is causing her to present frequently to the GP.

Discuss psychological treatment (grief counselling or grief therapy) and explain what this will involve.

Antidepressants are not recommended for normal grief.

Addressing other problem areas can also help, including advice with sleep or hypnotics for short-term use.

Practical support can be helpful. What was the deceased's role in day-to-day activities (dealing with bills, finances, health issues, dependants, cooking, cleaning, etc.)? Exploring this and the need for help is important. Her mother is close to her and may be able to provide her with practical and emotional support.

PROBLEM SOLVING

Exclude major mental illness in this patient. Although grief is most likely, consider an affective or psychotic illness and use screening questions during the assessment.

Grief and depression share many features; however, they are considered as separate syndromes. The pervasiveness of low mood in depression versus the fluctuations in grief, with windows of light-heartedness, often helps to distinguish between them. Feelings of hopelessness and worthlessness tend to be more pronounced in depression, with the belief that there is no chance of 'getting better'.

ADDITIONAL POINTS

A grief reaction can occur for the loss of a body part or a pet. Abnormal grief is more likely to occur following a sudden, unexpected death or suicide. It can also occur when the survivor was dependent on the deceased, where there is a psychiatric history or where there is an inability to grieve because of dependants e.g. children.

FURTHER READING

Bonanno, G.A. & Kaltman, S. (2001) The varieties of grief experience. *Clinical Psychology Review*, 21, 705–34.

STATION 3: SSRIs and sexual dysfunction

KEY POINTS
Communication
Consent issues
Empathy and rapport
History of dysfunction
Explanation and advice to the couple

INTRODUCE YOURSELF

'Hello, my name is Dr_____, I'm one of the psychiatrists.'

SET THE SCENE

'I understand from the GP that your husband has had some problems, is that correct?'

'First, I would like to ask whether your husband knows you've come to talk to me today and whether he is happy for us to discuss this?' (Considering consent issues)

'Ok, would you please tell more about what has been happening?'

COMPLETING THE TASKS

Gather information in an empathic fashion. Sexual side effects are distressing, and have the potential to damage relationships.

Explain that you would also need to see her partner to discuss with him his concerns (if any!) and problems from his perspective. It would also be important to take a detailed history from him and plan what to do.

SSRIs

Explain that the side effects should have been explained to her partner and apologize if this did not happen.

SSRIs can affect any or all of the phases of the sexual cycle, causing reduced libido, impaired arousal, erectile dysfunction, and absent or delayed orgasm. SSRIs are most commonly associated with delayed ejaculation and absent or delayed orgasm.

Which medication the patient has been taking is important, as some SSRIs are less likely to cause sexual side effects.

Timing

It is important to establish whether the sexual side effects were present before the medication was started. Ask when the antidepressant was started and when the side effects began. Ask about other side effects associated with SSRIs (e.g. dyspepsia, nausea, vomiting and insomnia).

Sexual dysfunction occurs in depression itself and existing dysfunction could worsen with treatment. How long have they been together as a couple? Is this the first episode of sexual dysfunction?

Ask if anything has been done to date about the side effects.

Physical health

The patient would need to be present, but the collateral history would also be useful. Explain that you might need to order some physical investigations (liver function tests (LFTs), glucose, hormone levels).

It is important to ask about possible organic causes:

Genital: structural abnormalities, prostatectomy, sexually transmitted infections (STIs)

Cardiovascular: myocardial infarction (MI), angina, peripheral vascular disease

Neurological: peripheral nerve damage, spinal injury, epilepsy

Endocrine: diabetes, hypogonadism, hyperprolactinaemia

Musculoskeletal: arthritis

Medication: many, including antidepressants, steroids, antipsychotics.

Plan

Although drug holidays can be a sensible approach, the partner should be warned that stopping antidepressants suddenly can cause withdrawal effects. Features of the discontinuation syndrome could be elaborated on here.

Treatment should consider the psychological factors and normal fluctuation of sexual functioning. The medication can be stopped, the dose lowered or an alternative started with less propensity to sexual adverse effects, with careful consideration of the type of sexual dysfunction, comorbid medical and psychiatric illness and other prescribed medications. Despite an unconvincing evidence base, cognitive behavioural therapy (CBT) can help these patients cope with the dysfunction, reduce symptom severity, or help prevent worsening. Sex therapy or referral to a sex therapy service can also be of benefit.

Promoting a better lifestyle, a healthy weight, regular exercise and smoking cessation will be of benefit. Some patients will have pre-existing sexual dysfunction, perhaps related to chronic substance misuse or alcohol. Addressing these factors may improve sexual function.

There is an evidence base for the use of phosphodiesterase-5 inhibitors such as sildenafil for the management of SSRI-associated erectile dysfunction and for decreased libido, possibly adding or switching to bupropion.

PROBLEM SOLVING

This station usually involves an extremely upset or angry partner. She is angry at the doctors for 'causing the problem' with the medication. She is upset because she feels her partner no longer finds her attractive and she is desperate to start a family. You must be empathetic and not enter into a confrontational approach. There is nothing wrong with apologizing where appropriate and then try to help her find solutions.

ADDITIONAL POINTS

According to DSM-IV-TR definitions and criteria, sexual dysfunction associated with medications or other substances is characterized by a disturbance in the processes that characterize the sexual response cycle (desire/arousal–excitement–orgasm–resolution) or by pain associated with sexual intercourse. The dysfunction results in marked distress or interpersonal difficulties, and it is fully explained by use of medication; the symptoms develop within 1 month of use of the medication, or the use of the medication is aetiologically related to the disturbance.

FURTHER READING

Balon, R. (2006) SSRI-associated sexual dysfunction. *American Journal of Psychiatry, 163,* 1504–9.

STATION 4: Body dysmorphic disorder

KEY POINTS
Communication
Empathy and rapport
History of complaint
Overvalued or delusional
Explanation of diagnosis
Management discussion

INTRODUCE YOURSELF

'Hello, my name is Dr___, I'm one of the psychiatrists.'

SET THE SCENE

'Thank you for seeing me today. I understand you have some concerns about your eyes. Could you please tell me more about this?'

COMPLETING THE TASKS

Body dysmorphic disorder (BDD) is a clinical condition where there is a preoccupation with a defect that is imaginary and generally not present. If a minor defect is present, it is significantly less obvious than the patient perceives. Commonly, the area of concern involves some part of the head, e.g. nose, ears, hairline.

History taking

Establish what his beliefs about his appearance are and whether they are held with poor insight (overvalued ideas) or no insight (delusional). Ask about how his belief affects his day-to-day life. How long does he spend looking at himself? What does he do to hide or mask his features? What does he avoid doing? What has he considered doing to put himself right?

Enquire about risk. Ask about thoughts of self-mutilation, deliberate self-harm (DSH) and suicidality.

The DSM-IV diagnostic criteria state that if preoccupation with a minor physical anomaly is present then the person's concern is regarded as markedly excessive. To distinguish BDD from normal concerns about appearance, a preoccupation must cause significant distress or handicap. Some suggest that in BDD, preoccupation with 'imagined' defects lasts at least an hour a day. The 'distress or handicap' might be avoiding social situations to escape feeling uncomfortable in front of others.

Management

The NICE guidelines on BDD recommend two treatments: CBT and SSRIs. CBT involves learning alternative ways to think about their appearance and to move their attention away from 'self'. They learn to stop comparing their appearance and ruminating. They have to learn to face their fears without concealment and stop rituals such as checking and excessive grooming. Anxiety usually occurs in the short term, but facing up to the fear leads to the anxiety gradually subsiding.

Antidepressants are the medication of choice. Often antidepressants are used in combination with CBT, although they can be used alone. A number of studies claim limited efficacy of the antipsychotics as sole treatment, even in patients with delusions, although there have been no randomized controlled trials (RCTs) of SSRIs versus antipsychotics. SSRIs are indicated when BDD patients have obviously depressed mood. Treatment guidelines are as for obsessive–compulsive disorder (OCD): a higher-dose SSRI for a prolonged period of time.

PROBLEM SOLVING

This presentation could be part of another disorder, e.g. a greater delusional disorder, OCD, social phobia or a major depressive disorder. Generally there is low self-esteem and patients consider themselves unattractive and ugly.

Individuals with BDD often repeatedly seek treatment from dermatologists and cosmetic surgeons. Individuals may resort to surgery in an attempt to correct the supposed abnormality. This usually makes no difference and repeats the cycle of preoccupation, checking in mirrors and grooming, seeking reassurance, and ruminating. When psychiatric input is finally sought, the outcome is improved for most people. Others may function reasonably well for a time and then relapse. For many, despite the best treatment available, symptoms persist for years.

ADDITIONAL POINTS

The older term for BDD is 'dysmorphophobia', which is still used. Complaints usually surround perceived or trivial flaws on the face or head. Sometimes there is a feeling of 'ugliness' rather than a specific feature. Other more usual body image distortions include thinning hair, wrinkles, increased vascularity or redness.

FURTHER READING

Veale, D. (2001) Cognitive-behavioural therapy for body dysmorphic disorder. *Advances in Psychiatric Treatment*, 7, 125–32.

STATION 5: Seasonal affective disorder

KEY POINTS
Communication skills and empathy
History of affective symptoms
Excluding important differentials
Diagnosis and explanation
Treatment options

INTRODUCE YOURSELF

'Hello my name is Dr____, I'm one of the psychiatrists.'

SET THE SCENE

'I've had a letter from your GP who informs me that your sleep and mood seem to worsen during the winter months, is that correct?'

'Could you tell me a little bit more about what's been happening?'

COMPLETING THE TASKS

History of SAD features:

Low mood

Duration of episodes of low mood (can be of varying severity)

Is mood persistently low?

Anhedonia?

Associated symptoms (worrying, low self-esteem, hopelessness, helplessness)

Fatigueability should be present

Hyperphagia and hypersomnia are also noticeable

Weight gain

Ask about a history of manic or hypomanic symptoms and explore these.

Ask about an association with season, especially re effect of living in different climate, timings of symptoms, onset each year, etc.

Elicit impact on functioning (work, relationships, family, etc.).

Any history of self-harm or suicidality?

Exclude important differentials

Ask about lifelong history of mood swings (cylothymia)

Alcohol or drug misuse

Anxiety disorders

Differential diagnoses in this man's case are:

1. seasonal affective disorder (SAD);
2. recurrent depressive disorder;
3. cyclothymia or even bipolar affective disorder (BPAD).

The most likely diagnosis is SAD. Explain that in cyclothymia the mood changes are not as prolonged as the ones he has experienced and are not as severe. In addition to this, his symptoms always begin in autumn and resolve in spring, which is typical of SAD. The story of mildly elevated mood in spring time also supports the diagnosis.

It would be helpful to get an informant's history to be more confident of the diagnosis and review the GP's records to ensure the timings are correct. In particular, you want to check with an informant (perhaps the partner) more about the times when he feels mildly elated, as people who are hypomanic may not be aware of this themselves and if this is the case, a diagnosis of BPAD would be more appropriate.

SAD is considered by some to be a form of recurrent depressive disorder in which sufferers consistently experience low mood in the winter months. It is not clear if the aetiology differs entirely from other depressive illnesses.

Treatment options

Light therapy: Involves sitting near a light box which mimics the effect of sun light each day. Light therapy has been shown to be more effective in the morning than the evening. Effects are seen within a few days but may take 2 weeks to reach full effect. Patients can hire a light box so that they can find out if it suits them before buying one. Patients should continue to use the light box for half an hour a day throughout the winter months once they feel well, to prevent relapse. 10,000-lux light is needed for any benefit. Treatment should be started in early autumn or late summer.

Antidepressant medication can also be helpful; a trial of an SSRI should be considered.

Psychological and social interventions such as CBT can also help if this has not already been tried (enquire what kind of psychotherapy he has already had) and also support and information for his partner.

You should explain that many patients experience a seasonal pattern to their depressive illness. People with winter depression or SAD can remain in remission with holidays to the sun and light therapy.

More information and support can be given by the SAD Association.

PROBLEM SOLVING

Be aware that seasonal affective disorder is a controversial diagnosis thought by some to be a temporal coincidence between regular depression and the time of year. Cynics suggest that it is a creation of psychiatrists and the media. On balance, there is a continuum of symptoms in winter months on which some individuals suffer much more than others.

ADDITIONAL POINTS

SAD is subsumed under recurrent depressive disorder in ICD-10 (F33).

SAD sufferers are thought to have circadian phase delay. The light therapy is thought to effect a phase advance which alleviates the unwanted symptoms.

Dawn-simulating light clocks are more recent developments thought to help symptoms.

FURTHER READING

Eagles, J.M. (2003) Seasonal affective disorder. *British Journal of Psychiatry*, 182, 174–6.

INDEX

Note: page numbers in italics denote tables and in bold, figures